The Neuman Systems Model

4th Edition

D1451529

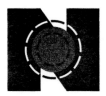

The Neuman Systems Model

4th Edition

Betty Neuman
Jacqueline Fawcett
Editors

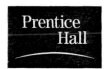

Upper Saddle River, New Jersey 07458

Library of Congress Cataloging-in-Publication Data

The Neuman systems model / Betty Neuman, Jacqueline Fawcett, editors.—4th ed.
    p. cm.
  Includes bibliographical references and index.
  ISBN 0-13-027856-4
  1. Nursing—Philosophy. 2. Nursing—Study and teaching. I. Neuman, Betty M. II.
Fawcett, Jacqueline.

RT84.5 .N474 2002
610.73—dc21

2001021852

Publisher: *Julie Alexander*
Executive Editor: *Maura Connor*
Director of Production and Manufacturing: *Bruce Johnson*
Managing Production Editor: *Patrick Walsh*
Manufacturing Manager: *Ilene Sanford*
Production Liaison: *Julie Boddorf*
Production Editor: *Linda Begley*
Creative Director: *Cheryl Asherman*
Cover Design Coordinator: *Maria Guglielmo*
Cover Designer: *Gary J. Sella*
Editorial Assistant: *Beth Romph*
Composition: *Rainbow Graphics*
Printing and Binding: *R. R. Donnelley & Sons*

Prentice-Hall International (UK) Limited, *London*
Prentice-Hall of Australia Pty. Limited, *Sydney*
Prentice-Hall Canada Inc., *Toronto*
Prentice-Hall Hispanoamericana, S.A., *Mexico*
Prentice-Hall of India Private Limited, *New Delhi*
Prentice-Hall of Japan, Inc., *Tokyo*
Prentice-Hall Singapore Pte. Ltd.
Editora Prentice-Hall do Brasil, Ltda., *Rio de Janeiro*

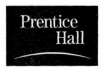

10 9 8 7 6 5 4 3 2
ISBN 0-13-027856-4

I continue to be most grateful for the love and support I always received from my late husband, Kree, for the experiences of being the mother of Nancy, and for the joy I have experienced as Alissa's grandmother.

Betty Neuman

I am forever grateful to my husband, John S. Fawcett, for his steadfast love and support. He always has helped me to do whatever was required to write, and teach, and learn more about nursing knowledge.

Jacqueline Fawcett

Contents

Contributors

Maria Alvarez Amaya, PhD, RNC
University of Texas at El Paso
School of Nursing
El Paso, Texas

Diane Breckenridge, PhD, RN
Research Fellow
University of Pennsylvania
School of Nursing
Philadelphia, Pennsylvania

Barbara Scott Cammuso, PhD, EdD, RNCS
Department of Nursing
Fitchburg State College
Fitchburg, Massachusetts

John A. Crawford, RPN, BA, MA (Educ), PhD
(Candidate)
Department of Psychiatric Nursing
Faculty of Health Sciences, Douglas College
New Westminster, British Columbia, Canada

Diane Fashinpaur, MSN, RN, CFNP
Director, Health Services
The University of Akron
Akron, Ohio

Jacqueline Fawcett, PhD, FAAN
College of Nursing
University of Massachusetts–Boston
Boston, Massachusetts

Barbara T. Freese, PhD, RN
Lander University
School of Nursing
Greenwood, South Carolina

Sandra K. Giangrande, MSN, CS, PhD
(Candidate)
University of Pennsylvania
School of Nursing
Philadelphia, Pennsylvania

Eileen Gigliotti, PhD, RN
The City University of New York
The College of Staten Island
Department of Nursing
Staten Island, New York

Jean A. Kelley, EdD, RN, FAAN
Professor Emeritus
School of Nursing
University of Alabama at Birmingham
Birmingham, Alabama

Marlou de Kuiper, RN, BEd, MN
Hogeschool van Utrecht
Master of Science in Nursing Degree Program
Utrecht, Holland

Margaret Louis, PhD, RN
Department of Nursing
University of Nevada, Las Vegas
Las Vegas, Nevada

Lois Lowry, RN, DNSc
East Tennessee State University
Johnson City, Tennessee

Ruud de Munck, BcPM, RN, RPN
Department of Personnel and Education
Emergis, Institute for Mental Health Care
Zeeland, Holland

André Merks, BcN, MScN, RN
Department of Prevention and Care Development
Emergis, Institute for Mental Health Care
Zeeland, Holland

Betty Neuman, PhD, FAAN
Theorist-Consultant
Founder/Director, Neuman Systems Model Trustee
Group, Inc.
Beverly, Ohio

Diana M. L. Newman, EdD, RN
Neumann College
Department of Nursing
Aston, Pennsylvania

Linchong Pothiban, DSN, RN
Faculty of Nursing
Chiang Mai University
Chian Mai, Thailand

Karen S. Reed, PhD, RN
School of Nursing
University of Akron
Akron, Ohio

Jan Russell, PhD, RN
University of Missouri
School of Nursing
Kansas City, Missouri

Nena F. Sanders, DSN, RN
Ida V. Moffett School of Nursing
Samford University
Birmingham, Alabama

Barbara F. Shambaugh, PhD, RN
President, Diogenes Ltd.
Brookline, Massachusetts

Michael A. Tarko, RPN, BA, PhD (Candidate)
Department of Psychiatric Nursing
Faculty of Health Sciences, Douglas College
New Westminster, British Columbia, Canada

Madelyn L. Torakis, RN, MSN
Children's Hospital of Michigan
Detroit, Michigan

Andrea J. Wallen, EdD, RN
Department of Nursing
Fitchburg State College
Fitchburg, Massachusetts

Preface

Since the mid-1970s, when the Neuman Systems Model was first used for nursing education and practice, the model has both led and followed evolving health care trends. During the 1980s, the model gained worldwide popularity as a valid and appropriate structure for care across cultural and health care disciplinary boundaries. Throughout the 1990s, use of the model as a guide for clinical practice, research, education, and administration increased. We anticipate that use of the Neuman Systems Model will continue throughout the twenty-first century, given the increasing recognition of the need for a wholistic, systems approach to global health care concerns.

This fourth edition of *The Neuman Systems Model* continues the tradition established with the previous three editions by including contributions that clearly reflect the broad, cross-cultural applicability of the model. Part One of this edition presents a detailed description of the Neuman Systems Model. Chapter 1 represents a reorganization of earlier presentations of the Neuman Systems Model. No changes in the content of the model have been made for this edition of the book.

Part Two focuses on the Neuman Systems Model and Clinical Practice. Chapter 2 is a discussion of guidelines for Neuman Systems Model–based clinical practice. Chapter 3 is an integrative review of the Neuman Systems Model–based clinical practice literature. Chapter 4 is a presentation and discussion of clinical tools that have been derived from the Neuman Systems Model. Chapters 5 and 6 present specific applications of the Neuman Systems Model in nursing practice in the United States (Chapter 5) and Canada (Chapter 6).

Part Three focuses on the Neuman Systems Model and Nursing Research. Chapter 7 presents guidelines for Neuman Systems Model–based nursing research. Chapter 8 is an integrative review of the Neuman Systems Model–based research literature. Chapter 9 is a presentation and discussion of research instruments that have been derived from or linked with the Neuman Systems Model. Chapters 10 and 11 present specific applications of the Neuman Systems Model in nursing research in the United States (Chapter 10) and Thailand (Chapter 11).

Part Four focuses on the Neuman Systems Model and Nursing Education. Chapter 12 presents guidelines for Neuman Systems Model–based nursing education. Chapter 13 is an integrative review of the literature about the use of the Neuman Systems Model as a guide for nursing education. Chapter 14 is a presentation and discussion of educational tools that have been derived from the Neuman Systems Model. Chapters 15 and 16 present specific applications of the Neuman Systems Model in nursing education in the United States (Chapter 15) and Holland (Chapter 16).

Part Five focuses on the Neuman Systems Model and Nursing Administration. Chapter 17 is a discussion of guidelines for Neuman Systems Model–based administration of nursing services. Chapter 18 is an integrative review of the Neuman Systems Model–based nursing administration literature. Chapters 19 and 20 present specific applications of the Neuman Systems Model as a guide for administration of nursing services in the United States (Chapter 19) and Holland (Chapter 20).

Part Six addresses the Neuman Systems Model and the Future. In Chapter 21, Betty Neuman presents ideas about the future of the Neuman Systems Model.

This edition also includes five appendices. Appendix A provides the definition of each Neuman Systems Model concept. Appendix B presents Betty Neuman's autobiography and a chronology of the development and utilization of the Neuman Systems Model. Appendix C includes the Neuman Systems Model Nursing Process Format and the Neuman Systems Model Assessment and Intervention Tool, as well as a family case study that illustrates the wellness-focused, comprehensive, and flexible features of the Neuman Systems Model. Appendix D is a description of the Neuman Systems Model Trustees Group and a list of current Trustees. Appendix E presents a comprehensive bibliography of Neuman Systems Model literature, including primary sources, commentaries, and applications in clinical practice, research, education, and administration.

This fourth edition is suitable as a text for all levels of nursing education in all clinical specialties, as well as for continuing education programs. This edition also is a useful text for students, educators, clinicians, researchers, and administrators in all health care disciplines.

We acknowledge the enthusiasm of users and would-be users of the Neuman Systems Model worldwide. Their interest in and questions about practical uses of the model provided the motivation for this edition.

We offer our gratitude to all contributing authors for their willingness to share their most creative work with us and with the readers of this edition. We are grateful also for the continuing support of the Neuman Systems Model Trustees. Their commitment to the Neuman Systems Model certainly will assure its continuing contributions to the advancement of health care knowledge in general and nursing knowledge in particular.

We extend our appreciation to Maura Connor, Executive Editor, Nursing, and Beth Ann Romph, Editorial Assistant, Nursing, of Prentice Hall Health, for their support, encouragement, and assistance throughout the preparation of this edition. We also acknowledge the essential contributions of all the people who facilitated the production of this edition, with special appreciation to Linda Begley.

Betty Neuman, PhD, FAAN
Jacqueline Fawcett, PhD, FAAN

The Neuman
Systems Model

4th Edition

PART I

THE NEUMAN SYSTEMS MODEL

one

The Neuman Systems Model

Betty Neuman

The Neuman Systems Model is a unique, systems-based perspective that provides a unifying focus for approaching a wide range of nursing concerns. A system acts as a boundary for a single client, a group, and even a number of groups; it can also be defined for a social issue. The client system in interaction with the environment delineates the domain of nursing concern. The model is dynamic because it is based on the client's continuous relationship to environmental stress factors, which have potential for causing a reaction, or obvious symptomatic reaction to stress, or could affect reconstitution following treatment of a stress reaction. In particular, the model takes into account all variables affecting a client's possible or actual response to stressors and explains how system stability is achieved in relation to environmental stressors imposed upon the client. The main nursing goal is to facilitate optimal wellness for the client through retention, attainment, or maintenance of client system stability. Optimal wellness represents the greatest possible degree of system stability at a given point in time. Thus, wellness is a matter of degree, a point on a continuum running from the greatest degree of wellness to severe illness or death. Nursing action or intervention is based on a synthesis of comprehensive client data and relevant theory that is appropriate to the client's perception of need and is related to functional competence or possibility within the client's environmental context.

The content of this chapter is a revision of earlier presentations of the Neuman Systems Model and its relationship to systems theory (Neuman, 1982, 1989b, 1995). The revisions are primarily ones of organization of content rather than changes in the basic ideas comprising the model. The wholistic perspective, concepts, and processes of the Neuman Systems Model remain equally applicable to any health care discipline, which increases the value of the model for interdisciplinary and multidisciplinary use. Moreover, the Neuman Systems Model is not in conflict with other nursing conceptual models; rather, it has been shown to be complementary to other nursing models because of its broad, comprehensive systemic wholistic perspective.

In this chapter, the content of the Neuman Systems Model is explicitly related to the

3

four concepts of nursing's metaparadigm—person, environment, health, and nursing. The definition of each Neuman Systems Model concept is given in Appendix A, at the end of this book. Betty Neuman's autobiography and a chronology of the development and utilization of the Neuman Systems Model are given in Appendix B. The Neuman Systems Model Nursing Process Format and the Neuman Systems Model Assessment and Intervention Tool are presented in Appendix C. The members of the Neuman Systems Model Trustees Group are listed in Appendix D. A comprehensive Neuman Systems Model bibliography is presented in Appendix E.

SYSTEMS THEORY AND NURSING

Systems theory has the potential for development of a totally new posture toward health care professionalism. All scientific disciplines, including nursing, benefit from use of a systemic structure for organization, specification, and cohesion of their increasingly complex components.

The significance of systems theory for nursing has been recognized for many years. Hazzard (1975), for example, noted: "General system theory is a theory of organized complexity, where all the elements are in interaction. Such a theory can be utilized well in nursing. Nursing is a system because it consists of elements in interaction" (p. 383). Systems theory continues to be used as a unifying force for scholarly exploration in various scientific disciplines, as well as in the fields of business and finance. Yet a major question lingers: Will nursing fully recognize and accept the exciting potential for and inevitable challenge of developing its scientific professional base within the breadth of a systems perspective? New frontiers are possible for the discipline through research validation of systems use in continually evolving practice roles.

The growing complexity of nursing demands that an organizational system is able to change as required, while preserving and even enhancing its inherent character. The systems approach has the potential for such organization, while allowing the assimilation of new demands through adjustive processes, which are requisite if new qualities are to emerge. Aydelotte's comments remain as valid today as when they were published in 1972. She stated:

> Nursing leadership must reorient itself and restructure itself in such a way that nursing education and practice are inseparable, are symbolic, and are united in purpose. We must put aside inertia, apathy, competitiveness, personal animosities, and censorship. We must restructure a set of social relationships [that] will enable society to receive that which it has charged us to provide. If we do not do this, society will surely place the charge they have given us elsewhere. Portions of nursing leadership, in resisting change, have boldly overlooked the fact that nursing as an occupation is a social institution and social institutions, many of long standing, are crumbling and changing today as a result of the reordering of priorities and of values and services by current day society. There is a great need to accelerate the progressive movements now occurring in nursing: striking changes in levels of nursing practice; greater development of clinical specialization; and significant alterations in the reciprocal roles held by nurses and other health personnel, particularly the physicians. There is increasing evidence that these movements are responsive to what society wants and are the directions that society will support. (p. 23)

Rapid societal changes, with concomitant new creative expectations, roles, functions, and conditions, create stress areas for nursing practice. A great challenge for nursing will continue as the discipline attempts to remain stable yet flexible enough to meet the action and reaction effects of both internal and external environmental demands. As nursing functions become more diversified and complex, the traditional linkages or structures that hold all of nursing together are being severely challenged. Thus, nursing professional inconsistencies need closure to prevent others from making decisions.

The discipline of nursing has become a complex system, if measured only by the diversity of roles and functions. A systems perspective adds to our appreciation of the system's complexity and to the exploration and valuing of its parts. Portions of the domain of nursing can be dealt with either as organized wholes within the larger superstructure or as parts or subparts of the defined whole system.

For example, a nurse manager is concerned with the broad, all-encompassing domain, whereas a clinical nurse specialist gives priority of function to a specific area as a part or subpart of the larger system. Using this example, the roles and functions of both the clinical specialist and the manager would contribute to the development of new alliances, providing truly wholistic client care. Other examples could be provided of new alliances that benefit the nursing discipline and that enhance both education and practice. A reorientation to the functional domain of nursing, with subsystems clearly defined, is required; we must view structurally the logical overall system within which nursing education and practice take place. After the boundaries of the larger system are established, the parts and subparts inherent within it must be clearly defined. The use of systems theory can help nursing define itself in relation to new health mandates and care reform issues, such as major emphasis on wellness promotion and disease prevention.

As nursing roles and functions expand, they become more complex and comprehensive, and a broader structure will be required to encompass them. Expansiveness as a result of assimilation of change is a characteristic of the systems concepts. Complex nursing phenomena can be placed within a logical and empirically valid open systems perspective; as the number of parts or subparts increases, the whole expands. Regardless of the size of an identified system, its boundaries, as well as the characteristics of the interrelating parts, must be defined for analysis and utilization. With an expansive systems perspective as a nursing base, we must overlook neither scientific exploration nor the crossing of interdisciplinary boundaries where cooperation and collaboration are requisites.

Banathy (1973) acknowledged that solutions to increasingly more complex technological and social problems are not found in the thinking and tools of single analytically oriented disciplines. We have had to evolve a new way of thinking and a new approach to disciplined inquiry: systems science. Systems science has demonstrated its effectiveness in attacking highly complex and large-scale problems. It evolves models constructed of systems concepts that are applicable to several traditional fields of knowledge. It also develops strategies that can be applied to the solution of problems. The integration of systems concepts into our thinking leads us to acquire the systems view, and the systems view enables us to think of ourselves, our environment, and the entities that surround us (and of which we are a part) in a new way. This new way of thinking can be applied to analysis, design, or development, and management of systems for the solution of complex problems. Adapting systems thinking to nursing demands a high degree of flexibility, which in turn allows for much creativity. A great risk for the nursing profession lies in failing to measure up to the flexibility required by rapid societal changes and demands and instead maintaining a tragic semblance of stability through defensive rigidity. Maintenance of a quasi-homeostatic or stability state through use of the systems approach also must be guarded against.

For nursing to mature as a discipline and expand through a systems perspective, a wide variety of creative approaches to client care must be examined. A possible beginning point might be to rethink two major functional components of nursing—education and practice. In the systems approach, the two are interdependent and mutually affected by environmental changes. The forming of a cooperative, collaborative relationship between these two interdependent parts of the system creates favorable conditions for enhancement of the system. The ability to form meaningful relationships is requisite for the growth of any system.

Miller (1965) identified the dimensions of the system as structure, process, and function. *Structure* refers to the arrangement of parts and subparts of a system at any given point in time. *Process* and *function* refer to matter, energy, and information exchanges with interaction between the parts and subparts. Living systems are open systems, and a steady state exists when the composition of a system is relatively constant despite continuous exchanges between the system and its environment. In systems thinking, the "whole" is the structure; sharing is the function.

Inherent within the systems perspective are guidelines for system enhancement and expansion. This feature is particularly significant to nursing, which is becoming an increasingly complex system within the general health care system. Some advantages of the use of systems theory in nursing are the integration of systems concepts with the increasing complexity of nursing phenomena, leading to new perspectives for nursing, and the clarification and definition of nursing knowledge related to the social sciences. This is congruent with Fawcett's (1999) assertion that only a strong link between theory and research will advance nursing knowledge. Moreover, Orem (1971) maintained that a general concept of nursing is essential for knowledge production within the field because an adequate general concept of nursing makes explicit the proper object of the profession.

Inherent in all systems are structure and dynamic organization, principles and laws, and terms affecting the constraints of their environments. Bertalanffy (1968) described general system theory as consisting of the scientific exploration of "wholes" and "wholeness." The interdisciplinary nature of concepts, models, and principles applying to systems provides a logical approach toward the unification of science. Beckstrand (1980) suggested that further development of nursing knowledge occurs by rigorous application of the methods of science, ethics, and philosophy to problems encountered in the professional experience of nurses. Inasmuch as conceptual models represent reality, they are basic to any attempt at theory development. A model facilitates deductions from premises, explanations, and predictions, often with unexpected results. Oakes (1978) maintained that general system theory will prove to be the step toward the ultimate goal of improvement in the quality of client care. As nursing continues to use systems components knowledgeably over time, to the benefit of the client/client system, it should evolve into a logically defensible, wholistic, and scientific discipline.

In the change process, a stress war always is being waged between the rigidity required to retain valued elements of the past and the uncertainty and flexibility required for new structures to emerge. Lazlo (1972) claimed that without synthesis of the items of knowledge held valid in a society, neither individual nor long-term purposes can be identified or rationally pursued. Inherent in nursing, as within any other system, are factors for either maintenance or growth through change (Figure 1-1).

The more complex the nursing system becomes, the more difficult it is to maintain the status quo, and the greater is the need for a viable organizational structure that can maintain relative stability during the process of change. As the boundaries of nursing roles and functions continue to broaden and expand, nurses are gaining freedom to assert themselves, while paradoxically and simultaneously increasing their need for a valid organizational base or structure.

Implicit in the goal of attaining stability through use of systems is the risk of coordination and control to a degree that limits the flexibility necessary for adjusting the nursing system to the changing environment, thus producing a closed rather than the desired open system. An open system is one in which there is a continuous flow of input and process, output, and feedback. Within the open systems approach is the potential for self-determinative, creative, and adjustive effects in relation to internal and external environmental stressors imposed upon nursing, and a tangible structure within which change can safely take place. Although some alteration in the conception of and approaches to nursing is inherent in the use of the systems approach, the requisite structure allowing for flexibility exists for meeting the challenge of tomorrow's new nursing posture.

Discovering order is a major challenge of the systems approach. Florence Nightingale could well have been the first pioneer in systems thinking for nursing when she demanded that nursing laws be discovered and defined (Riehl & Roy, 1974). In determining these laws, we must carefully consider nursing as a rapidly evolving system. Ashby (1972) noted that we must treat systems as wholes composed of related parts between which interaction occurs. In analyzing the system, nursing could use general system theory, defined by Klir (1972) as a collection of concepts, principles, tools, problems, methods, and techniques associated with systems.

The whole of nursing as a system must be clearly identified with boundaries defined before its parts can be properly analyzed. Then we can identify the interacting parts or subparts and their relationship to the whole system. The ways in which the combination of interacting system parts form the structure of the whole is significant.

The organization of nursing in relation to systems thinking may be classified as follows. The health care system is the larger system; it includes the discipline of nursing. The discipline of nursing includes two major functional components—nursing education and nursing practice. Nursing education and nursing practice contain many subparts, with specialized areas of concern.

By systemically considering specific interactions occurring within as well as among each of the parts and subparts of the nursing discipline, we can deal appropriately with

	Maintenance	**Growth**	
Rigidity and maintenance	Safety Security Certainty Familiarity Rigidity	Risk Anxiety Uncertainty Difference Flexibility	Flexibility and change

FIGURE 1-1. Choice factors in change.

the constraints the environment places on nursing, thus assuring that the profession meets its commitment both to the client and to the larger client system. Accelerated development and integration of nursing as a science can take place within the context of such an organized yet flexible structure. As a whole system, nursing must have a reciprocal relationship with the environment of the larger health care system and with the larger social system surrounding it, while sharing with the parts and subparts of its own system (Figure 1-2). For example, nursing as a component of the health care system is related to other disciplines with the common goal of maintaining the integrity of the client/client system. The actions of nursing affect the health care system and in turn are affected by it. These sharing relationships of parts and subparts of the health care system represent a type of interdependency and accountability requisite for optimal system functioning and, in fact, for the evolutionary survival of the whole system.

The whole system is bound by the available environment and constraints, whether it is nursing, the client, or other systems, as illustrated in Figure 1-2. A first constructive step in conceptualizing a system is to analyze processes occurring within the arbitrarily defined system. The next step is to relate wholes to their environment. A system is defined when its parts or subparts can be organized into an interrelating whole. Although organization is logical, structural differences may exist from system to system. The implied concept of wholistic organization is one of keeping parts intact or stable in their intimate relationships. The nature and number of parts and their relationships determine the complexity of the system. Both systems processes and nursing actions are purposeful and goal directed. That is, nursing vigorously attempts to control variables affecting client care, for example, toward the general improvement of client system capability or performance, better adjustment of behavior patterns, or perhaps better skill performance of a specific task. An inherent danger in the use of a systems model is oversimplification, especially when the phenomena and definition of entities under consideration are very complex. When used correctly, however, a systems model dramatically and convincingly demonstrates the nature of a process, which leads to better understanding and more accurate prediction of outcomes.

The concept of system—something consisting of interacting components—is not lim-

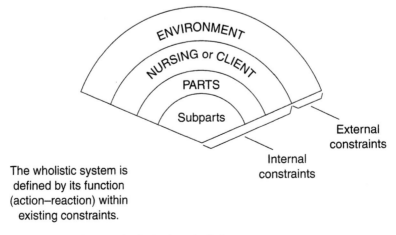

The wholistic system is defined by its function (action–reaction) within existing constraints.

FIGURE 1-2. Nursing, or client, or both, in the wholistic system.

ited and can apply to any defined whole. It is relevant to nursing in dealing with varied client system interrelationships, because the same terms and principles can be applied to facts in either system parts or the whole. A clear conception of systems organization requires skill in viewing client situations abstractly; that is, client system boundaries and related variables may lose some clarity because they are dynamic and constantly changing, presenting differing appearances according to time, place, and the significance of events. The uniqueness of the characteristic response of each system part implies that each must be studied and understood at its own level if we are to understand its significance in relationships and to the stability of the whole systems organization.

Dunn (1961) described the state of wellness as the integration of social, cultural, psychological, and biological functioning in a manner that is oriented to maximize the potential capabilities of the identified system. Components of a system, from a wholistic viewpoint, are not significantly connected except with reference to the whole. A system, then, can be defined as a pervasive order that holds together its parts. With this definition, nursing can readily be conceptualized as a complete whole with identifiable smaller wholes or parts. The whole structure is maintained by interrelationships of system components, through regulations that evolve out of the dynamics of the open system. As increasing organization becomes automatic in the course of development, regulations are ideally compensatory to system internal and external feedback.

The open systems concept increases understanding and has far-reaching implications for nursing; it provides an important working hypothesis for the development of new insights and statements for verification of new theoretical perspectives. The open systems concept, with possibilities inherent for stability, has been found to be increasingly relevant particularly to the sciences, contributing greatly to the expansion of scientific theory. The systems concept has significant potential for nursing, simultaneously representing both a great challenge and an opportunity as health care reform evolves.

For professional nursing to grow, expand, become relevant to rapidly changing social demands, and best articulate its future direction, all nurses must subscribe to a broadly based organizing structure. The unifying effects of a systems approach adequately provide the necessary structure for relatedness within the nursing discipline and point the way for discovery of commonalities and cooperative relationships with other health care disciplines, while allowing nursing to declare emphatically its unique professional profile. Inasmuch as the members of all health care disciplines understand systems terminology, important interdisciplinary sharing and communication should improve significantly.

In contrast to past mechanistic views in science is the newer concern with wholeness, dynamic interaction, and organization. Working terms derived from general system theory, such as *wholeness, order, differentiation, goal directedness, stressors, stability,* and *feedback* are homologous to nursing concepts. Principles and terminology can be readily transferred from one discipline to another, having a unifying effect on all the sciences. The trend toward cooperative interdisciplinary alliances is becoming increasingly clear.

New insights and principles for professional nursing are possible as new areas amenable to research and resolution are discovered. Valid, realistic, and operational systems principles can advance nursing toward becoming a scientific discipline bearing a new professional image. The systems perspective points the way for nursing to discover its own uniqueness, which lies in the way it organizes and uses knowledge rather than in its fund of knowledge per se. The use of systems thinking should help clarify how the bridge is made between knowledge and nursing action; it should identify which nursing actions are beneficial to the client and should support research efforts that advance nursing science.

The staggering yet noble movement toward professionalism in nursing is at best arduous, prolonged, and often divisive; however, new tools are being acquired to meet this continuous and provocative challenge. Nurse theorists continue to expand their conceptual model components to include a more wholistic perspective. The rapid acceleration of model usage, a significant development for organizing nursing phenomena, is the precursor of the development of the profession into a recognized scientific discipline. The systems perspective offers new hope for those who seek professionalism in nursing and provides a basis for continued creativity in relatively unexplored arenas made possible by worldwide evolving health reform issues and opportunities.

Wholism is both a philosophical and a biological concept, implying relationships and processes arising from wholeness, dynamic freedom, and creativity in adjusting to stressors in the internal and external environments. Using a wholistic systems approach to both protect and promote client welfare, nursing action must be skillfully related to meaningful and dynamic organization of the various parts and subparts of the whole affecting the client. The various interrelationships of the parts and subparts must be appropriately identified and analyzed before relevant nursing action can be taken. A system implies dynamic energy exchange, moving either toward or away from stability, which has a direct relationship to prediction of outcomes.

Basically, nursing functions within accepted, familiar, and often singular concepts. It is now imperative that the discipline articulates its function within a comprehensive structure. That is, we must conceptualize nursing action in wellness–illness and organization–disorganization states more broadly. Consideration of a more broadly based organizing structure will help facilitate the professional goal of enabling clients to move toward optimal wellness in any setting.

The open systems approach permits a reorientation to a scientific, thinking approach to studying people. Bertalanffy (1968) maintained that a different image of the person in society is needed. That is, the client must be considered an unlimited entity with an active personality system, whose evolution follows principles, symbolism, and systemic organizations, and it is not always possible to see the potential expansions of this entity and the ramifications of its actions.

The open systems approach begins by identifying and mapping repeated cycles of input, process, and output, which serves as feedback for further input; these cycles comprise the dynamic organizational pattern. Bertalanffy (1968, 1980) brought systems to the biological and social sciences through a convergence of regular pattern blends with their evolutionary history.

A living open system is never at rest but rather tends to move cyclically toward differentiation and elaboration for further growth and survival of the organism. The continuous dynamism and energy flow implicit within the systems concept adequately provide the most tangible structure within which the plethora of phenomena in nursing can meet the desired goal of protecting client/client system integrity.

Heslin (1986) claimed that a revitalization occurs when a living open system achieves stability in an equifinal process. She considers every restorative process and reconstitution following a reaction, interaction, and intervention to be the reestablishment of an equifinal steady state. She related system output to the end product of the process and also viewed it as input to further cycles, resulting in a redefined pattern of stability. Based on open systems theory, variables are interrelated and organized in various patterns that serve as sources of system input and output alike. Her view that processed input provides output as feedback for further input, creating an organized pattern within the open system, supports the open systems theory of both Bertalanffy's (1980) and Lazarus's (1981) systemic views.

Emery (1969) explained that in adapting to its environment, an open system will attempt to cope with external environmental stressors by ingesting them or acquiring control over them for survival purposes. At the simplest level, a steady state, governed by a dynamic interaction of parts and subparts, is one of stability over time. At more complex levels, a steady state preserves the character of the system through growth and expansion. As a system becomes progressively more organized, conditions of regulation or constraints become more complex. For example, as social organizations increase, their roles become more specialized in function. The process of development, evolution, and increasing order are beyond homeostasis or stability, just as the lack of development results in regression to lesser states and ultimately to extinction. Gray and colleagues (1969) found Menninger's notion of a continuum—a circular motion in all living activity, regardless of limitation—highly useful. Examples may be the cycle of wellness to illness to wellness again or the balance process of homeostatic and heterostatic mechanisms.

Putt (1972) noted that systems theory focuses attention on variables inherent in the client's adaptation to the environment, as well as on the effects of each system on other systems. She pointed out that as one system articulates with another system, the relationship of both is changed. In addition, Putt viewed systems theory as a relevant framework for the assessment of client needs, the development of nursing care plans, and the determination of nursing actions. Maintaining that the assessment of client needs is the first step in providing professional nursing care, she found that, guided by systems models, one can more easily achieve a desired level or quality of nursing care.

SYSTEMS THEORY AND THE NEUMAN SYSTEMS MODEL

The complexity of health care systems requires comprehensive conceptual models that provide the needed structure and direction for information processing, goal-directed activities, and a socially acceptable quality of care. Furthermore, the conceptualization of health care as systems of care requires the use of conceptual models that reflect systems theory. The Neuman Systems Model meets both of these requirements—it is a comprehensive conceptual model and it is derived from systems theory. Furthermore, as a systems model, the Neuman Systems Model is relevant for use by members of all health care disciplines. In addition, its systems orientation facilitates understanding of the diverse systems of health care that are found throughout the world. Thus, the Neuman Systems Model is applicable to clients of all cultures worldwide.

The intent of the Neuman Systems Model is to set forth a structure that depicts the parts and subparts and their interrelationship for the whole of the client as a complete system. The same fundamental idea or concept would apply equally well to a small group or community, a larger aggregate, or even the universe. The model provides the structure, organization, and direction for nursing action; it is flexible enough to deal adequately with the client's infinite complexity. Putt (1972) describes the concept of "living system" as open to the environment, freely interchanging energy and information with surrounding matter, maintaining itself, and seeking a steady state while existing in an interlocking hierarchy ranging in size from cosmic to microscopic.

The Neuman Systems Model focuses attention on living open systems. It is an open systems model that views nursing as being primarily concerned with defining appropriate action in stress-related situations or in possible reactions of the client/client system; since environmental exchanges are reciprocal, both client and environment may be positively or negatively affected by each other. More specifically, the Neuman Systems Model is a systemic perspective of health and wellness, defined as the condition or the degree of system stability, that is, the condition in which all parts and subparts (variables) are in balance or harmony with the whole of the client/client system. The client is an interacting open system in total interface with both internal and external environmental forces or stressors. Furthermore, the client is in constant change, with reciprocal environmental interaction, at all times moving either toward a dynamic state of stability or wellness or toward one of illness in varying degrees. Health is reflected in the level of wellness: when system needs are met, a state of optimal wellness exists. Conversely, unmet needs reduce the client wellness condition.

Environment has been generally conceptualized as all factors affecting and affected by the system. Environment is that viable arena that has relevance to the life space of the system, including a created environment. Consideration of environment is critical because health and wellness vary as to the needs, predisposition, perception, and goals of all identifiable systems. Consideration of the environment also is critical because, as nursing practice focuses more and more on the community, nurses realize that they cannot control or directly manage the client's environment, as they can in inpatient settings. It therefore becomes a necessity rather than an option to view the client as part of other systems, such as the family and the community.

THE NEUMAN SYSTEMS MODEL

The philosophic base of the Neuman Systems Model encompasses wholism, a wellness orientation, client perception and motivation, and a dynamic systems perspective of energy and variable interaction with the environment to mitigate possible harm from internal and external stressors, while caregivers and clients form a partnership relationship to negotiate desired outcome goals for optimal health retention, restoration, and maintenance. This philosophic base pervades all aspects of the model.

The Neuman Systems Model is predominantly wellness oriented and wholistic. The content of the model draws from and is related to Gestalt, stress, and dynamically organized systems theories (de Chardin, 1955; Cornu, 1957; Edelson, 1970; Lazarus, 1981, 1999; Selye, 1950). It is based on stress and reaction or possible reaction to stressors within the total environment of the defined client as a system.

More specifically, the Neuman Systems Model has some similarity to Gestalt theory, which implies that each client/client system is surrounded by a perceptual field that is in dynamic equilibrium. The model also relates to field theories endorsing the molar view that all parts of the system are intimately interrelated and interdependent (Edelson, 1970). Emphasis is placed on the total organization of the field. In the wholistic Neuman Systems Model, the organization of the field or system considers the occurrence of stressors, the reaction or possible reaction of the client to stressors, and the particular client as a system, taking into consideration the simultaneous effects of the interacting variables—physiological, psychological, sociocultural, developmental, and spiritual. This is similar to Gestalt theorists' view of insight as the perception of relationships in a total situation.

De Chardin (1955) and Cornu (1957) suggest that in all dynamically organized systems the properties of a part are determined to an extent by the wholes that contain it. This means that no part can be considered in isolation; each must be viewed as part of the whole. The single part influences our perception of the whole, and the patterns or features of the whole influence our awareness of each system part.

The specific components of the Neuman Systems Model and their connections are depicted in Figure 1-3. The definition of each component is given in Appendix A. Figure 1-3 depicts the Neuman Systems Model as a comprehensive systems-based conceptual framework for nursing and other health care disciplines that is concerned with stressors, reactions to stressors, and the prevention interventions that address potential and actual reactions to stressors. The figure depicts the client within a systems perspective wholistically and multidimensionally. Moreover, it illustrates the composite of five interacting variables—physiological, psychological, sociocultural, developmental, and spiritual—that ideally function harmoniously or are stable in relation to internal and external environmental stressor influences upon the client, as a system, at a given point in time.

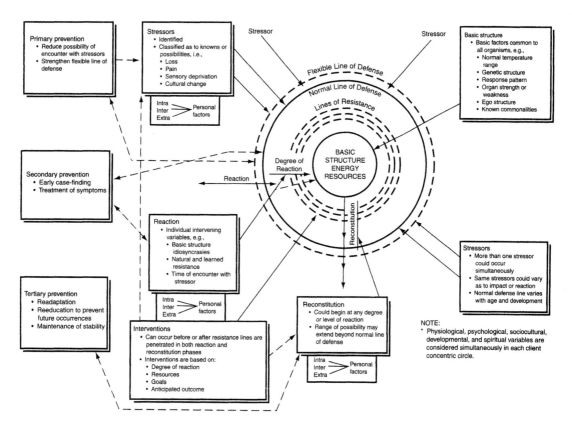

FIGURE 1-3. The Neuman Systems Model. *(Original diagram copyright © 1970 by Betty Neuman.)*

The unique perspective of the Neuman Systems Model is summarized in the following statements:

- Each individual client or group as a client system is unique; each system is a composite of common known factors or innate characteristics within a normal, given range of response contained within a basic structure.
- The client as a system is in dynamic, constant energy exchange with the environment.
- Many known, unknown, and universal environmental stressors exist. Each differs in its potential for disturbing a client's usual stability level, or normal line of defense. The particular interrelationships of client variables—physiological, psychological, sociocultural, developmental, and spiritual—at any point in time can affect the degree to which a client is protected by the flexible line of defense against possible reaction to a single stressor or a combination of stressors.
- Each individual client/client system has evolved a normal range of response to the environment that is referred to as the normal line of defense, or usual wellness/stability state. It represents change over time through coping with diverse stress encounters. The normal line of defense can be used as a standard from which to measure health deviation.
- When the cushioning, accordionlike effect of the flexible line of defense is no longer capable of protecting the client/client system against an environmental stressor, the stressor breaks through the normal line of defense. The interrelationships of variables—physiological, psychological, sociocultural, developmental, and spiritual—determine the nature and degree of system reaction or possible reaction to the stressor.
- The client, whether in a state of wellness or illness, is a dynamic composite of the interrelationships of variables—physiological, psychological, sociocultural, developmental, and spiritual. Wellness is on a continuum of available energy to support the system in an optimal state of system stability.
- Implicit within each client system are internal resistance factors known as lines of resistance, which function to stabilize and return the client to the usual wellness state (normal line of defense) or possibly to a higher level of stability following an environmental stressor reaction.
- Primary prevention relates to general knowledge that is applied in client assessment and intervention in identification and reduction or mitigation of possible or actual risk factors associated with environmental stressors to prevent possible reaction. The goal of health promotion is included in primary prevention.
- Secondary prevention relates to symptomatology following a reaction to stressors, appropriate ranking of intervention priorities, and treatment to reduce their noxious effects.
- Tertiary prevention relates to the adjustive processes taking place as reconstitution begins and maintenance factors move the client back in a circular manner toward primary prevention.

The unique perspective of the Neuman Systems Model is elaborated in the following discussion of the model components, which is organized by the nursing metaparadigm concepts—person, environment, health, and nursing.

Person as Client/Client System

The person is viewed as a client or client system (Figure 1-4). The term *client* was selected out of respect for newer client–caregiver collaborative relationships, as well as the wellness perspective of the model. The Neuman Systems Model considers the client, whether one or many, proximal or distal, as a system. Each system boundary must be identified or defined, along with the parts contained within it. What is defined or included within the boundary of the system must have relevance to a particular health care discipline and represent the reality of its domain of concern.

Within the Neuman Systems Model the client or client system may be an individual, a family, a group, a community, or a social issue. More specifically, the client as a system represents an "individual," a "person," or "man." The client system also may represent more than one person in environmental interaction, for example, in groups of various sizes (e.g., family, community, or a social issue). The model components are equally applicable to narrowly defined systems and to those defined as broadly as situations dictate, that is, ranging from one client as a system to the global community as a system.

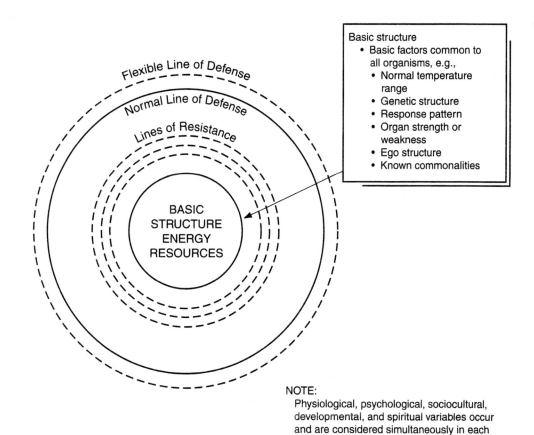

Basic structure
- Basic factors common to all organisms, e.g.,
  - Normal temperature range
- Genetic structure
- Response pattern
- Organ strength or weakness
- Ego structure
- Known commonalities

Flexible Line of Defense

Normal Line of Defense

Lines of Resistance

BASIC STRUCTURE ENERGY RESOURCES

NOTE:
Physiological, psychological, sociocultural, developmental, and spiritual variables occur and are considered simultaneously in each client concentric circle.

FIGURE 1-4. Client/client system.

The Five Variables. The client system is a composite of five interacting variable areas, which are in varying degrees of development and have a wide range of interactive styles and potential. The five client system variables are defined broadly and generally; the first four are commonly understood by nurses and members of other health professions. Inasmuch as the spiritual variable is more open to interpretation, it is described in more detail in Table 1-1. The variables are:

- *Physiological*—refers to bodily structure and internal function.
- *Psychological*—refers to mental processes and interactive environmental effects, both internally and externally.
- *Sociocultural*—refers to combined effects of social cultural conditions, and influences.

TABLE 1-1. THE SPIRITUAL VARIABLE

Spiritual variable considerations are necessary for a truly wholistic perspective and a truly caring concern for the client/client system. An analogy of the "seed" can be used to further qualify and clarify the statement that the spirit controls the mind and the mind controls the body as it relates to the Neuman Systems Model spiritual variable.

It is assumed that each person is born with a spiritual energy force, or "seed," within the spiritual variable, as identified in the basic structure of the client system. The seed or human spirit with its enormous energy potential lies on a continuum of dormant, unacceptable, or undeveloped to recognition, development, and positive system influence. Traditionally, a seed must have environmental catalysts, such as timing, warmth, moisture, and nutrients, to burst forth with the energy that transforms it into a living form that then, in turn, as it becomes further nourished and developed, offers itself as sustenance, generating power as long as its own source of nurture exists.

The human spirit combines with the power of the Holy Spirit as a gift from God when the innate human force, or "seed," becomes catalyzed by some life event such as humility, joy, or crisis; this energy begins to magnify and becomes recognizable within the thought patterns as something whose truths must become known and tested in life situations. Ideally in the testing, mental and physical expressions such as understanding, compassion, and love become manifested.

As thought patterns are positively affected, the body becomes increasingly nourished and sustained through positive use of spiritual energy empowerment. For example, it has been proven that a joyous thought enhances the immune system; the opposite also is true, with a negative outcome for the body.

Thus, it is assumed that spiritual development in varying degrees empowers the client system toward well-being by positively directing spiritual energy for use first by the mind and then by the body.

The beginning of spiritual awareness and development can take place at any stage of the life cycle. The supply of spiritual energy, when understood and positively used by the client system, is inexhaustible except for the death of the living system as we know it. The human spirit returns to the God source to live on into eternity when death occurs and it is no longer needed to empower the living mind, soul, and body.

The spiritual variable positively or negatively affects or is affected by the condition and interactive effect of the other client system variables, such as grief or loss (psychological states), which may arrest, decrease, initiate, or increase spirituality. The potential exists for movement in either direction on a continuum.

Through careful assessment of client needs in the spiritual area, followed by purposeful intervention, such as fostering hope that affects the will to live, the relation between the spiritual variable and wellness may be better understood and utilized as an energy source in achieving client change and optimal system stability.

- *Developmental*—refers to age-related development processes and activities.
- *Spiritual*—refers to spiritual beliefs and influences.

The five client system variables are considered simultaneously. Ideally, the five variables function harmoniously or are stable in relation to internal and external environmental stressor influences. The five client system variables are within the basic structure, as well as within the flexible line of defense, the normal line of defense, and the lines of resistance.

The Basic Structure. As can be seen in Figure 1-4, the client or client system is represented by a series of concentric rings or circles surrounding a basic structure. The basic structure or central core consists of basic survival factors common to the species, such as variables contained within it, innate or genetic features, and strengths and weaknesses of the system parts. Examples for the client as an individual are innate mechanisms for the maintenance of a normal temperature range, genetic response patterns, and the strength or weakness of body organs. In relation to the five client system variables, certain unique features or baseline characteristics also exist for each client or client system; an example is cognitive ability. The concentric circles—the flexible and normal lines of defense and the lines of resistance—function essentially as protective mechanisms for the basic structure to preserve client system integrity.

The Flexible Line of Defense. The flexible line of defense forms the outer boundary of the defined client system, whether a single client, a group, or a social issue. Each line of defense and resistance contains similar protective elements related to the five variables—physiological, psychological, developmental, sociocultural, and spiritual—while being distinguished by their specific protective functions. The flexible line of defense is depicted in Figure 1-4 as the outer, broken circle surrounding the normal (solid) line of defense. It acts as a protective buffer system for the client's normal or stable state. That is, it ideally prevents stressor invasions of the client system, keeping the system free from stressor reactions, or symptomatology. It is accordionlike in function. As it expands away from the normal defense line, greater protection is provided; as it draws closer, less protection is available. It is dynamic rather than stable and can be rapidly altered over a relatively short time period or in a situation like a state of emergency or a condition like undernutrition, sleep loss, or dehydration. Single or multiple stressor impact has the potential for reducing the effectiveness of this buffer system. When the normal line of defense is rendered ineffective in relation to a particular stressor impact, a reaction will occur within the client system. That is, when the normal line of defense has been penetrated, the client presents with symptoms of instability or illness, caused by one or more stressors. In all lines of defense and resistance are found elements that are similar but specific functionally, related to the five client system variables. Some examples are coping patterns, lifestyle factors, and developmental, sociocultural, and belief system influences.

The Normal Line of Defense. The flexible line of defense protects the normal line of defense. The normal line of defense is depicted as the solid boundary line that encircles the broken internal lines of resistance (Figure 1-4). This line represents what the client has become, the state to which the client has evolved over time, or the usual wellness level. The adjustment of the five client system variables to environmental stressors determines client stability or usual wellness level. The normal defense line is a standard against which deviancy from the usual wellness state can be determined. It is the result of previous system behavior, defining the stability and integrity of the system and its ability to maintain them. Influencing factors are the system variables, coping patterns, lifestyle factors, developmental and spiritual influences, and cultural considerations. Any stressor can create a reaction within the client by invading the normal line of defense when it is insufficiently protected by the flexible line of defense. A client reaction may reduce the ability of the system to withstand additional stressor impact, especially if the effectiveness of the lines of resistance is reduced. The normal line of defense is considered dynamic in that it can expand or contract over time. For example, the usual wellness level or system stability may remain the same, become reduced, or expand following treatment of a stressor reaction. It is also dynamic in terms of its ability to become and remain stabilized to deal with life stresses over time, thus protecting the basic structure and system integrity.

Lines of Resistance. The series of concentric broken circles surrounding the basic structure are identified as lines of resistance for the client (Figure 1-4). These lines are activated following invasion of the normal line of defense by environmental stressors. The lines of resistance protect the basic structure. These resistance lines contain certain known and unknown internal and external resource factors that support the client's basic structure and normal defense line, thus protecting system integrity. An example is the body's mobilization of white blood cells or activation of immune system mechanisms. Effectiveness of the lines of resistance in reversing the reaction to stressors allows the system to reconstitute; ineffectiveness leads to energy depletion and death.

The Lines of Defense and Resistance. A functionally interactive relationship exists jointly among all lines of defense and resistance, as each line individually contains the five system variables and protects the system components pertaining to it. Lifestyle, coping patterns, client expectations, and motivation are all inherent within the lines of defense and resistance, ultimately protecting the basic structure. Input, output, and feedback across these boundary lines provide corrective action to change, enhance, and stabilize the system, with the goal of achieving the optimal wellness level. Additional information about the lines of defense and resistance is given in Table 1-2.

Environment

The environment is broadly defined as all internal and external factors or influences surrounding the identified client or client system (Figure 1-5). The Neuman Systems Model identifies three relevant environments: the internal environment, which is intrapersonal in nature; the external environment, which is interpersonal and extrapersonal in nature; and the created environment, which is intrapersonal, interpersonal, and extrapersonal in nature.

Internal Environment. The internal environment consists of all forces or interactive influences internal to or contained solely within the boundaries of the defined client/client system. It correlates with the Neuman Systems Model intrapersonal factors or stressors.

External Environment. The external environment consists of all forces or interactive influences external to or existing outside the defined client/client system. It correlates with both the inter- and extrapersonal factors or stressors.

TABLE 1-2. THE NEUMAN SYSTEMS MODEL LINES OF DEFENSE AND RESISTANCE

This narrative is presented to further clarify use of the circular diagram of the Neuman Systems Model as a dynamic guide for relevant client care (Figure 1-3). The five Neuman Systems Model client system variables—physiological, psychological, sociocultural, developmental, and spiritual—define the nature of a chosen client system through their interaction patterns with each other and with both internal and external environmental influences, thereby creating a dynamic client system energy flow.

The client system basic energy or central core structure, consisting of the five client system variables, must be protected by the lines of defense and resistance to keep the system viable. Each of these lines of defense and resistance is similar in purpose, that is, to keep the system stable. Each contains the five client system variables.

The flexible line of defense ideally protects the system from immediate or short-term environmental stressors that could destabilize the normal line of defense, that is, the usual client system wellness condition. It is important to assess the strength and nature of each interacting variable within the flexible line of defense to determine how well it functions as a protective shield or composite. Examples are effects of sleep patterns, perception of events, nature of perceived social support, age-related energy expenditure, and spiritual beliefs.

The same basic principles of assessment are inherent in the normal line of defense, which should be viewed as a long-term adjustment to stressors, or the client system's usual stressor coping patterns and lifestyle influences. Client system adjustment within the normal line of defense develops over time. The normal line of defense defines the current health status of the client system, thereby acting as a standard for assessment of the normal or usual health condition and/or variance from wellness. Ideally, the pattern of interactions between the five client system variables and the environment keeps the system stable. However, when this fails and the normal line of defense is penetrated by one or more stressors, a reaction or system destabilization occurs, which requires assessment of the degree of deviation from the normal wellness condition.

When a reaction or destabilization occurs, the lines of resistance are called into play as both internal and external resources. The lines of resistance, based on the assessment of the interaction between the five client system variables and the environment, as well as system support, must deal with the degree of system destabilization (illness symptoms). Ideally, the available system resources within the lines of resistance are adequate to reconstitute the system energy flow and return it to its optimal wellness level. When the system fails to respond to use of available resources, decreased system wellness or death may result.

By assessing the effects of all five client system variables in interaction with the environment, the client system's health status becomes known and clarifies for the caregiver appropriate use of the three prevention-as-intervention modalities to facilitate an optimal client system wellness condition.

Created Environment. Another important environment is the created environment, which represents an open system exchanging energy with both the internal and external environment (Neuman, 1989b, 1990). This environment, developed unconsciously by the client, is a symbolic expression of system wholeness. That is, it acts as an immediate or long-range safe reservoir for existence or the maintenance of system integrity expressed consciously, unconsciously, or both simultaneously.

The created environment is dynamic and represents the client's unconscious mobilization of all system variables (particularly the psychosociocultural), including the basic structure energy factors, toward system integration, stability, and integrity. It is inherently purposeful. Though unconsciously developed, its function is to offer a protective

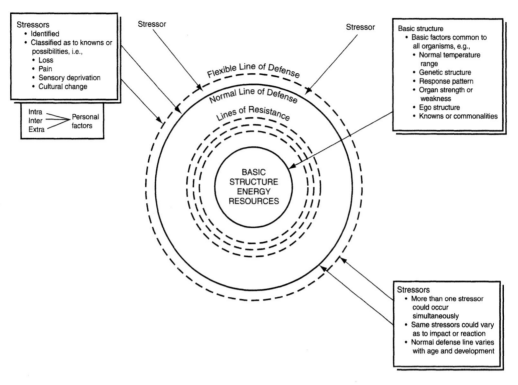

FIGURE 1-5. Environment.

perceptive coping shield (Lazarus, 1981) or safe arena for system function as the client is usually cognitively unaware of the host of existing psychosocial and physiological influences. It pervades all systems, large and small, at least to some degree; it is spontaneously created, increased, or decreased, as warranted by a special condition of need. It supersedes or goes beyond the internal and external environments, encompassing both.

The insulating effect of the created environment changes the response or possible response of the client to environmental stressors, for example, the use of denial or envy (psychological), physical rigidity or muscular constraint (physiological), life-cycle continuation of survival patterns (developmental), required social space range (socio-cultural), and sustaining hope (spiritual). Perception has a direct relationship to coping (Lazarus, 1981); the client's perception may be faulty in his or her creation of a "special" reality, thus binding energy for optimal function. All basic structure factors and system variable influences are identified by the created environment, which is developed and maintained through binding available energy in varying degrees of protectiveness; at any given place or point in time or over time, it may be necessary to change a situation or the self to cope with perceived system threat. The caregiver will need to determine through assessment (1) what has been created (nature of it), (2) the outcome of it (extent of its use and client value), and (3) the ideal that has yet to be created (the protection that is needed or possible, to a lesser or greater degree). These are all important areas for determination to best understand and support the client's created environment. After the nature and quality of the client's created environment is accurately assessed, further integration and synthesis of it may be desirable for optimal client wellness. The created environment is based on unseen, unconscious knowledge, as well as self-esteem, beliefs, energy exchanges, system variables, and predisposition; it is a process-based concept of perpetual adjustment within which a client may either increase or decrease available energy affecting the wellness state. The caregiver's goal is to guide the client in the conservation and use of energy as a force to move beyond the present condition, ideally preserving and enhancing the wellness level. What was originally created to safeguard the health of the system may have a negative outcome effect in the binding of available energy. The client should be treated in a gentle, nonjudgmental manner, allowing his or her control and choice as to change. One can assume that self-introspective ability is poor requiring careful search for factors that bind energy and help in movement toward increasing levels of self actualization and optimal health.

A major objective of the created environment is to stimulate the client's health. It has been well documented that a diseased condition is often created by cognitive distortions on the part of the client or the caregiver, although intervention traditionally focuses on physical and observable symptoms, overlooking causal factors like unexplored beliefs and fears. For example, a client's fear of job loss, with resultant lowered self-esteem and role conflict because of the inability to meet financial obligations, may lead to spinal problems. A client's ideas based on past experiences also may influence a current health state; for example, the belief in the length of time required to cure the common cold may have a positive or negative health outcome.

In wellness and illness states, all causal factors must be evaluated as to internal, innate, and external factors (known as variables and stressors) affecting the client; known or potential interrelationships, interactions, and interdependencies that may have created a given health state must be identified and correlated. Optimal client wellness is dependent on the evaluation of all causal factors, along with nursing action through relevant nursing intervention. Client awareness of the created environment and its relationship to health is a key concept that nursing may wish to pursue and further develop through research-based practice. As the caregiver recognizes the value of the client-created environment and purposely intervenes, the interpersonal relationship can become one of important mutual exchange.

Stressors. A tendency exists within any system to maintain a steady state or balance among the various disruptive forces operating within or upon it. The Neuman Systems Model identifies these forces as stressors. Stressors are defined as tension-producing stimuli with the potential for causing system instability. More specifically, stressors are tension-producing stimuli or forces occurring within the internal and external environmental boundaries of the client system. More than one stressor may be imposed on the client system at any given time. According to Gestalt theory, any stressor to some degree influences the client's reaction to all other stressors.

Stressors may have either a positive or negative outcome effect. This largely depends on the client's perception and ability to negotiate the effects of the stressor. In particular, within the context of the Neuman Systems Model, stressors are regarded as inherently neutral or inert; the client's perception of each stressor and the nature of the encounter with the stressor determine whether the outcome or effect is beneficial or noxious (Lazarus, 1999).

Neuman Systems Model environmental stressors are classified as intrapersonal, interpersonal, and extrapersonal in nature. They are present within as well as outside the client system.

- Intrapersonal stressors are internal environmental forces that occur within the boundary of the client system (e.g., conditioned response or autoimmune response).
- Interpersonal stressors are external environmental interaction forces that occur outside the boundaries of the client system at the proximal range (e.g., between one or more role expectations or communication patterns).
- Extrapersonal stressors are external environmental interaction forces that occur outside the boundaries of the client system at the distal range (e.g., between one or more social policies or financial concerns).

Stressors may be present in situational or maturational crises, whether or not experienced as such by the client. The five client systems variables within the flexible line of defense ideally protect the client system from possible instability caused by stressors. Determining factors would include the client's physiologic condition, cognitive skills, sociocultural influences, developmental state, and spiritual considerations. It is important to view the whole client system as dealing not with one or a few of the variables, but rather to view all variables as affecting the client at any given point in time. The wholeness concept is based on appropriate consideration of the interrelationships of variables, which determine the amount of resistance an individual has to any environmental stressors, whether or not a reaction has occurred.

Stressors have potential for reaction with the client or can cause a reaction with defined symptoms, and can influence reconstitution following treatment of symptoms. The time of stressor occurrence, past and present condition of the client system, nature and intensity of the stressor, and the amount of energy required by the client to adjust all are important considerations. The caregiver may be able to predict possible client adjustment based on past coping behavior or patterns in a similar situation, all conditions being equal. Coping is directly related to client perception and cognition. Cognitive appraisal determines the degree of stress felt, while coping functions mediate the reaction (Lazarus, 1981).

Critical to system analysis is the identification of stressors as to type, time of encounter, and nature of a reaction or possible reaction to them. Stressors may have a positive outcome, with the potential for beneficial, temporary, or even ultimate system change. For example, in an avoidance condition such as agoraphobia, anxiety may be clinically imposed as a stressor for the possible longer-term gain of mitigating the phobia, allowing for higher-level functioning. Various conditions and constraints accompany stressors. For example, a stressor may create a series of effects in more than one part or subpart of the client system and in response to these effects may itself in turn be affected.

The Client System and the Environment

Environmental exchanges must be identified as to their nature and possible or actual outcome for the client or client system. As an open system, the client system is in interaction and total interface with the environment. The client is a system capable of both input and output related to intrapersonal, interpersonal, and extrapersonal environmental influences, interacting with the environment by adjusting to it, or as a system, adjusting the environment to itself. The process of interaction and adjustment results in varying degrees of harmony, stability, or balance between the client and environment. Ideally, there is optimal client system stability. The client may influence or be influenced by environmental forces either positively or negatively at any given point in time. A particular stressor with a negative outcome for a client at a particular point in time may not always be noxious. The adjustment of the system may alter the client response pattern. Input, output, and feedback between the client and the environment is of a circular nature; client and environment have a reciprocal relationship, the outcome of which is corrective or regulative for the system.

A system receives suitable satisfaction only by interacting with the available environment in order to take on its parts for fulfillment of survival needs. Energy flow is continuous between the client and the environment even when a relatively stable state is maintained.

Health

The Neuman Systems Model conceptualization of health is illustrated in Figure 1-6. Health, or wellness, is viewed as a continuum; wellness and illness are on opposite ends of the continuum. Health for the client is equated with optimal system stability, that is, the best possible wellness state at any given time (Figure 1-7). The health of the client is envisioned as being at various, changing levels within a normal range, rising or falling throughout the life span because of basic structure factors and satisfactory or unsatisfactory adjustment by the client system to environmental stressors. Health is a manifestation of living energy available to preserve and enhance system integrity.

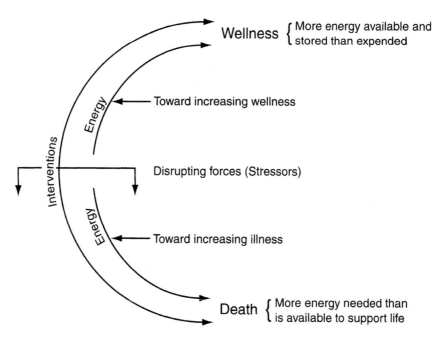

FIGURE 1-6. Neuman Systems Model wellness–illness continuum.

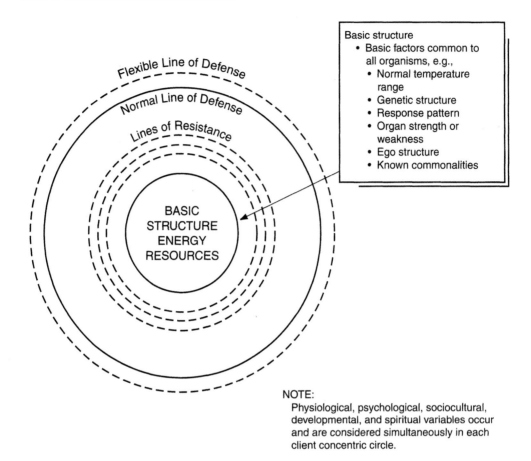

Basic structure
- Basic factors common to all organisms, e.g.,
  - Normal temperature range
  - Genetic structure
  - Response pattern
  - Organ strength or weakness
  - Ego structure
  - Known commonalities

Flexible Line of Defense

Normal Line of Defense

Lines of Resistance

BASIC STRUCTURE ENERGY RESOURCES

NOTE:
Physiological, psychological, sociocultural, developmental, and spiritual variables occur and are considered simultaneously in each client concentric circle.

FIGURE 1-7. Health.

The Neuman Systems Model wellness–illness continuum (Figure 1–6) implies that energy flow is continuous between the client system and the environment. To conceptualize wellness, then, is to determine the actual or possible effects of stressor invasion in terms of *existing client system energy levels*. Client movement is toward wellness when more energy is being generated than used; when more energy is required than is being generated, movement is toward illness and possible death. Variances from wellness or varying degrees of system instability are caused by stressor invasion of the normal line of defense.

The condition of the flexible line of defense determines whether a reaction might be likely to take place in an encounter with a stressor (Figure 1-7). Ideally, the flexible line of defense is strong enough to prevent or reduce the magnitude of a possible stressor reaction. A dynamic stability state can exist within the system along the internal lines of resistance, following a reaction to a stressor. However, a violent energy flow occurs when the client system is disrupted from its normal or stable state; that is, it expends energy to cope with system changes. When more energy is used by the system than is built and stored, the outcome may be death. The degree of wellness is determined by the amount of energy required to return to and maintain system stability. When more energy is available than is being used, the system is stable.

Stability implies a state of balance or harmony requiring energy exchange between the system and environment to cope adequately with imposing stressors. Stability preserves the character of the system. An adjustment in one direction is countered by a movement in the opposite direction, both movements being approximately rather than precisely compensatory. With opposing forces in effect, the process of stability is an example of the regulatory capacity of a system. Feedback of output into input makes the system self-regulatory in relation to either maintenance of a desired health state or goal outcome. For example, much research is needed to determine client health status by identification of compensatory actions among one or more system variables. Interaction of parts can fuse the client/environment into a unit relationship as a system. Health, within a systemic perspective is viewed as a continuum from wellness to illness. The two end states are opposites; wellness is a state of saturation or inertness, one free of disrupting needs; illness is a state of insufficiency with disrupting needs unsatisfied.

Nursing

The nursing component of the model (Figure 1-8) illustrates that the major concern for nursing is in keeping the client system stable through accuracy in assessing the effects and possible effects of environmental stressors and in assisting client adjustments required for an optimal wellness level. Optimal means the best possible health state achievable at a given point in time. Nursing actions are initiated to best retain, attain, and maintain optimal client health or wellness, using the three preventions as interventions to keep the system stable. In keeping the system stable, the nurse creates linkages among the client, the environment, health, and nursing.

Prevention as Intervention. The point of entry into the health care system for both the client and the caregiver is at the primary prevention level (before a reaction to stressors has occurred), at the secondary prevention level (after a stressor reaction has occurred), or at the tertiary prevention level (following treatment of a stressor reaction). The prevention-as-intervention format or modes (Figures 1-9, 1-10, and 1-11; see also Appendix C, Table C-6) are a typology of interventions that not only identify the entry point condition for the client into the health care system, but also indicate the general type of intervention or action required. This intervention modality allows for multilevel intervention, because more than one of the prevention-as-intervention modes can be used simultaneously, as the client condition warrants.

The Neuman Systems Model prevention-as-intervention typology provides an intervention typology. First considered is *primary prevention as intervention*. This modality (Figure 1-9) is used for primary prevention as wellness retention, that is, to protect the client system normal line of defense or usual wellness state by strengthening the flexible line of defense. The goal is to promote client wellness by stress prevention and reduction of risk factors. This includes a variety of strategies for health promotion.

Intervention can begin at any point at which a stressor is either suspected or identified. Primary prevention as intervention is provided when the degree of risk or hazard is known but a reaction has not yet occurred. The caregiver may choose to reduce the possibility of stressor encounter or in some manner attempt to strengthen the client's flexible

Primary prevention
- Reduce possibility of
  encounter with stressors
- Strengthen flexible line of
  defense

Secondary prevention
- Early case finding
- Treatment of symptoms

Tertiary prevention
- Readaptation
- Reeducation to prevent
  future occurrences
- Maintenance of stability

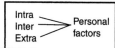

Intra
Inter   Personal
Extra   factors

Interventions
- Can occur before or after resistance lines are
  penetrated in both reaction and
  reconstitution phases
- Interventions are based on:
  - Degree of reaction
  - Resources
  - Goals
  - Anticipated outcome

FIGURE 1-8. Nursing.

line of defense to decrease the possibility of a reaction. Ideally, primary prevention is also considered concomitant with secondary and tertiary preventions as interventions.

Assuming that either the above intervention was not provided or that it failed and a reaction occurred, intervention known as secondary prevention as intervention or treatment would be provided in terms of existing symptoms. The *secondary prevention-as-intervention* modality (Figure 1-10) is used for secondary prevention as wellness attainment, that is, to protect the basic structure by strengthening the internal lines of resistance. The goal is to provide appropriate treatment of symptoms to attain optimal client system stability or wellness and energy conservation.

Treatment could begin at any point following the occurrence of symptoms. Maximum use of existing client internal and external resources would be considered in an attempt to stabilize the system by strengthening the internal lines of resistance, thus reducing the reaction. Relevant goals are established, based on use of the Neuman Systems

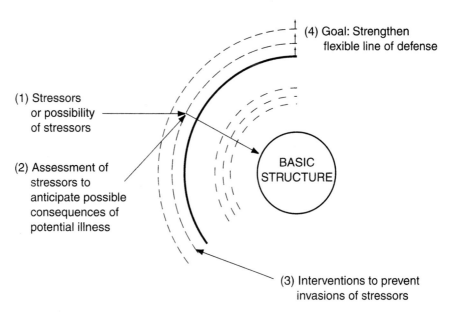

FIGURE 1-9. Format for primary prevention-as-intervention mode. *(Copyright © 1980 by Betty Neuman.)*

Model Nursing Process Format (Appendix C, Table C-1), which has been designed to implement the model. Through its use, the meaning of the experience to the client is discovered, as well as existing needs and resources for meeting them. Through the synthesis of comprehensive client data and relevant theory, an umbrellalike, or comprehensive,

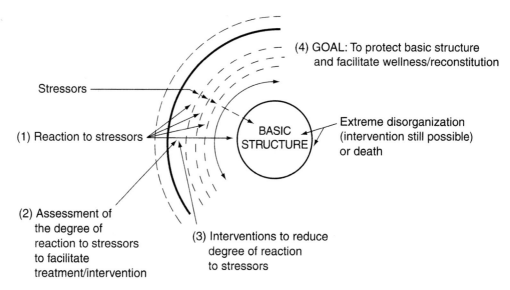

FIGURE 1-10. Format for secondary prevention-as-intervention mode. *(Copyright © 1980 by Betty Neuman.)*

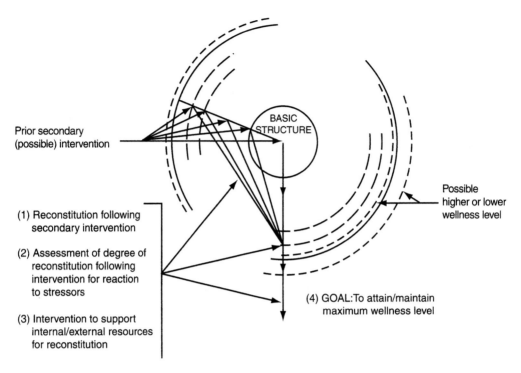

Prior secondary
(possible) intervention

BASIC
STRUCTURE

Possible
higher or lower
wellness level

(1) Reconstitution following
    secondary intervention

(2) Assessment of degree of
    reconstitution following
    intervention for reaction
    to stressors

(4) GOAL:To attain/maintain
    maximum wellness level

(3) Intervention to support
    internal/external resources
    for reconstitution

FIGURE 1-11. Format for tertiary prevention-as-intervention mode. *(Copyright © 1980 by Betty Neuman.)*

nursing diagnostic statement is made, from which nursing goals for nursing intervention can be readily determined in collaboration with clients can be readily determined for nursing intervention.

If, following treatment, secondary prevention as intervention fails to reconstitute the client, death occurs as a result of failure of the basic structure to support the intervention. Reconstitution is identified as beginning at any point following treatment; it is the determined energy increase related to the degree of reaction. Complete reconstitution may progress well beyond the previously determined normal line of defense or usual wellness level, it may stabilize the system at a lower level, or it may return to the level prior to illness.

The *tertiary prevention-as-intervention* modality (Figure 1-11) is used for tertiary prevention as wellness maintenance, that is, to protect client system reconstitution or return to wellness following treatment. Reconstitution may be viewed as feedback from the input and output of secondary intervention. The goal is to maintain an optimal wellness level by supporting existing strengths and conserving client system energy. Tertiary prevention as intervention can begin at any point in client reconstitution following treatment, that is, when some degree of system stability has occurred. Reconstitution at this stage is dependent on the successful mobilization of client resources to prevent further stressor reaction or regression; it represents a dynamic state of adjustment to stressors and integration of all necessary factors towards optimal use of existing resources for client system stability or wellness maintenance.

This dynamic view of tertiary prevention tends to lead back, in circular fashion, toward primary prevention. An example of this circularity is either avoidance of specific known hazardous stressors or desensitization to them. In using this intervention typology, the client condition, in relation to environmental stressors, becomes readily apparent. One or all three prevention modalities give direction to, or may be simultaneously used for, nursing action, with possible synergistic benefits.

Health Promotion. Health promotion based on the Neuman Systems Model is a component of the primary prevention-as-intervention modality. This contradicts Pender's (1987) view that the two areas should be considered separate entities. In the Neuman Systems Model, health promotion is subsumed within the area of primary prevention and becomes one of the specific goals within it for nursing action. For example, following need determination, intervention goals would include education and appropriate supportive actions toward achieving optimal client wellness, that is, augmenting existing strengths related to the flexible line of defense and thus decreasing the possibility of risk or threat of client reaction to potential or actual stressors. The major goal for nursing is to reduce stressor impact, whether actual or potential, and to increase client resistance. Ideally, health promotion goals should work in concert with both secondary and tertiary prevention as interventions to prevent recidivism and to promote optimal wellness, since the Neuman Systems Model is wellness oriented. Health promotion, in general, and within the primary prevention concept, relates to activities that optimize the client wellness potential or condition.

Inasmuch as the Neuman Systems Model always has considered environmental stressors as having a continuous impact on the client system, health promotion is inherently a major area of concern for both client and caregiver, not only in retention, but also in attainment and maintenance of optimal client/client system wellness (Neuman, 1974, pp. 104–106). Primary prevention as intervention with inherent health promotion is an expanding futuristic, proactive concept with which the nursing field must become increasingly concerned. It has unlimited potential for major role development that could shape the future image of nursing as world health care reform continues to evolve in the twenty-first century.

The Nursing Process and the Neuman Systems Model. Insufficient methodology exists for truly scientific approaches to complex and rapidly changing nursing concerns. Nurses largely conceptualize and utilize their social science knowledge for nursing in their own unique way, thus contributing to general inadequacy in professional communication and often poorly defined client goals. The need is critical for meaningful definitions and conceptual frames of reference for nursing practice if the profession is to be established as a science. For example, though considerable progress has been made in the past few years, the profession is still without definitive criteria for establishing a nursing diagnosis within the nursing process. It is considered to be in an evolving state from its present North American Nursing Diagnosis Association (NANDA) guidelines. There is major concern that these criteria relate only in part to various nursing conceptual frameworks. Therefore, the Neuman Systems Model concepts should be used for Neuman Systems Model nursing diagnoses.

The Neuman Systems Model Nursing Process Format was designed specifically for nursing implementation of the Neuman Systems Model (Appendix C, Table C-1). The nursing process format has been developed within the following three categories: nursing diagnosis, nursing goals, and nursing outcomes. These categories best fit the systemic perspective of the Neuman Systems Model. The utility of the format was first validated by doctoral students at the University of Alabama in 1982; its validity and social utility have since been documented in a wide variety of international nursing education and practice areas.

In using the Neuman Systems Model, the nurse is concerned with acquiring significant and comprehensive client system data to determine the impact or the possible impact of environmental stressors. Selected, prioritized client information is related to or is synthesized with relevant social science and nursing theories. This process fully explains the client condition, providing the logic or rationale for subsequent nursing action. That is, it provides the basis for a broad, comprehensive (umbrellalike) diagnostic statement concerning the entire client condition, from which logically defensible goals are easily and accurately derived. The Neuman Systems Model Nursing Process Format is elaborated by the Neuman Systems Model Assessment and Intervention Tool: Client Assessment and Nursing Diagnosis (Appendix C, Table C-3), the Neuman Systems Model Assessment and Intervention Tool: Summary of Goals with Rationale (Appendix C, Table C-4), the Neuman Systems Model Assessment and Intervention Tool: Intervention Plan to Support Stated Goals (Appendix C, Table C-5), and the Neuman Systems Model Assessment and Intervention Tool: Format for Prevention as Intervention (Appendix C, Table C-6).

A unique feature of the Neuman Systems Model nursing process is determination of the perceptions of both client system and caregiver (see the Neuman Systems Model Assessment and Intervention Tool: Client Assessment and Nursing Diagnosis, Appendix C, Table C-3). Another important feature is the mutual determination of client intervention goals (see Neuman Systems Model Nursing Process Format, Appendix C, Table C-1). These characteristics follow current mandates within the health care system for client rights in health care issues.

Although many authors have set forth various characteristics as integral components of the nursing process as a whole and in each of its phases, Phaneuf (1976) pointed out that there is little to support assumptions concerning the outcomes of the nursing process unless they are made from an adequate database. The Neuman Systems Model Nursing Process Format attempts to offer some resolution to the awkward dilemma in the following manner. Sufficient client data are obtained to make a comprehensive diagnostic statement and objectively determine client variance from wellness. Relevant goal setting is then defensible in terms of the theoretical synthesis with client data. Through the use of this specially designed nursing format, analytical outcomes are possible since they are based on purposeful prevention-as-intervention modalities.

THE NEUMAN SYSTEMS MODEL AND MIDDLE-RANGE THEORY DEVELOPMENT

The author and a valued nursing colleague, Audrey Koertvelyessy (Neuman & Koertvelyessy, 1986), jointly identified the major theory for the model as the Theory of Optimal Client System Stability. The theory asserts that stability represents health for the system. Several other theories inherent within the model could be identified and clarified with the goal of optimizing health for the client; for example, nursing is prevention as intervention and the client as a system is wholistic.

Koertvelyessy (personal communication, fall 1987) also proposed the Theory of Prevention as Intervention. She views the concept of prevention—primary, secondary, or tertiary—as prevalent and significant in the Neuman Systems Model, linked to each of the broad concepts of the model, that is, client, environment, health, and nursing. Inasmuch as the prevention strategies are the modes instituted to retain, attain, or maintain stability of the client's health status, she considers the development of a theory statement linking these concepts as a necessary next step.

CONCLUSION

The Neuman Systems Model is a comprehensive guide for nursing practice, research, education, and administration that is open to creative implementation. Although creative interpretations and implementation of the model are valued, structural changes that could alter its original meaning and purpose are not sanctioned. Indeed, fundamental changes in the meaning or purpose or content of the model would reflect the development of a new conceptual model that should be identified as such.

The Neuman Systems Model helps nurses to organize the nursing field within a broad systems perspective as a logical way of dealing with its growing complexity. Earlier, the Neuman Systems Model was criticized as being too broad, as were other conceptual models of nursing; now, this quality has become a major reason for increasing acceptance of the model and its documented utility.

The Neuman Systems Model has the potential for unifying various health-related theories, clarifying the relationships of variables in nursing care and role definitions at various levels of nursing practice. Nursing practice goals should enable the client to create and shape reality in a desired direction, related to retention, attainment, or maintenance of optimal client system wellness, or a combination of these, through purposeful prevention interventions. Nursing prevention interventions should mitigate or reduce stress factors and adverse conditions that affect or could affect optimal client functioning at any given point in time. The Neuman Systems Model Nursing Process Format and the Assessment and Intervention Tool (Appendix C) were designed to implement the Neuman Systems Model by incorporating its terminology and encompassing its breadth of purpose.

Although nurse theorists have increasingly added system components to their models, initially they viewed man or the client collectively or the person singularly as a behavioral composite, a biological system, an organism at a particular stage of development, or as part of an interactive process. As befits a wholistic perspective, the Neuman Systems Model has always considered all of these factors simultaneously and comprehensively within a systems perspective. That is, the client is viewed as a composite of interacting variables—physiological, psychological, developmental, sociocultural, and spiritual—that are, ideally, functioning harmoniously or are stable in relation to both internal and external environmental stressor influences. This approach to the client/client system prevents possible fragmentation and failure to interrelate various aspects of the client system as the nursing goal becomes that of facilitating optimal client system stability.

A great need exists to clarify and make explicit not only the relationship of variables affecting a client during and following an illness, but also those related to wellness retention for ambulatory and evolving high-risk groups. Inasmuch as health care is shifting increasingly toward primary prevention, including health promotion, an understanding of how these variables interface with those of secondary and tertiary prevention is important. These relationships are illustrated in the Neuman Systems Model diagram (Figure 1-3). The Neuman Systems Model fits well with the wholistic concept of optimizing a dynamic yet stable interrelationship of spirit, mind, and body of the client in a constantly changing environment and society (Neuman & Young, 1972). The Neuman Systems Model has fulfilled the World Health Organization mandate for the year 2000 and reaches far beyond, seeking unity in wellness states—wellness of spirit, mind, body, and environment. The Neuman Systems Model also is in accord with the views of the American Nursing Association, sharing its concern about potential stressors and its emphasis on primary prevention, as well as world health care reform concern for preventing illness.

The multidimensionality and wholistic systemic perspective of the Neuman Systems Model is increasingly demonstrating its relevance and reliability in a wide variety of clinical and educational settings throughout the world. Its comprehensive approach accommodates a variety of health-related theories. It also has the potential for generating important nursing theory through research into its components and by the unification of existing theories to serve world health care concerns well into the future.

REFERENCES

Ashby, W. (1972). Systems and their informational measures. In G. J. Klir (Ed.), *Trends in general systems theory.* New York: Wiley.

Aydelotte, M. (1972). Nursing education and practice: Putting it all together. *Journal of Nursing Education, 2*(4), 23.

Banathy, B. (1973). Models of educational information systems. In M. D. Rubin (Ed.), *Systems in society.* Washington, DC: Society for General Systems Research.

Beckstrand, J. (1980). A critique of several conceptions of practice theory in nursing. *Research in Nursing and Health, 3,* 69–70.

Bertalanffy, L. (1968). *General system theory.* New York: Braziller.

Bertalanffy, L. (1980). *General systems theory* (rev. ed.). New York: Braziller.

Cornu, A. (1957). *The origins of Marxist thought.* Springfield, IL.: Thomas.

DeChardin, P. T. (1955). *The phenomenon of man.* London: Collins.

Dunn, H. (1961). *High-level wellness.* Arlington, VA: Beatty.

Edelson, M. (1970). *Sociotherapy and psychotherapy.* Chicago: University of Chicago Press.

Emery, F. (Ed.). (1969). *Systems thinking.* Baltimore: Penguin.

Fawcett, J. (1999). *The relationship of theory and research* (3rd ed.). Philadelphia: Davis.

Gray, W., Rizzo, N. D., & Duhl, F. D. (Eds.). (1969). *General systems theory and psychiatry.* Boston: Little, Brown.

Hazzard, M. (1975). An overview of systems theory. *Nursing Clinics of North America, 6,* 383–84.

Heslin, K. (1986). A systems analysis of the Betty Neuman model. Unpublished student paper, University of Western Ontario, London, Ontario, Canada.

Klir, G. J. (1972). Preview: The polyphonic general systems theory. In G. J. Klir (Ed.), *Trends in general systems theory.* New York: Wiley.

Lazarus, R. (1981). The stress and coping paradigm. In C. Eisdorfer, D. Cohen, A. Kleinman, &

P. Maxim (Eds.), *Models for clinical psychopathology* (pp. 177–214). New York: SP Medical and Scientific Books.

Lazarus, R. (1999). *Stress and emotion: A new synthesis.* New York: Springer.

Lazlo, E. (1972). *The systems view of the world: The natural philosophy of the new development in the sciences.* New York: Braziller.

Miller, J. (1965). Living systems: Structure and process. *Behavioral Science, 10,* 337–79.

Neuman, B. (1974). The Betty Neuman health-care systems model: A total person approach to patient problems. In J. P. Riehl & C. Roy (Eds.), *Conceptual models for nursing practice* (pp. 99–114). New York: Appleton-Century-Crofts.

Neuman, B. (1982). *The Neuman Systems Model: Application to nursing education and practice.* Norwalk, CT: Appleton-Century-Crofts.

Neuman, B. (1989a). The Neuman nursing process format: Family. In J. P. Riehl & C. Roy (Eds.), *Conceptual models for nursing practice* (3rd ed., pp. 49–62). Norwalk, CT: Appleton & Lange.

Neuman, B. (1989b). *The Neuman Systems Model* (2nd ed.). Norwalk, CT: Appleton & Lange.

Neuman, B. (1990). Health on a continuum based on the Neuman Systems Model. *Nursing Science Quarterly, 3,* 129–35.

Neuman, B. (1995). *The Neuman Systems Model* (3rd ed.). Norwalk, CT: Appleton & Lange.

Neuman, B., & Koertvelyessy, A. (1986, August). The Neuman Systems Model and nursing research. Paper presented at Nursing Theory Congress, Toronto, Ontario, Canada.

Neuman, B., & Young, R. J. (1972). A model for teaching total person approach to patient problems. *Nursing Research, 21,* 264–69.

Oakes, K. L. (1978). A critique of general theory. In A. Putt (Ed.), *General systems theory applied to nursing.* Boston: Little, Brown.

Orem, D. E. (1971). *Nursing: Concepts of practice.* New York: McGraw-Hill.

Pender, N. J. (1987). *Health promotion in nursing practice* (2nd ed.). Norwalk, CT: Appleton & Lange.

Phaneuf, M. (1976). *The nursing audit: Self-regulation in nursing practice* (2nd ed.). New York: Appleton-Century-Crofts.

Putt, A. (1972). Entropy, evolution and equifinality in nursing. In J. Smith (Ed.), *Five years of cooperation to improve curricula in western schools of nursing.* Boulder, CO: Western Interstate Commission for Higher Education.

Riehl, J. P., & Roy, C. (1974). *Conceptual models for nursing practice.* New York: Appleton-Century-Crofts.

Selye, H. (1950). *The physiology and pathology of exposure to stress.* Montreal: ACTA.

PART II

THE NEUMAN SYSTEMS MODEL AND CLINICAL PRACTICE

two

Guidelines for Neuman Systems Model–Based Clinical Practice

Barbara T. Freese, Betty Neuman, Jacqueline Fawcett

The Neuman Systems Model was developed as a way to organize the content of clinical nursing courses (Neuman & Young, 1972). The use of the model as a guide for nursing practice was recognized almost immediately. Later, the use of the model as a guide for clinical practice in the full array of health care disciplines was recognized (Neuman, 1982). When the Neuman Systems Model is used as a guide for clinical practice, the nursing metaparadigm concept *person* is the client system, which may be an individual, a family, or a community. The metaparadigm concept *environment* encompasses the internal, external, and created environments. The metaparadigm concept *health* refers to optimal client system stability. And, the metaparadigm concept *nursing*—or the concept that refers to another health care discipline, such as *physical therapy*—focuses on utilization of primary, secondary, and tertiary prevention as intervention.

This chapter identifies guidelines for Neuman Systems Model–based clinical practice. These guidelines are applicable to clinical practice in any health care discipline. The chapter includes a discussion of each guideline and an explanation of how the Neuman Systems Model facilitates wholistic, multidisciplinary clinical practice.

THE NEUMAN SYSTEMS MODEL CLINICAL PRACTICE GUIDELINES

Rudimentary guidelines for Neuman Systems Model–based nursing practice were extracted from the content of the model several years ago (Fawcett, 1989) and were refined over time (Fawcett, 1995a, 2000). The most recent refinements, which are the result of dialogue among the three authors of this chapter, are presented in Table 2-1. Although the guidelines initially were targeted to nursing, our interest in the multidisciplinary use

TABLE 2-1. Guidelines for Neuman Systems Model–Based Clinical Practice

1. Purpose of Clinical Practice	The purpose of clinical practice is to assist clients to retain, attain, or maintain optimal system stability.
2. Clinical Problems of Interest	Clinical problems encompass actual or potential reactions to intrapersonal, interpersonal, and extrapersonal stressors.
3. Settings for Clinical Practice	Clinical practice occurs in virtually any health care or community-based setting, such as clinics, hospitals, hospices, homes, and the streets and sidewalks of the community.
4. Characteristics of Legitimate Participants in Clinical Practice	Legitimate participants in clinical practice are those individuals, families, groups, and communities who are faced with actual or potential intrapersonal, interpersonal, and extrapersonal stressors.
5. The Process of Clinical Practice	The process of clinical practice is the Neuman Systems Model Process Format, which encompasses three components—diagnosis, goals, and outcomes.
6. Client–Caregiver Relationship	The Neuman Systems Model Process Format engages the client system and the caregiver in a mutual partnership to determine diagnosis, goals, and outcomes.
7. Diagnostic Taxonomy	Diagnoses may be classified into a Neuman Systems Model diagnostic taxonomy that is organized according to client system (individual, family, group, community), level of response (primary, secondary, tertiary), client subsystem responding to the stressor (physiological, psychological, sociocultural, developmental, spiritual), source of the stressor (intrasystem, intersystem, extrasystem), and type of stressor (physiological, psychological, sociocultural, developmental, spiritual).
8. Typology of Clinical Interventions	Clinical interventions occur as primary, secondary, and tertiary prevention interventions, in accord with the degree to which stressors have penetrated the client system's lines of defense and resistance.
9. Typology of Outcomes	General outcomes are derived from the content of the Neuman Systems Model. Client system–specific outcomes involve application of the general outcomes to particular clinical situations.
10. Contributions of Clinical Practice to Participants' Well-Being	Neuman Systems Model–based clinical practice contributes to client system well-being by facilitating the highest possible level of stability achievable at a given point in time.
11. Clinical Practice and Research	Clinical practice is linked to research through the use of research findings to direct practice. In turn, problems encountered in clinical practice give rise to new research questions.

of the Neuman Systems Model called for the extrapolation of the guidelines to other disciplines concerned with the health of individuals, families, and communities. Consequently, the guidelines listed in Table 2-1 have been written for clinicians in all health care disciplines.

The first guideline stipulates that the purpose of clinical practice is to assist clients to retain, attain, or maintain optimal system stability. *Optimal stability* means that there is harmony among the five client system variables—physiological, psychological, sociocultural, developmental, and spiritual. The client's potential for optimal system stability varies with time and across the life span.

The second guideline stipulates that the clinical problems of interest are the actual or potential reactions to intrapersonal, interpersonal, and extrapersonal stressors. Stressors are fundamentally neutral but typically are perceived as positive or negative by a client. The stressors already may have occurred or may be threatening or possible. The client's perception of and reaction to stressors determines the extent of system stability.

The third guideline stipulates that clinical practice occurs in virtually any health care or community-based setting, such as clinics, hospitals, hospices, homes, and the streets and sidewalks of the community. Thus, practice is not limited to designated health care settings, such as a hospital or nursing home, but occurs in any setting in which nurses or other members of the multidisciplinary health care team are engaged in helping clients to retain, attain, or maintain optimal system stability.

The fourth guideline stipulates that legitimate participants in clinical practice are those individuals, families, groups, and communities who are faced with actual or potential or intrapersonal, interpersonal, and extrapersonal stressors. Just as the setting for nursing practice is not limited to designated health care settings, so the participants in clinical practice are not limited to clients who seek care in such settings. Moreover, individuals, families, groups, and communities are regarded as equally legitimate clients.

The fifth guideline stipulates that the process for clinical practice is the Neuman Systems Model Process Format, which encompasses three components—diagnosis, goals, and outcomes. The term *Process Format* is used to connote the multidisciplinary use of the Neuman Systems Model Nursing Process Format (see Appendix C, Table C-1). When particularized for a certain health care discipline, the name of that discipline is added as the modifier for each process component. For example, the components are nursing diagnosis, nursing goals, and nursing outcomes for nursing practice. Similarly, the components are physical therapy diagnosis, physical therapy goals, and physical therapy outcomes for physical therapy practice. The Process Format is compatible with use of the scientific method to solve problems and to achieve desired outcomes across the array of clinical practices of a multidisciplinary team.

The sixth guideline stipulates that the Neuman Systems Model Process Format engages the client system and the caregiver in a mutual partnership to determine diagnosis, goals, and outcomes. Inclusion of both client and caregiver in all components of the Process Format is based on the belief that ownership of the client's health belongs to the client. Consequently, health care must involve the client as an active participant, to the extent possible, if it is to be effective.

The seventh guideline stipulates that the diagnoses may be classified in a taxonomy, using organizing principles derived from the Neuman Systems Model. A taxonomy of diagnoses establishes a common language for communication among health care providers across disciplines, and can provide a uniform approach for computer-based client information systems. The five organizing principles of the Neuman Systems Model diagnostic taxonomy are: (1) client system (individual, family, group, community), (2) level of response (primary, secondary, tertiary), (3) client subsystem responding to the stressor (physiological, psychological, sociocultural, developmental, spiritual), (4) source of the stressor (intrasystem, intersystem, extrasystem), and (5) type of stressor (physiological, psychological, sociocultural, developmental, spiritual) (D.M.L. Newman, personal communication, June 15, 2000; Ziegler, 1982).

The eighth guideline stipulates that clinical interventions occur as primary, secondary, or tertiary prevention interventions, in accord with the degree to which stressors have penetrated the client system's lines of defense and resistance. From the Neuman Systems Model perspective, prevention interventions vary in accord with the degree to which stressors have threatened or affected client system stability. That is, prevention interventions are selected based on the actual or potential impact of stressors on client system stability. When stressors that have not yet occurred threaten the client, primary prevention interventions should help the client to retain optimal system stability. When the client has experienced stressors, secondary or tertiary prevention interventions should help to attain and maintain optimal system stability.

The ninth guideline stipulates that general outcomes are derived from the content of the Neuman Systems Model. General outcomes are statements about the concepts of the Neuman Systems Model, such as "Strengthened Flexible Line of Defense" or "Higher Level of Client System Stability." A comprehensive list of general outcomes remains to be developed. Client system–specific outcomes involve application of the general statements to particular clinical situations, such as "The client drank additional fluid with replacement electrolytes prior to exercise on a hot day."

The tenth guideline stipulates that Neuman Systems Model–based clinical practice contributes to client system well-being by facilitating the highest possible level of stability achievable at a given point in time. Client system stability potential varies with time and across the life span. Clinicians use the Neuman Systems Model Process Format to assist clients to reach their unique system stability level at a particular time point in the life span.

The eleventh guideline stipulates that clinical practice is linked to research through the use of research findings to direct practice. Neuman Systems Model–based studies should advance nursing knowledge by increasing understanding of how the model can be used in clinical practice to promote optimal client system stability (Fawcett, 1995b). More specifically, research findings can serve as the basis for recommendations regarding use of particular prevention interventions in clinical practice (Louis, 1995). In turn, problems encountered in clinical practice give rise to new research questions. If, for example, a prevention intervention did not have the expected outcome, a retrospective case study could be done to determine what factors in the internal, external, or created environment might have contributed to the unexpected outcome.

IMPLEMENTING THE NEUMAN SYSTEMS MODEL IN MULTIDISCIPLINARY CLINICAL PRACTICE

Multidisciplinary use requires a conceptual model to be a comprehensive and systematic approach to the care of client systems. The Neuman Systems Model is ideal because its wholistic systems focus allows multidisciplinary health care team members to coordinate their separate efforts.

Three of the many issues that have an impact on the delivery of care in the current health care arena support and even mandate the use of the Neuman Systems Model in clinical practice. These issues are an emphasis on productivity and efficiency, perspectives that represent functional diversity rather than unity, and fragmented specialization instead of wholistic care.

These issues make it difficult for clinicians to implement an approach to practice that requires a considerable amount of time for comprehensive assessment and determination of client system goals. The Neuman Systems Model can be used to advantage in such a situation because it enables health care team members to work within a common perspective to motivate and empower the client to retain, attain, and maintain optimal system stability over time. Furthermore, the Neuman Systems Model makes it possible for each team member to focus on concepts of particular interest, such as one of the five client system variables or a particular type of stressor. The nurse, acting as the care manager or care coordinator (Anderson, 1999), ensures that all five client system variables and all stressors are taken into account in a coordinated manner.

Consider, for example, a 13-year-old boy who was hospitalized due to orthopedic trauma and now is being discharged to home care. His physician, respiratory therapist, and physical therapist, respectively, are concerned with his physical injuries, respiratory status, and physical rehabilitation *(physiological variable)*. His counselor is concerned with helping him deal with the experience as a situational crisis *(psychological variable)*. His social worker is concerned with home care planning and discharge coordination *(sociocultural variable)*. His minister is concerned with pastoral care for the young boy and his family *(spiritual variable)*. His teacher is concerned with helping him adjust to home schooling and achieve age-appropriate academic progress *(developmental variable)*. The nurse's role as care manager or coordinator is to ensure that his care is coordinated appropriately to deal with the multiple stressors that have affected all five client system variables.

CONCLUSION

Application of the guidelines for Neuman Systems Model–based clinical practice that were presented in this chapter is evident in Chapters 5 and 6. An integrated review of the published reports of use of the Neuman Systems Model in clinical practice is the subject matter of Chapter 3, and the clinical tools that have been derived from the Neuman Systems Model are discussed in Chapter 4.

REFERENCES

Anderson, C. A. (1999). Hitting the wall. *Nursing Outlook, 47,* 153–54.

Fawcett, J. (1989). *Analysis and evaluation of conceptual models of nursing* (2nd ed.). Philadelphia: Davis.

Fawcett, J. (1995a). *Analysis and evaluation of conceptual models of nursing* (3rd ed.). Philadelphia: Davis.

Fawcett, J. (1995b). Constructing conceptual–theoretical–empirical structures for research. In B. Neuman (Ed.), *The Neuman Systems Model* (3rd ed., pp. 459–71). Norwalk, CT: Appleton & Lange.

Fawcett, J. (2000). *Analysis and evaluation of contemporary nursing knowledge: Nursing models and theories.* Philadelphia: Davis.

Louis, M. (1995). The Neuman model in nursing research: An update. In B. Neuman (Ed.), *The Neuman Systems Model* (3rd ed., pp. 473–80). Norwalk, CT: Appleton & Lange.

Neuman, B. (1982). *The Neuman Systems Model: Application to nursing education and practice.* Norwalk, CT: Appleton-Century-Crofts.

Neuman, B., & Young, R. J. (1972). A model for teaching total person approach to patient problems. *Nursing Research, 21,* 264–69.

Ziegler, S. M. (1982). Taxonomy for nursing diagnosis derived from the Neuman systems model. In B. Neuman (Ed.), *The Neuman Systems Model: Application to nursing education and practice* (pp. 55–68). Norwalk, CT: Appleton-Century-Crofts.

three

The Neuman Systems Model and Clinical Practice: An Integrative Review, 1974–2000

Maria Alvarez Amaya

A conceptual model of nursing reflects its author's philosophy of nursing, as well as his or her individual values. The function of a conceptual model in nursing practice is to provide a distinctive frame of reference that guides approaches to patient care (Fawcett, 1997). A conceptual model of nursing specifies person, environment, health, and nursing. An ideal practice model makes provisions for all actual and potential client needs that arise in particular clinical situations in concordance with the goals of nursing (Fawcett et al., 1992). The value of the Neuman Systems Model for organizing clinical nursing practice is evident in the large and diverse body of literature that has emerged in the 28 years since its inception. This chapter presents an integrative review of literature addressing application of the Neuman Systems Model to clinical practice.

CRITERIA FOR RETRIEVAL OF THE LITERATURE

The review encompassed Neuman Systems Model–based literature about clinical nursing practice that was published through May 2000. Hand searches of several journals, including all issues through 1998 of *Advances in Nursing Science, Image: Journal of Nursing Scholarship*, and *Nursing Science Quarterly*, were conducted. Hand searches of all volumes of the printed versions of the *International Nursing Index (INI)* and *Cumulative Index to Nursing and Allied Health Literature (CINAHL)* from the mid-1970s through the early 1990s were done. This period was before the widespread availability of the CD-ROM and online versions of those databases. Computer-assisted searches were done using the CD-ROM and then the online versions of *Index Medicus (Medline)*, *INI* (available online as part of *Medline*), through May 2000 and *CINAHL* through March 2000. A list of 115 publications with practice-related titles was generated. Eight publications were omitted because they were in a foreign language (n = 1), or were unrelated to clinical practice (n = 7). The remaining 107 publications were reviewed.

Criteria for Classification of the Literature

The Neuman Systems Model identifies a structure for client system development and the wholistic process. The client system may be an individual, family, group, or community. The range and diversity of clinical situations used to demonstrate the overall applicability of the Neuman Systems Model is broadly categorized by client system.

INDIVIDUAL CLIENT SYSTEMS

Neuman defines the individual client as a total person (or a total system). According to the Neuman Systems Model, *wholistic nursing practice* refers to the simultaneous consideration of all relevant factors that have meaning for client wellness in a given clinical situation. The individual client system is in dynamic interaction with its environment. Wellness is the state of balance between the client and the environment, and is mediated by the interrelationships of multiple factors. Illness results from imbalance between available energy and energy output. Illness states (system disequilibrium) are preceded by disruptions in the lines of defense and resistance that surround the basic core, a breakdown of the client's ability to counteract the effects, or both. Nurses caring for individual clients can apply the Neuman Systems Model to a variety of clinical situations in diverse settings to prevent or treat actual and potential responses, devise strategies to prevent further negative effects, and assist clients to return to optimal wellness (Neuman, 1982, 1989, 1995).

The review of literature revealed that Neuman Systems Model applications to individual client care varied, ranging from simple comparisons of model concepts to complex, detailed descriptions. The publications discussed in this section are representative of that range. Table 3-1 presents a list of literature about individual client system applications. The table is arranged as a chronology by clinical specialty to facilitate readability.

Trépanier, Dunn, and Sprague (1995) applied Neuman Systems Model concepts to define the perinatal client as a synergistic maternal–fetal unit that becomes two separate but interacting biological entities by the third trimester. Wholistic assessment and wellness in the antepartum, intrapartum, and neonatal periods were emphasized. Actual and potential stressors in the internal maternal–fetal environment and the external environment that resulted in low birth weight were identified. The resulting database facilitated nursing diagnosis and formed the basis for comprehensive individualized perinatal care.

Pierce and Hutton (1992) applied the spiritual variable and created environment concepts to enhance wholistic care. The client system was defined as a 30-year-old man with human immunodeficiency virus (HIV). The client was seen as a composite of physiologic, psychological, developmental, sociocultural, and spritual variables. The spiritual

TABLE 3-1. Application of the Neuman Systems Model to Individual Clients

Year	Author	Clinical Area	Brief Description
1980	Utz	Medicine and Surgery	Hypertension
1982	Echlin	Medicine and Surgery	Palliative care of terminally ill clients
1983	Cunningham	Medicine and Surgery	Tertiary management after cerebral hemorrhage
1984	Bigbee	Women's Health	Health needs of rural women
1985	Redheffer	Medicine and Surgery	Myocardial infarction (MI) in emergency settings
1985	Ross & Bourbonnais	Medicine and Surgery	Post-MI rehabilitation
1986	Sullivan	Medicine and Surgery	Spinal cord injury in critical care settings
1988	Brown	Medicine and Surgery	Risk reduction of cardiovascular disease
1988	Torkington	Pediatric Nursing	Nutritional needs of infants
1989	Biley	Medicine and Surgery	Stress management in critical care settings
1989	Smith	Medicine and Surgery	Complicated MI
1989	Wallingford	Medicine and Surgery	Family-centered critical care
1989	Herrick & Goodykoontz	Psychiatric Mental Health	Family-centered care of a disturbed adolescent
1990	Foote, Piazza, & Schultz	Medicine and Surgery	Spinal cord injury
1990	Hoeman & Winters	Medicine and Surgery	Long-term care of spinal cord injury clients
1990	Hiltz	Gerontology	Rehabilitation of elders with chronic obstructive pulmonary disease (COPD)
1990	Moore & Munro	Gerontology	Mental health assessment
1991	Baerg	Medicine and Surgery	Transcultural assessment of a 77-year-old Cree Indian in a preop setting
1991	Kido	Medicine and Surgery	Psychosis in critical care settings
1991	Shaw	Medicine and Surgery	Conceptual model for orthopedic practice
1991	Weinberger	Medicine and Surgery	Management after colostomy
1991	Lindell & Olsson	Women's Health	Oral contraceptive counseling
1992	Bergstrom	Medicine and Surgery	Pathologic hypermetabolism in critically ill clients
1992	Piazza et al.	Pediatric Nursing	Child with leukemia
1993	Bullock	Women's Health	Abused women
1993	Galloway	Pediatric Nursing	Professional and personal growth while caring for an infant with bronchopulmonary dysplasia
1993	Orr	Pediatric Nursing	Hospitalized child
1993	Waters	Psychiatric Mental Health	Substance abuse
1995	Fawcett, Tulman, and Samarel	Medicine and Surgery	Conceptual framework for functional assessment
1995	Goodman	Medicine and Surgery	Assessment of client perspectives and quality of care
1995	Picton	Medicine and Surgery	Family-centered care in emergency settings

(continues)

TABLE 3-1. Application of the Neuman Systems Model to Individual Clients *(continued)*

Year	Author	Clinical Area	Brief Description
1995	Miner	Women's Health	Perinatal human immunodeficiency virus (HIV)
1995	Poole & Flowers	Women's Health	Perinatal substance abuse
1995	Ware & Shannahan	Pediatric Nursing	Neonatal intensive care unit (NICU) parent support group
1995	Wormald	Pediatric Nursing	Care of a child with tonsillitis
1996	Gibson	Gerontology	Health promotion in elders
1996	Hassell	Psychiatric Mental Health	Conceptual model for management of depression
1997	Black, Deeny, & McKenna	Medicine and Surgery	Neurosensory stress in critical care settings
1997	Cowperthwaite et al.	Medicine and Surgery	Latex allergies in operating room settings
1997	Mill	Medicine and Surgery	Long-term care of HIV clients
1997	Fawcett	Psychiatric Mental Health	Conceptual models for practice
1998	Wright	Medicine and Surgery	Spiritual care
1998	Fawcett	Psychiatric Mental Health	Conceptual models & therapeutic modalities
1998	Gigliotti	Women's Health	Nursing diagnoses in perinatal settings

variable influences all other client system variables, thereby affecting optimal wellness. The created environment is fabricated to buffer the ego structure and is a symbolic, yet purposeful expression of wholeness that encompasses both the internal and external environments. Assessment of the spiritual variable and created environment-guided nursing interventions that linked primary prevention and wellness.

Russell, Hileman, and Grant (1995) highlighted the needs of individual caregivers of clients with HIV and cancer in home settings. The focus was on the environment in relation to the caregiver as client system. The external environment included family structure and relationships. The internal environment emphasized the created environment. The caregiver was seen to function primarily in the realm of the created environment, particularly when providing care to the terminally ill. The created environment served as protective insulation of the caregiver's ego structure. The authors deemed it important to assess the caregiver's created environment first to identify potential stressors and effects. The nursing goal was to reduce possible stressor encounters and to strengthen the caregiver's flexible lines of defense.

In critical care settings, physiological needs that threaten the client's basic structure are often at the forefront. Fawcett and colleagues (1992) suggested that, among various conceptual models that may be appropriate in critical care settings, the Neuman Systems Model promotes both system stability and optimal wellness. Bueno and Sengin (1995) stated that the Neuman Systems Model helps nurses maintain focus on the interactive client system components that are critical to retaining and attaining stability. The Neuman Systems Model focuses the nurse's attention on the total clinical situation with its bio-psycho-social-spiritual domains while permitting scrutiny of parts and subparts. Bueno and Sengin (1995) maintained that the Neuman Systems Model has utility in complex critical care settings as an organizing framework for addressing physiological, psychological, sociocultural, developmental, and spiritual issues of the client system.

McInerney (1982) addressed several themes in the total person approach in critical care settings that she considered universal. She proposed that the Neuman Systems Model could address the health needs of cardiac surgery clients in the first 12 hours postoperatively. Although cardiac surgery was viewed as the major physiological stressor, the possibility of negative consequences and anticipated lifestyle changes were major psychological stressors influencing the client's total recovery.

Wright and colleagues (1994) compared and contrasted the Neuman Systems Model, Orem's General Theory of Nursing, and Roy's Adaptation Model in a pediatric oncology setting. Although all three conceptual models were found to be useful guides for clinical practice, Wright and colleagues pointed out that the Neuman Systems Model was the only one that addressed wellness and illness disease prevention.

Knight (1990) identified the chief strength of the Neuman Systems Model for the care of clients with multiple sclerosis as its emphasis on client perception, which has a significant effect on outcomes. Client management using the Neuman Systems Model was found to be congruent with a wholistic approach to the care of these clients because it focuses attention on the multiple complex interacting variables encountered during a lifetime with the disease.

Several authors emphasized the compatibility of the traditional nursing process and the Neuman Systems Model. The Neuman Systems Model contains all the steps of the nursing process organized into three steps—nursing problem identification, goals, and outcomes. Mayers and Watson (1982) analyzed the compatibility of the Neuman Systems Model and the nursing process and found that the linkage with theoretical terms translated into theory-based nursing process. In their analysis, assessment identified intra-, inter-, or extrapersonal stressors that disrupt normal lines of defense to produce system instability. They pointed out that nursing diagnosis is a process of inference, validation, and deduction, and that the Neuman Systems Model assessment tool validates assessment conclusions by its requirement for reconciliation between the client's and the caregiver's perceptions. Neal (1982) agreed that the use of a conceptual model, such as the Neuman Systems Model, provides a distinctive frame of reference for nursing process by identifying data collection parameters from which to make nursing diagnoses and identify expected outcomes.

Cunningham (1982) illustrated use of the Neuman Systems Model nursing process as an organizing framework to address pain in a client with trauma in a critical care setting. Pain was seen as the prime stressor. The client's current and predicted pain response was assessed from the perspective of intra-, inter-, and extrapersonal factors composed of physiological, psychological, sociocultural, and developmental variables. Primary, secondary, and tertiary prevention interventions to reduce pain were planned accordingly.

Chiverton and Flannery (1995) applied the Neuman Systems Model nursing process to assess cognitive function in an acute care setting using a neuroassessment tool. Traumatic brain injury was viewed as a stressor that disrupts the basic structure to an extent that renders the client completely without adaptive energy. Nursing interventions at the secondary level are necessary to maintain client system stability until the client's cognitive function returns.

Baker (1982) focused on secondary and tertiary preventions aimed at strengthening lines of defense and resistance of clients experiencing acute respiratory distress from chronic obstructive pulmonary disease (COPD). The author noted that the psychological concomitants of COPD, such as fear, anxiety, depression, and lowered self-esteem, could add to debilitation.

Cardona (1982) applied the Neuman Systems Model nursing process to plan and implement tertiary inpatient care. Rehabilitation was seen as a restorative process that affects the total person and requires a team approach to facilitate adaptation.

Lile (1990) emphasized primary prevention interventions directed at reducing encounters with stressors and strengthening defense mechanisms for risk reduction. She viewed risk factors for coronary heart disease in women as the result of exposure to chronic, habitual stressors that eventually disrupt the normal line of defense. Primary prevention interventions should emphasize health information, support, and motivation of the client toward high-level wellness.

Breckenridge (1982) applied the Neuman Systems Model to prevention interventions in clients with renal disease. The dynamic circular schematic of primary, secondary, and tertiary prevention interventions in the Neuman Systems Model was found to be useful for fostering wholistic approaches on a continuum of care (Breckenridge, 1982, 1989). She recommended that care plans include prevention interventions at all levels because of the chronic nature of renal disease (Breckenridge, 1982).

Molassiotis (1997) described Neuman Systems Model–guided assessment of quality of life in clients with cancer who had a bone marrow transplant. Adaptation to illness/treatment and quality of life were seen as a five-stage process that is influenced by physiological, psychological, social, and developmental variables. Nursing intervention can take place at any point in the process. The goals of nursing interventions are to prevent ineffective coping or maladjustment, and to promote adjustment to illness.

Narsavage (1997) focused on strengthening lines of resistance in clients with COPD. Shared nurse–client perceptions form the basis for interventions. Inasmuch as the client's perception of self-control influences quality of life in clients with COPD, Narsavage discussed various methods to change perception of control as a mode to strengthen lines of resistance.

According to the Neuman Systems Model, the state of wellness achieved after every restorative process, or equifinal steady state, may be the same or different. The equifinal steady-state components become input for other cycles. Death results when the energy requirements to maintain survival mechanisms exceed that which is readily available. Rice (1982) explained that efforts to strengthen internal lines of resistance might fail when clients are unable to reconstitute following penetration of stressors that produce severe disequilibrium. She applied the Neuman Systems Model to assessment and care of a 78-year-old client with cerebrovascular accident whose condition gradually deteriorated. Using Neuman Systems Model concepts, Rice described the final stressor as the client's loss of independent function and his transfer to a long-term care facility.

Herrick, Goodykoontz, and Herrick (1992) present therapeutic modalities for psychiatric mental health nursing based on the Neuman Systems Model. Therapeutic modalities were selected to care for a severely disturbed boy based on three components of the Neuman Systems Model—sources of stressors (extra-, inter-, and intrasystem), level of response (primary, secondary, or tertiary), and system of focus (group, family, or individual). The assessment revealed the strategies within a modality that were most appropriate, such as individual counseling, play therapy, and behavior therapy.

Francine Clark (1982) described the Neuman Systems Model as an instrument to guide the integration of psychiatric and developmental theories and the nursing process. She maintained that the Neuman Systems Model is a useful tool for psychiatric mental health nurse practitioners who are concerned with increased professional accountability and the concomitant need for client participation in the therapeutic process.

Extending the application of the Neuman Systems Model to health care systems, Hinton-Walker (1993) advocated a paradigmatic change in approaches to chronic care from the current acute care–oriented model to a participatory and resource-driven primary care model. She further stated that nurse practitioners are the best equipped to provide the wide range of services needed by the chronically ill.

Stuart and Wright (1995) described the challenges faced by psychiatric mental health nurses due to emerging mental health needs of diverse groups. Psychiatric clients are more acutely ill when hospitalized, are treated more aggressively to shorten their length of stay, and are discharged with higher acuities than in the past. The Neuman Systems Model provides a conceptual map to organize total care in cost-constrained mental health settings, and not merely to target symptomatic relief.

Herrick and colleagues (1991) pointed out that the case manager role in a child psychiatric setting provided opportunities for wholistic care in a climate of cost constraints. Short inpatient stays require planning for a continuum of care after discharge. Neuman Systems Model concepts were integrated to organize a therapeutic modality for comprehensive care along a continuum, with clear links to the nursing process.

THE FAMILY CLIENT

Few publications address the application of the Neuman Systems Model applications to family clients. Systems approaches are evident in these publications, with their emphasis on the complex, interdependent, dynamic, and interactive processes within a client system.

Neuman (1983) views the family as a composite of individual members in harmonious relationships that form a cluster of related meanings and values. Wellness is synonymous with family system stability, and implies harmonious function. A family system encounters stressors of intra-, inter-, and extrafamily nature and is influenced by physiological, psychological, developmental, and spiritual variables. Culture often is a factor as well. The family nursing goal is to aid in stabilizing families, and their individual members, within their environment.

Reed (1989, 1993) interpreted the Neuman Systems Model in noting that families have both a composite identity and an individual member profile. She further noted the lack of a discrete nursing conceptual base for family nursing practice and proposed the Neuman Systems Model to fill this gap. The traditional theoretical foundations of family nursing are multidisciplinary in nature and emphasize family theory. These theories are not entirely acceptable to nursing because they lack wholistic approaches, and because underlying belief systems may be compromised when frameworks are combined. Inasmuch as the Neuman Systems Model is process oriented, it can be used to integrate family theory into a distinct nursing practice framework.

The Neuman Systems Model places family theory process concepts on the flexible line of defense and structure concepts on the normal line of defense (Reed, 1989, 1993). Therefore, assessment of the flexible and normal lines of defense encompasses assessment of family process and structure concepts. Reed (1989) stated that lines of resistance are internal factors that protect both the family as a system and each individual within the family system following disruptions by stressors. Internal factors that correlate with the lines of resistance are the concepts of interrelatedness, interdependence, values, and beliefs. These concepts are, in turn, related to the five Neuman Systems Model variables. Reed (1989) further operationalized the Neuman Systems Model by dividing the family into five domains corresponding to the five client system variables. The flexible and normal lines of defense, lines of resistance, and basic structure were then identified within each domain (Reed, 1993).

Cross (1995) agreed with Neuman's (1983) view of family wellness when she stated that successful transactions with the environment were reflective of a family's adjustment to that environment. She demonstrated this in the application of a systems approach to plan family-centered care for a client with Hodgkin's disease. The nursing care plan demonstrated assessment of intra-, inter-, and extrapersonal stressors within the context of physiological, psychological, developmental, sociocultural, and spiritual variables over time (Cross, 1995).

Quayhagen and Roth (1989) facilitated theory-based family assessment of selected Neuman Systems Model concepts. Family stressors were assessed using matched psychometrically sound research instruments. In this way, stressors that cause disruption in the family system were measured. The instruments provided empirical validation for clinical inferences based on the Neuman Systems Model.

Beckingham and Baumann (1990) integrated crisis theory and Neuman Systems Model concepts to develop an assessment and decision-making model to incorporate families in the decision-making process regarding the care of elders. The model is useful for elder families in crisis situations that may be encountered in either inpatient or community settings. A systematic approach to family assessment assured that as many factors as possible were considered in optimal decision making.

Delunas (1990) used the Neuman Systems Model as a framework for the clinical nurse specialist to utilize in developing a plan of care aimed at preventing intrafamily elder abuse while maintaining family integrity. The focus was on primary prevention interventions through systematic assessment of the family as a unit. Owens (1995) applied a similar approach in the family-centered approach to the care of a woman with Down's syndrome.

Goldblum-Graff and Graff (1982) recognized that the Neuman Systems Model, as a wholistic health care model, is analogous to Engel's biopsychosocial model, which is widely used by mental health therapists. They reported extensive experience with the Neuman Systems Model in their family therapy practice. Their therapeutic approach was based on assessment of intra-, inter-, and extrafamilial stressors. The goals of primary, secondary, and tertiary prevention interventions were considered throughout the therapeutic process.

Tomlinson and Anderson (1995) proposed a slightly different viewpoint in their family health systems nursing paradigm. The family was viewed as a separate entity in unique interaction with the environment. Family health is a wholistic function of the family system. Thus, although the Neuman Systems Model views the family more as context for the individual with a system interface, Tomlinson and Anderson recognized the potential for a clearer family system perspective in their paradigm. Their paradigm of family health embraces more than the health of individuals. It links family structure, function, and health variables, incorporates the biopsychosocial and contextual system aspects of nursing, and addresses the levels of family interaction with the nurse.

THE AGGREGATE/COMMUNITY CLIENT

Community health nursing practice is based on the integration of the nursing role and public health, epidemiology, environmental science, psychology, sociology, anthropology, economics, and political science, to name a few of the disciplines that contribute to the body of knowledge. According to Beddome (1989), the Neuman Systems Model promotes the development of a distinct body of knowledge for community health nursing practice through its dynamic view of the complex community client, which allows integration of theories from other disciplines. Several publications have addressed the application of the Neuman Systems Model to the community as the client system (Table 3-2).

According to Benedict and Sproles (1982), basic assumptions underlie community/ public health nursing practice. The community entity is reflected in a population's characteristics. These characteristics represent group-specific tendencies that define a population at risk or determine a priority high-risk group. High-risk populations may be viewed as composites of interacting variables with a basic core.

Spradley (1990) added that systems theory is the underlying base of community health nursing. Several authors agree that the Neuman Systems Model provides a framework for viewing the community from a systems perspective, and the model facilitates synthesis of a broad knowledge base for interdisciplinary practice (Anderson, McFarlane, & Helton, 1986; Benedict & Sproles, 1982; Buchanan, 1987; Haggart, 1993; Helland, 1995).

Spradley (1990) further described the compatibility of the Neuman Systems Model with a conceptual framework of community health nursing. Physiological, psychological, developmental, sociocultural, and spiritual variables were compared to biological and environmental factors, adequacies and inadequacies of the health care system, and psychosociocultural health determinants. Assessment of these variables reveals the unique response to stressors exhibited by each community client.

Spradley (1990) went on to describe the community client system. The core of basic survival of a community is its ability to make the best use of its natural resources. The lines of resistance include a community's sense of responsibility. The normal line of defense includes a community's police and firefighting systems. The flexible line of defense might include maintenance of roads and support of schools. Examples of intrapersonal

TABLE 3-2. Application of the Neuman Systems Model to Community Clients

Year	Author	Brief Description
1974	Balch	Application of Neuman Systems Model conceptual framework
1980	Craddock & Stanhope	Home health care
1988	Gavan, Hastings-Tolsma, & Troyan	Nutrition across the life span
1993	Coutu-Wakulczyk & Beckingham	Conceptual models for gerontologic nursing in the community
1993	Mynatt & O'Brien	Chemical dependency prevention program for the nursing community
1995	Procter & Cheek	Transcultural nursing of aggregates experiencing catastrophic events
1996	Cookfair	Assessment of high-risk aggregates

stressors might be poor system maintenance. An interpersonal stressor arising from interaction with other people or systems might include stressful intergroup relationships, inadequate support systems, or maladaptive cultural patterns. Extrapersonal stressors might arise from the environment itself, such as economic problems, tornado damage, or a nuclear spill. Nursing goals include removing or minimizing environmental stressors, strengthening clients' defenses, and promoting recovery or stability.

The community client has been defined as both an aggregate of clients and a geopolitical community. The community as client has an engrained core structure of survival mechanisms surrounded by lines of defense and resistance (Anderson, McFarlane, & Helton, 1986; Beddome, 1989; Benedict & Sproles, 1982; Buchanan, 1987; Haggart, 1993). The focus of nursing assessment determines what these boundaries are in a particular situation.

Accurate identification of subsystems in the environment is crucial to assessment and nursing diagnosis. Authors have viewed community subsystems as interdependent units of relationships, interactions, and influences that determine the degree of a community's health state or stability by their dynamic interactions, and which must be defined for assessment purposes. Beddome (1989) states that assessment of subsystems included within physiological, psychological, developmental, sociocultural, and spiritual variables works well when the client system is an individual. However, subsystems are less easily defined when applied to entities like buildings, roadways, and communication systems within the community. Nevertheless, identification of subsystems is deemed particularly useful for assessing inter- and extrasystems of both aggregate and geopolitical community clients. Community subsystems may include recreation, safety and transportation, communication, education, health and social services, economics, politics and government, and the physical environment (Anderson, McFarlane, & Helton, 1986).

Community stressors are defined as intra-, inter-, or extrasystem factors that affect the level of function and may cause disequilibrium. Stessors may be positive or negative, may be perceived at both the individual and community levels, and may be completely preventable or inherently prevalent (Benedict & Sproles, 1982). Physiological, psychological, developmental, and sociocultural variables interact with inter-, intra-, and extrasystem factors to produce a cumulative effect that acts on the flexible line of defense (Buchanan, 1987). Benedict and Sproles (1982) recommend assessment of intra-, inter-, and extracommunity factors as a logical beginning point for organizing a community assessment database. Community stressors then can be identified and levels of care for the community implemented to reduce actual or potential stressor effects (Benedict & Sproles, 1982).

The flexible line of defense is a dynamic buffer that mediates temporary responses, such as neighborhood coalitions formed to respond to a particular situation (Anderson, McFarlane, & Helton, 1986). The normal line of defense includes constant and relatively stable sources of support (Benedict & Sproles, 1982) that are reflective of a community's wellness level (Anderson, McFarlane, & Helton, 1986). The internal lines of resistance are intrasystem mechanisms that act to defend against stressors that have penetrated the normal line of defense (Anderson, McFarlane, & Helton, 1986). Anderson and colleagues (1986) also stated that internal lines of resistance might be thought of as relatively stable coping patterns designed to counteract the effects of a stressor after it has penetrated the normal lines of defense. An example is an evening recreational program that is established to prevent juvenile crime. The degree of reaction is the degree of disequilibrium or disruption that results from the stressors impinging on the community's lines of defense and resistance, such as morbidity and mortality, unemployment, and crime rates.

Community health is the degree of wellness (stability or equilibrium) resulting from adaptation processes. It involves the level of wellness of the individuals that constitute a community. Haggart (1993) defines community health as the level of harmonious interaction of subsystems within the internal and external environments, and Buchanan (1987) defines it as the availability of essential resources necessary for the wellbeing of individuals, whose lack thereof constitutes a stressor (Anderson, McFarlane, & Helton, 1986). Community assessment identifies conditions of relative balance or imbalance (or the range of wellness responses) within each subsystem (Buchanan, 1987).

The goal of community health nursing is a healthy community (system equilibrium). Nursing functions contribute to the regulation and control of system responses to stressors and help the community attain, maintain, retain, and promote optimal wellness (Anderson, McFarlane, & Helton, 1986). Haggart (1993) states that the level of community health is equivalent to the level of harmony with the internal and external environments. Thus, optimal community wellness may require nursing interventions that promote social change as well as those that facilitate a return to stability depending on the situation.

Helland (1995) demonstrated a practical application of the Neuman Systems Model to formulate a nursing diagnosis for the community client. In making a Neuman Systems Model–based nursing diagnosis for a community client, model concepts must be clearly delineated in the data collection phase. The process of developing nursing diagnoses for an aggregate of abused women was preceded by systematic identification of intra-, inter-, and extrapersonal stressors within the context of physiological, psychological, developmental, sociocultural, and spiritual variables.

Ross and Helmer (1988) adapted the Neuman Systems Model to the nursing process in community clients. Data were collected on the population's perception of its situation, stressors, responses, and lines of defense. These perceptions were compared to the nurse's self-identified perceptions. Data were interpreted and summarized from inter-, intra- and extrapersonal perspectives, and were organized into physiological, psychological, developmental, sociocultural, and spiritual categories.

Peirce and Fulmer (1995) conceptualized elders as aggregate cohorts in the community. Aging was seen as a normal process with both positive and negative outcomes that is especially suited to a wellness model such as the Neuman Systems Model. The aging process was conceptualized as a loss of flexibility and buffering ability in the lines of defense, resulting in inevitable and irreversible change, especially loss of physiological function. Although elders have a diminished ability to fend off stressors, other variables (psychological, sociocultural, developmental, and spiritual) may or may not vary. The goal of gerontological nursing is to differentiate between intrinsic and extrinsic reactions. Peirce and Fulmer outlined sources of physiological, psychological, sociocultural, developmental and spiritual stressors in the elderly within intra-, inter-, and extrapersonal dimensions.

Primary prevention interventions in community health nursing involve the identification of risk prior to the occurrence of a reaction. These interventions involve consideration of community-specific factors that contribute to public health (Buchanan, 1987). Primary prevention intervention in community health settings is interpreted as illness prevention and health promotion (Buchanan, 1987; Haggart, 1993). Nursing actions are aimed at strengthening lines of defense or removal of the stressor (Anderson, McFarlane, & Helton, 1986).

Secondary prevention intervention in community systems is dependent on resources for service delivery after a reaction has occurred. For example, after a hurricane, a community needs access to trauma care services and temporary shelters so that rescue workers can assist those in need. Nursing actions are aimed at supporting lines of defense and resistance to minimize the degree of reaction (Anderson, McFarlane, & Helton, 1986).

Tertiary prevention intervention supports reconstitution following disequilibrium, and may include legislative and political processes that aid in restoration (Beddome, 1989; Benedict and Sproles, 1982; Buchanan, 1987). Tertiary prevention intervention is aimed at preventing further disequilibrium and reestablishing the equilibrium of the community system (Anderson, McFarlane, & Helton, 1986).

Sohier (1989, 1995) elaborated on the thesis that culture in the care of clients holds special relevance for community clients, as well as for family and individual clients. Due to complex social trends such as "new wave" immigration, nurse–client interactions rarely occur within a common cultural context. Unless the nurse validates client perception, a variety of interpersonal cultural barriers arise that may contribute to noncompliance or nonadherence. Thus, through its requirement for cross-validation of nurse and client perceptions, the Neuman Systems Model is seen as a bridge across cultural gaps. The flexibility and dynamism of the systems approach helps to circumvent many nurse–client barriers that preempt expected outcomes in cross-cultural contexts.

The Neuman Systems Model has been applied to address a variety of other community health nursing practice problems, including cost constraints (Buchanan, 1987), increased demand for primary prevention for both general and special populations (Buchanan, 1987; Haggart, 1993), cross-cultural barriers (Anderson, McFarlane, & Helton, 1986; Haggart, 1993; Procter & Cheek, 1995; Sohier, 1989, 1995), increased demand for secondary-level services (Hinton-Walker, 1993), and home health care services (Craddock & Stanhope, 1980).

CONCLUSION

The review of the literature presented in this chapter illustrates diverse applications of the Neuman Systems Model to clinical practice with individual, family, and aggregate/community client systems in a variety of settings. The Neuman Systems Model is widely perceived to encompass a philosophy and values compatible with acknowledged roles and functions of nursing. Various authors described how the Neuman Systems Model provides a distinctive frame of reference to address particular health conditions within the context of clinical specialties and/or distinct settings. The publications specified client, environment, nursing, and health according to Neuman Systems Model concepts. Many centered on how the model guided wholistic approaches to patient care. Clearly, the Neuman Systems Model is capable of addressing actual and potential client needs within a broad spectrum of clinical situations. International use of the Neuman Systems Model provides additional evidence of its broad applicability (Cheung, 1997; J. Clark, 1982; Engberg, 1995; Millard, 1992; Salvage & Turner, 1989; Vaughan & Gough, 1995). However, there remains a dearth of Neuman Systems Model–based literature in many areas, including environmental health nursing, nursing administration, and interdisciplinary practice.

Neuman (1982) intended the model to provide a framework for interdisciplinary health care delivery that could be used by nurses to assist individuals, families, and groups to retain, attain, and maintain optimal wellness levels by purposeful interventions. Craddock and Stanhope (1980) recognized the value of the Neuman Systems Model for interdisciplinary interactions. However, there is very little mention in the literature about interdisciplinary applications.

In 1982, Stevens noted that the Neuman Systems Model practice-related literature demonstrated a range of interpretations of wholism. She explained that at one extreme, oversimplification of the concept was reflected by the mere use of a comparable method. At the other extreme, complex and detailed taxonomies made the concept overly complex. Curran (1995) stated that wholism is not merely the comprehensive accumulation of all essential parts, but also relates complex, interdependent, dynamic, and interactive processes within a client system. Neuman Systems Model applications to family and aggregate/community clients were more likely to emphasize system wholeness, whereas applications focusing on individual client systems tended to emphasize parts and subparts and relate them to the whole.

Neuman (1982) views nursing as a whole system with parts and subparts inherent within it. In any given setting, it is possible to establish relevant parts and subparts and the linkages between them. The literature provides ample evidence that certain portions within the domain of nursing can be selected and dealt with as organized wholes. The systems approach holds the promise envisioned by Neuman (1982) for increasing self-determination, creativity, and adaptive ability of the profession by providing a tangible structure within which change can take place.

REFERENCES

Anderson, E., McFarlane, J., & Helton, A. (1986). Community-as-client: A model for practice. *Nursing Outlook, 34,* 220–24.

Baerg, K. L. (1991). Using Neuman's model to analyze a clinical situation. *Rehabilitation Nursing, 16,* 38–39.

Baker, N. A. (1982). Use of the Neuman model in planning for the psychological needs of the respiratory disease patient. In B. Neuman (Ed.), *The Neuman Systems Model: Application to nursing education and practice* (pp. 241–51). Norwalk, CT: Appleton-Century-Crofts.

Balch, C. (1974). Breaking the lines of resistance. In J. P. Riehl & C. Roy (Eds.), *Conceptual models for nursing practice* (pp. 130–34). New York: Appleton-Century-Crofts.

Beckingham, A. C., & Baumann, A. (1990). The aging family in crisis: Assessment and decision-making models. *Journal of Advanced Nursing, 15,* 782–87.

Beddome, G. (1989). Application of the Neuman Systems Model to the assessment of community-as-client. In B. Neuman (Ed.), *The Neuman Systems Model* (2nd ed., pp. 363–74). Norwalk, CT: Appleton & Lange.

Benedict, M. B., & Sproles, J. B. (1982). Application of the Neuman model to public health nursing practice. In B. Neuman (Ed.), *The Neuman Systems Model: Application to nursing education and practice* (pp. 223–40). Norwalk, CT: Appleton-Century-Crofts.

Bergstrom, D. (1992). Hypermetabolism in multisystem organ failure: A Neuman systems perspective. *Critical Care Nursing Quarterly, 15*(3), 63–70.

Bigbee, J. (1984). The changing role of rural women: Nursing and health implications. *Health Care of Women International, 5,* 307–22.

Biley, F. C. (1989). Stress in high dependency units. *Intensive Care Nursing, 5,* 134–41.

Black, P., Deeny, P., & McKenna, H. (1997). Sensoristrain: An exploration of nursing interventions in the context of the Neuman Systems Model. *Intensive and Critical Care Nursing, 13,* 249–58.

Breckenridge, D. M. (1982). Adaptation of the Neuman Systems Model for the renal client. In B. Neuman (Ed.), *The Neuman Systems Model: Application to nursing education and practice* (pp. 267–77). Norwalk, CT: Appleton-Century-Crofts.

Breckenridge, D. M. (1989). Primary prevention as an intervention modality for the renal client. In B. Neuman (Ed.), *The Neuman Systems Model* (2nd ed., pp. 397–406). Norwalk, CT: Appleton & Lange.

Brown, M. W. (1988). Neuman's systems model in risk factor reduction. *Cardiovascular Nursing, 24*(6), 43.

Buchanan, B. F. (1987). Human–environment interaction: A modification of the Neuman Systems Model for aggregates, families, and the community. *Public Health Nursing, 4,* 52–64.

Bueno, M. M., & Sengin, K. K. (1995). The Neuman Systems Model for critical care nursing: A framework for practice. In B. Neuman (Ed.), *The Neuman Systems Model* (3rd ed., pp. 275–91). Norwalk, CT: Appleton & Lange.

Bullock, L. F. C. (1993). Nursing interventions for abused women on obstetrical units. *AWHONN's Clinical Issues in Perinatal and Women's Health Nursing, 4*(3), 371–77.

Cardona, V. D. (1982). Client rehabilitation and the Neuman model. In B. Neuman (Ed.), *The Neuman Systems Model: Application to nursing education and practice* (pp. 278–90). Norwalk, CT: Appleton-Century-Crofts.

Cheung, Y. L. (1997). The application of Neuman Systems Model to nursing in Hong Kong. *Hong Kong Nursing Journal, 33*(4), 17–21.

Chiverton, P., & Flannery, J. C. (1995). Cognitive impairment: Use of the Neuman Systems Model. In B. Neuman (Ed.), *The Neuman Systems Model* (3rd ed., pp. 249–61). Norwalk, CT: Appleton & Lange.

Clark, F. (1982). The Neuman Systems Model: A clinical application for psychiatric nurse practitioners. In B. Neuman (Ed.), *The Neuman Systems Model: Application to nursing education and practice* (pp. 335–53). Norwalk, CT: Appleton-Century-Crofts.

Clark, J. (1982). Development of models and theories on the concept of nursing. *Journal of Advanced Nursing, 7,* 129–34.

Cookfair, J. M. (1996). Community as client. In J. M. Cookfair (Ed.), *Nursing care in the community* (2nd ed., pp. 19–37). St. Louis: Mosby–Year Book.

Coutu-Wakulczyk, G., & Beckingham, A. C. (1993). Selected nursing models applicable to gerontological practice. In A. C. Beckingham & B. DuGas (Eds.), *Promoting healthy aging: A nursing and community perspective* (pp. 80–110). St. Louis: Mosby–Year Book.

Cowperthwaite, B., LaPlante, K., Mahon, B., & Markowski, T. (1997). Latex allergy in the nursing population. *Canadian Operating Room Nursing Journal, 15* (2), 23–24, 26–28, 30–32.

Craddock, R. B., & Stanhope, M. K. (1980). The Neuman health-care systems model: Recommended adaptation. In J. P. Riehl & C. Roy (Eds.), *Conceptual models for nursing practice* (2nd ed., pp. 159–69). New York: Appleton-Century-Crofts.

Cross, J. R. (1995). Nursing process of the family client: Application of Neuman's Systems Model. In P. J. Christensen & J. W. Kenney (Eds.), *Nursing process: Application of conceptual models* (4th ed., pp. 246–69). St. Louis: Mosby–Year Book.

Cunningham, S. G. (1982). The Neuman model applied to an acute care setting: Pain. In B. Neuman (Ed.), *The Neuman Systems Model: Application to nursing education and practice* (pp. 291–96). Norwalk, CT: Appleton-Century-Crofts.

Cunningham, S. G. (1983). The Neuman Systems Model applied to a rehabilitation setting. *Rehabilitation Nursing, 8*(4), 20–22.

Curran, G. (1995). The Neuman Systems Model revisited: In B. Neuman (Ed.), *The Neuman Systems Model* (3rd ed., pp. 93–99). Norwalk, CT: Appleton & Lange.

Delunas, L. R. (1990). Prevention of elder abuse: Betty Neuman health care systems approach. *Clinical Nurse Specialist, 4,* 54–58.

Echlin, D. J. (1982). Palliative care and the Neuman model. In B. Neuman (Ed.), *The Neuman Systems Model: Application to nursing education and practice* (pp. 257–59). Norwalk, CT: Appleton-Century-Crofts.

Engberg, I. B. (1995). Brief abstracts: Use of the Neuman Systems Model in Sweden. In B. Neuman (Ed.), *The Neuman Systems Model* (3rd ed., pp. 653–56). Norwalk, CT: Appleton & Lange.

Fawcett, J. (1997). Conceptual models as guides for psychiatric nursing practice. In A. W. Burgess (Ed.), *Psychiatric mental health nursing: Promoting mental health* (pp. 627–42). Stamford, CT: Appleton & Lange.

Fawcett, J. (1998). Conceptual models and therapeutic modalities in advanced psychiatric mental health nursing practice. In A. W. Burgess (Ed.), *Advanced practice psychiatric mental health nursing* (pp. 41–48). Stamford, CT: Appleton & Lange.

Fawcett, J., Archer, C. L., Becker, D., et al. (1992). Guidelines for selecting a conceptual model of nursing: Focus on the individual patient. *Dimensions of Critical Care Nursing, 11,* 268–77.

Fawcett, J., Tulman, L., & Samarel, N. (1995). Enhancing function in life transitions and serious illness. *Advanced Practice Nursing Quarterly, 1*(3), 50–57.

Foote, A. W., Piazza, D., & Schultz, M. (1990). The Neuman Systems Model: Application to a patient with a cervical spinal cord injury. *Journal of Neuroscience Nursing, 22,* 302–306.

Galloway, D.A. (1993). Coping with a mentally and physically impaired infant: A self-analysis. *Rehabilitation Nursing, 18,* 34–36.

Gavan, C. A. S., Hastings-Tolsma, M. T., & Troyan, P. J. (1988). Explication of Neuman's model: A holistic systems approach to nutrition for health promotion in the life process. *Holistic Nursing Practice, 3*(1), 26–38.

Gibson, M. (1996). Health promotion for a group of elderly clients. *Perspectives, 20*(3), 2–5.

Gigliottti, E. (1998). You make the diagnosis. Case study: Integration of the Neuman Systems Model with the theory of nursing diagnosis in postpartum nursing. *Nursing Diagnosis: The Journal of Nursing Language and Classification, 9,* 14, 34–38.

Goldblum-Graff, D., & Graff, H. (1982). The Neuman model adapted to family therapy. In B. Neuman (Ed.), *The Neuman Systems Model: Application to nursing education and practice* (pp. 217–22). Norwalk, CT: Appleton-Century-Crofts.

Goodman, H. (1995). Patients' views count as well. *Nursing Standard, 9*(40), 55.

Haggart, M. (1993). A critical analysis of Neuman's Systems Model in relation to public health nursing. *Journal of Advanced Nursing, 18,* 1917–22.

Hassell, J. S. (1996). Improved management of depression through nursing model application and critical thinking. *Journal of the American Academy of Nurse Practitioners, 8,* 161–66.

Helland, W. Y. (1995). Nursing diagnosis: Diagnostic process. In P. J. Christensen & J. W. Kenney (Eds.), *Nursing process: Application of conceptual models* (4th ed., pp. 120–38). St. Louis: Mosby–Year Book.

Herrick, C. A., & Goodykoontz, L. (1989). Neuman's Systems Model for nursing practice as a conceptual framework for a family assessment. *Journal of Child and Adolescent Psychiatric and Mental Health Nursing, 2,* 61–67.

Herrick, C. A., Goodykoontz, L., & Herrick, R. H. (1992). Selection of treatment modalities. In

P. West & C. L. Evans (Eds.), *Psychiatric and mental health nursing with children and adolescents* (pp. 98–115). Gaithersburg, MD: Aspen.

Herrick, C. A., Goodykoontz, L., Herrick, R. H., & Hackett, B. (1991). Planning a continuum of care in child psychiatric nursing: A collaborative effort. *Journal of Child and Adolescent Psychiatric and Mental Health Nursing, 4*, 41–48.

Hiltz, D. (1990). The Neuman Systems Model: An analysis of a clinical situation. *Rehabilitation Nursing, 15*, 330–32.

Hinton-Walker, P. (1993). Care of the chronically ill: Paradigm shifts and directions for the future. *Wholistic Nursing Practice, 8*(1), 56–66.

Hoeman, S. P., & Winters, D. M. (1990). Theory-based case management: High cervical spinal cord injury. *Home Healthcare Nurse, 8*, 25–33.

Kido, L. M. (1991). Sleep deprivation and intensive care unit psychosis. *Emphasis: Nursing, 4*(1), 23–33.

Knight, J. B. (1990). The Betty Neuman Systems Model applied to practice: A client with multiple sclerosis. *Journal of Advanced Nursing, 15*, 447–55.

Lile, J. L. (1990). A nursing challenge for the 90s: Reducing risk factors for coronary heart disease in women. *Health Values: Achieving High-Level Wellness, 14*(4), 17–21.

Lindell, M., & Olsson, H. (1991). Can combined oral contraceptives be made more effective by means of a nursing care model? *Journal of Advanced Nursing, 16*, 475–79.

Mayers, M. A., & Watson, A. B. (1982). Nursing care plans and the Neuman Systems Model. In B. Neuman (Ed.), *The Neuman Systems Model: Application to nursing education and practice* (pp. 69–84). Norwalk, CT: Appleton-Century-Crofts.

McInerney, K. A. (1982). The Neuman Systems Model applied to critical care nursing of cardiac surgery clients. In B. Neuman (Ed.), *The Neuman Systems Model: Application to nursing education and practice* (pp. 308–15). Norwalk, CT: Appleton-Century-Crofts.

Mill, J. E. (1997). The Neuman Systems Model: Application in a Canadian HIV setting. *British Journal of Nursing, 6*, 163–66.

Millard, J. (1992). Health visiting an elderly couple. *British Journal of Nursing, 1*, 769–73.

Miner, J. (1995). Incorporating the Betty Neuman Systems Model into HIV clinical practice. *AIDS Patient Care, 9*(1), 37–39.

Molassiotis, A. (1997). A conceptual model of adaptation to illness and quality of life for cancer patients treated with bone marrow transplants. *Journal of Advanced Nursing, 26*, 572–79.

Moore, S. L., & Munro, M. F. (1990). The Neuman Systems Model applied to mental health nursing of older adults. *Journal of Advanced Nursing, 15*, 293–99.

Mynatt, S. L., & O'Brien, J. (1993). A partnership to prevent chemical dependency in nursing using Neuman's Systems Model. *Journal of Psychosocial Nursing and Mental Health Services, 31*(4), 27–34.

Narsavage, G. L. (1997). Promoting function in clients with chronic lung disease by increasing their perception of control. *Wholistic Nursing Practice, 12*(1), 17–26.

Neal, M. C. (1982). Nursing care plans and the Neuman Systems Model: II. In B. Neuman (Ed.), *The Neuman Systems Model: Application to nursing education and practice* (pp. 85–93). Norwalk, CT: Appleton-Century-Crofts.

Neuman, B. (1982). The Neuman health-care systems model: A total approach to client care. In B. Neuman (Ed.), *The Neuman Systems Model: Application to nursing education and practice* (pp. 8–28). Norwalk, CT: Appleton-Century-Crofts.

Neuman, B. (1983). Family intervention using the Betty Neuman health-care systems model. In I. W. Clements & F. B. Roberts (Eds.), *Family health: A theoretical approach to nursing care* (pp. 239–54). New York: Wiley.

Neuman, B. (1989). The Neuman Systems Model. In B. Neuman (Ed.), *The Neuman Systems Model* (2nd ed., pp. 3–64). Norwalk, CT: Appleton & Lange.

Neuman, B. (1995). The Neuman Systems Model. In B. Neuman (Ed.), *The Neuman Systems Model* (3rd ed., pp. 3–62). Norwalk, CT: Appleton & Lange.

Orr, J. P. (1993). An adaptation of the Neuman Systems Model to the care of the hospitalized preschool child. *Curationis, 16*(3), 37–44.

Owens, M. (1995). Care of a woman with Down's syndrome using the Neuman Systems Model. *British Journal of Nursing, 4,* 752–58.

Piazza, D., Foote, A., Wright, P., & Holcombe, J. (1992). Neuman Systems Model used as a guide for the nursing care of an 8-year-old child with leukemia. *Journal of Pediatric Oncology Nursing, 9*(1), 17–24.

Peirce, A. G., & Fulmer, T. T. (1995). Application of the Neuman Systems Model to gerontological nursing. In B. Neuman (Ed.), *The Neuman Systems Model* (3rd ed., pp. 293–308). Norwalk, CT: Appleton & Lange.

Picton, C. E. (1995). An exploration of family-centered care in Neuman's model with regard to the care of the critically ill adult in an accident and emergency setting. *Accident and Emergency Nursing, 3*(1), 33–37.

Pierce, J. D., & Hutton, E. (1992). Applying the new concepts of the Neuman Systems Model. *Nursing Forum, 27,* 15–18.

Poole, V. L., & Flowers, J. S. (1995). Care management of pregnant substance abusers using the Neuman Systems Model. In B. Neuman (Ed.), *The Neuman Systems Model* (3rd ed., pp. 377–86). Norwalk, CT: Appleton & Lange.

Procter, N. G., & Cheek, J. (1995). Nurses' role in world catastrophic events: War dislocation effects on Serbian Australians. In B. Neuman (Ed.), *The Neuman Systems Model* (3rd ed., pp. 119–31). Norwalk, CT: Appleton & Lange.

Quayhagen, M. P., & Roth, P. A. (1989). From models to measures in assessment of mature families. *Journal of Professional Nursing, 5,* 144–51.

Reed, K. S. (1989). Family theory related to the Neuman Systems Model. In B. Neuman (Ed.), *The Neuman Systems Model* (2nd ed., pp. 385–96). Norwalk, CT: Appleton & Lange.

Reed, K. S. (1993). Adapting the Neuman Systems Model for family nursing. *Nursing Science Quarterly, 6,* 93–97.

Redheffer, G. (1985). Application of Betty Neuman's Health Care Systems Model to emergency nursing practice: Case review. *Point of View, 22*(2), 4–6.

Rice, M. J. (1982). The Neuman Systems Model applied in a hospital medical unit. In B. Neuman (Ed.), *The Neuman Systems Model: Application to nursing education and practice* (pp. 316–23). Norwalk, CT: Appleton-Century-Crofts.

Ross, M., & Bourbonnais, F. (1985). The Betty Neuman Systems Model in nursing practice: A case study approach. *Journal of Advanced Nursing, 10,* 199–207.

Ross, M. M., & Helmer, H. (1988). A comparative analysis of Neuman's model using the individual and family as the units of care. *Public Health Nursing, 5,* 30–36.

Russell, J., Hileman, J. W., & Grant, J. S. (1995). Assessing and meeting the needs of home caregivers using the Neuman Systems Model. In B. Neuman (Ed.), *The Neuman Systems Model* (3rd ed., pp. 331–41). Norwalk, CT: Appleton & Lange.

Salvage, J., & Turner, C. (1989). Brief abstracts: The Neuman model use in England. In B. Neuman (Ed.), *The Neuman Systems Model* (2nd ed., pp. 445–50). Norwalk, CT: Appleton & Lange.

Shaw, M. C. (1991). A theoretical base for orthopaedic nursing practice: The Neuman Systems Model. *Canadian Orthopaedic Nurses Association Journal, 13*(2), 19–21.

Smith, M. C. (1989). Neuman's model in practice. *Nursing Science Quarterly, 2,* 116–17.

Sohier, R. (1989). Nursing care for the people of a small planet: Culture and the Neuman Systems Model. In B. Neuman (Ed.), *The Neuman Systems Model* (2nd ed., pp. 139–54). Norwalk, CT: Appleton & Lange.

Sohier, R. (1995). Nursing care for the people of a small planet: Culture and the Neuman Systems Model. In B. Neuman (Ed.), *The Neuman Systems Model* (3rd ed., pp. 101–17). Norwalk, CT: Appleton & Lange.

Spradley, B. W. (1990). *Community health nursing: Concepts and practice* (3rd ed., pp. 72–74). Glenview, IL: Scott, Foresman/Little, Brown Higher Education.

Stevens, B. (1982). Foreward. In B. Neuman (Ed.), *The Neuman Systems Model: Application to nursing education and practice* (pp. xii–xiv). East Norwalk, CT: Appleton-Century-Crofts.

Stuart, G. W., & Wright, L. K. (1995). Applying the Neuman Systems Model to psychiatric nursing practice. In B. Neuman (Ed.), *The Neuman Systems Model* (3rd ed., pp. 263–73). Norwalk, CT: Appleton & Lange.

Sullivan, J. (1986). Using Neuman's model in the acute phase of spinal cord injury. *Focus on Critical Care, 13*(5), 34–41.

Tomlinson, P. S., & Anderson, K. H. (1995). Family health and the Neuman Systems Model. In B. Neuman (Ed.), *The Neuman Systems Model* (3rd ed., pp. 133–44). Norwalk, CT: Appleton & Lange.

Torkington, S. (1988). Nourishing the infant. *Senior Nurse, 8*(2), 24–25.

Trépanier, M. J., Dunn, S. I., & Sprague, A. E. (1995). Application of the Neuman Systems Model to perinatal nursing. In B. Neuman (Ed.), *The Neuman Systems Model* (3rd ed., pp. 309–20). Norwalk, CT: Appleton & Lange.

Utz, S. W. (1980). Applying the Neuman model to nursing practice with hypertensive clients. *Cardio-Vascular Nursing, 16,* 29–34.

Vaughan, B., & Gough, P. (1995). Use of the Neuman Systems Model in England: Abstracts. In B. Neuman (Ed.), *The Neuman Systems Model* (3rd ed., pp. 599–605). Norwalk, CT: Appleton & Lange.

Wallingford, P. (1989). The neurologically impaired and dying child: Applying the Neuman Systems Model. *Issues in Comprehensive Pediatric Nursing, 12,* 139–57.

Ware, L. A., & Shannahan, M. K. (1995). Using Neuman for a stable parent support group in neonatal intensive care. In B. Neuman (Ed.), *The Neuman Systems Model* (3rd ed., pp. 321–30). Norwalk, CT: Appleton & Lange.

Waters, T. (1993). Self-efficacy, change, and optimal client stability. *Addictions Nursing Network, 5*(2), 48–51.

Weinberger, S. L. (1991). Analysis of a clinical situation using the Neuman Systems Model. *Rehabilitation Nursing, 16,* 278, 280–81.

Wormald, L. (1995). Samuel—the boy with tonsillitis: A care study. *Intensive and Critical Care Nursing, 11,* 157–60.

Wright, K B. (1998). Professional, ethical, and legal implications for spiritual care in nursing. *Image: Journal of Nursing Scholarship, 30,* 81–83.

Wright, P. S., Piazza, D., Holcombe, J., & Foote, A. (1994). A comparison of three theories of nursing used as a guide for the nursing care of an 8-year-old child with leukemia. *Journal of Pediatric Oncology Nursing, 11,* 14–19.

four

The Neuman Systems Model and Clinical Tools

Jan Russell

T he Neuman Systems Model was developed in 1970 as a total person approach to patient problems (Neuman & Young, 1972). The entire conceptual model is, in effect, a clinical tool for assessment and intervention of individuals, families, and communities (Neuman, 1982). The development of specific clinical tools based on the Neuman Systems Model has been a natural evolution of this wholistic perspective. The purpose of this chapter is to present and discuss the clinical tools that have been derived from the Neuman Systems Model for use with and for individuals, families, communities, and organizations (Table 4-1).

CLIENT AS INDIVIDUAL

The first clinical tools derived from the Neuman Systems Model emphasized systematic, wholistic assessment of individual clients. The goal of assessment was identification of prevention interventions. Neuman first presented the Neuman Systems Model Assessment and Intervention Tool in 1974, and she has continued to use the tool ever since (Neuman, 1974, 1982, 1989, 1995). The tool includes guidelines for assessment of stressors; a form for documenting goals and the rationale for those goals, categorized by type of prevention intervention (primary, secondary, tertiary); and a form for documenting the prevention-as-intervention plan.

Beitler, Tkachuck, and Aamodt's (1980) Assessment and Intervention Tool was the first of several assessment and intervention tools to be developed as modifications of the original Neuman Systems Model Assessment and Intervention Tool (Neuman, 1974). The purpose of their tool is to guide assessment of mental health, community, and medical–surgical patients and to facilitate development and documentation of appropriate prevention interventions. Beitler and colleagues provided an example of the use of their

61

TABLE 4-1. Clinical Tools Derived from the Neuman Systems Model

Tool and Citation	Description
Tools for Individuals	
Neuman Systems Model Assessment and Intervention Tool (Mirenda, 1986; Neuman, 1974, 1982, 1989, 1995)	Guides client system assessment and permits documentation of goals, intervention plan, and outcomes from the perspective of both clients and caregivers
Nursing Assessment Guide (Beckman et al., 1998)	A modification of the Neuman Systems Model Assessment and Intervention Tool
Assessment/Intervention Tool (Beitler, Tkachuck, & Aamodt, 1980)	Guides assessment, using an interview format, and documents associated interventions
Modified Assessment/Intervention Tool for Critical Care (Dunbar, 1982)	A modification of the Neuman Systems Model Assessment and Intervention Tool for use in the critical care setting
Client Perception of Transfer as a Stressor Tool (Dunbar, 1982)	Measures the client's perception of readiness for transfer from a surgical intensive care unit
Clinical Evaluation of the Nursing Care Plan Tool (Dunbar, 1982)	Measures the nurse's perception of a nursing care plan
Theoretical Evaluation of the Nursing Care Plan (Dunbar, 1982)	Measures the nurse's perception of a nursing care plan in terms of the concepts of the Neuman Systems Model
Format of Care Planning for the Acute Cardiac Surgical Client Using the Neuman Systems Model (McInerney, 1982)	Presents a comprehensive nursing care plan for clients who have had cardiac surgery
Depression Symptom Assessment Checklist (Clark, 1982)	Guides assessment and documentation of depression
Summary of Practitioner–Client Goals and Rationale in Treating Depressed Clients (Clark, 1982)	Presents a list of goals and associated prevention intervention goals for the depressed client
Intervention Plan to Support Goals (Clark, 1982)	Presents a list of prevention interventions for the depressed client
Systematic Nursing Assessment Tool for the CAPD Client (Breckenridge, Cupit, & Raimondo, 1982)	Guides assessment of continuous ambulatory peritoneal dialysis (CAPD) clients
Assessment/Intervention Tool for Postrenal Transplant Clients (Breckenridge, 1982)	Guides assessment of stressors and lists appropriate interventions for clients who have had a renal transplant
Nursing Assesment of the Elderly Form (Gunter, 1982)	A modification of the Neuman Systems Model Assessment and Intervention Tool for use with elderly clients
Nursing Assessment Form (Burke et al., 1989)	Guides identification of client's and nurse's perceptions of stressors and coping mechanisms, using open-ended questions; used at Mercy Catholic Medical Center in Pennsylvania

TABLE 4-1. Clinical Tools Derived from the Neuman Systems Model *(continued)*

Tool and Citation	Description
Tools for Individuals (continued)	
Assessment Tool (Fulbrook, 1991)	Guides assessment and documentation of client's (or advocate's) and nurse's perceptions and provides a framework for nursing diagnoses; fosters assessment of client and family
Care Plan (Fulbrook, 1991)	Permits documentation of problems, goals, interventions, and evaluation of interventions
Maternal/Fetal Assessment Tool (Dunn & Trépanier, 1989; Trépanier et al., 1995)	Guides assessment of a pregnant woman and her fetus; Used at a clinic in Ontario, Canada
Neonatal/Family Assessment Tool (Dunn & Trépanier, 1989; Trépanier, Dunn, & Sprague, 1995)	Guides assessment of the neonate and family; used at a clinic in Ontario, Canada
Perinatal Risk-Grading Tool (Trépanier, Dunn, & Sprague, 1995)	Permits categorization of perinatal risks; used at a clinic in Ontario, Canada
Early Weaning Risk Screening Tool (Murphy, 1990)	Permits identification of pregnant women at high risk for early weaning from breast feeding
Occupational Health Nursing Risk Profile (McGee, 1995)	Guides assessment of environmental stressors and stressor impact on workers' lines of defense and resistance, along with calculation of relative risk and attributable risk
Decision Matrix for Nursing Intervention (McGee, 1995)	Facilitates planning of nursing interventions
Format for Evaluation (McGee, 1995)	Permits documentation of evaluation of outcomes of nursing interventions
Patient Classification Worksheet (Hinton-Walker & Raborn, 1989)	Permits classification of patients in terms of personnel required for treatments within the context of physiological, sociocultural, and developmental variables; used at Jefferson Davis Memorial Hospital in Mississippi
Nursing Health Assessment Tool and Nursing Care Plan (Felix et al., 1995)	A modification of the Neuman Systems Model Assessment and Intervention Tool for use with elderly residents of chronic care facilities
Interdisciplinary High Risk Assessment Tool for Rehabilitation Inpatient Falls (Cotten, 1993)	Permits prediction of adult rehabilitation in patients at risk for falling
Minimum Data Set Format (Schlentz, 1993)	Presents a minimum data set for prevention interventions in long-term care facilities
Spiritual Care Scale (Carrigg & Weber, 1997)	Measures spiritual care for clients and distinguishes spiritual care from psychosocial care
Grid for Stressor Identification (Johnson et al., 1982)	Guides assessment of types and sources of stressors

(continues)

TABLE 4-1. Clinical Tools Derived from the Neuman Systems Model *(continued)*

Tool and Citation	Description
Tools for Individuals (continued)	
Guide for Assessment of Structural Components of a System (Johnson et al., 1982)	Permits documentation of the status of the basic structure, and the lines of defense and resistance across variable areas for individuals, groups, families, or communities
Guide for Data Synthesis to Derive Nursing Diagnosis (Johnson et al., 1982)	Permits documentation of client system responses to stressors and etiology of each stressor
Guide for Planning Theoretically Derived Nursing Practice (Johnson et al., 1982)	Premits documentation of nursing diagnoses; theoretically derived plan, goals, and intervention; and expected outcomes and evaluation
Format for Evaluation of Theoretically Derived Nursing Practice (Johnson et al., 1982)	Permits documentation of evaluation of expected and actual outcomes in terms of each nursing diagnosis, goal, and intervention
Neuman Systems Model Nursing Diagnosis Taxonomy (Ziegler, 1982)	Provides a taxonomy nursing diagnosis directly derived from the Neuman Systems Model; permits documentation of nursing diagnoses based on the Neuman Systems Model
Assessment and Analysis Guideline Tool (McHolm & Geib, 1998)	Guides health assessment and formulation of nursing diagnoses
Protocol of Potential Interventions for the Psychological Needs of the Patient with COPD (Baker, 1982)	Presents a list of psychological needs and associated nursing interventions for the client with chronic obstructive pulmonary disease
Nursing Protocol for Management of Immobilization (Cardona, 1982)	Presents a list of goals and associated interventions, rationale, and outcomes for clients at risk for complications from immobilization due to skeletal traction for treatment of a hip fracture
Nursing Protocol for Management of Mental Confusion (Cardona, 1982)	Presents a list of goals and associated interventions, rationale, and outcomes for clients who are mentally confused
Protocol for Pain (Cunningham, 1982)	Presents a list of interventions, rationale, and outcomes for reduction of pain experienced by clients who do not request pain relief due to attitudes toward pain relief measures and cultural group affiliation
Tools for Families	
Guide for Family Assessment (Reed, 1982)	A modification of the Neuman Systems Model Assessment and Intervention Tool for use with Families
Family Health Assessment/Intervention Tool (Mischke-Berkey, Warner, & Hanson, 1989)	Guides assessment and documentation of family and caregiver perceptions of family health
Family Systems Stressor–Strength Inventory: Family Form (Mischke-Berkey & Hanson, 1991)	Guides assessment of the family's perceptions of general and specific family system stressors and family system strengths

TABLE 4-1. Clinical Tools Derived from the Neuman Systems Model *(continued)*

Tool and Citation	Description
Tools for Families (continued)	
Family Systems Stressor–Strength Inventory: Clinician Form (Mischke-Berkey & Hanson, 1991)	Guides assessment of the clinician's preceptions of general and specific family system stressors and family system strengths
FAMLI-RESCUE (Flannery, 1991)	Guides collection and evaluation of data on family functioning and resources for use by neuroscience nurses working in acute care settings
Tools for Communities	
Community Assessment Guide (Benedict & Sproles, 1982)	Guides assessment of communities, including intracommunity, intercommunity, and extracommunity factors; and the community's and health planner's perceptions of stressors
Community-as-Client Assessment Guide (Beddome, 1989, 1995)	Guides collection of data about geopolitical and aggregate needs, community resources, and resource utilization patterns from the perspective of clients and caregivers
Tools for Organizations	
A Systems-Based Assessment Tool for Child Day-Care Centers (Bowman, 1982)	Guides assessment of stressors in child day-care centers
Neuman Systems-Management Tool for Nursing and Organizational Systems (Kelley & Sanders, 1995; Kelley, Sanders, & Pierce, 1989; Neuman, 1995)	Permits the nurse administrator to assess, resolve, prevent, and evaluate stressors in any type of administrative setting; measures the total system response to an environmental stressor

tool that focused on assessment of a client's interpersonal, intrapersonal, and extrapersonal stressors and development of goals for and outcomes of relevant prevention interventions. The example illustrated how easy it is to use the Neuman Systems Model and how comprehensive Neuman Systems Model–based clinical practice is.

In the early 1980s, clinicians developed Neuman Systems Model–based assessment tools for a wide variety of individual clients, including critical care clients (Dunbar, 1982; McInerney, 1982), psychiatric clients (Clark, 1982), clients with renal problems (Breckenridge, 1982; Breckenridge, Cupit, & Raimondo, 1982), and the elderly (Gunter, 1982). Most of those assessment tools focused on assessment of client system strengths and weaknesses, identification of stressors, and development of prevention interventions. Dunbar's (1982) Client Perception of Transfer as a Stressor Tool and her Modified Assessment/Intervention Tool for Critical Care are particularly sophisticated. Dunbar modified the original Neuman Systems Model Assessment and Intervention Tool (Neuman, 1974) for use in the critical care setting and also developed a new Neuman Systems Model–based tool that enables the nurse to determine the client's perception of readiness for transfer from the surgical intensive care unit.

In 1986, Mirenda described the use of the Neuman Systems Model Assessment and Intervention Tool (Neuman, 1974) by students enrolled in the Neumann College bac-calaureate nursing program. She claimed that use of this tool "truly directs an assessment of the 'total' person and unified and goal-directed interventions" (Mirenda, 1986, p. 27).

Based on a decade of use and experience, Neuman (1989) altered the content of the Neuman Systems Model in four important ways. First, she added the spiritual variable, which originally was subsumed within the sociocultural variable. Second, she expanded the concept of environment to include the created environment, as well as the internal and external environments. Third, she explicitly identified health promotion as a part of primary prevention as intervention. Fourth, she described a process of determining a nursing diagnosis that is consistent with the Neuman Systems Model. These changes facilitated clear and more comprehensive client system assessment and data for relevant prevention interventions.

Subsequently, clinicians developed several new tools that were tailored for the specific client populations served by particular clinical agencies. Burke and colleagues (1989) described the implementation of the Neuman Systems Model at Mercy Catholic Medical Center in Pennsylvania. Their Nursing Assessment Guide was designed for use with the client population served by that clinical agency. Burke and colleagues noted that the use of the Nursing Assessment Guide, which was a focal point of the implementation of the Neuman Systems Model, promoted a high quality of nursing care for all patients; facilitated a unified, goal-directed nursing care approach; increased the professionalism of nursing practice by enhancing responsibility, autonomy, and accountability for registered nurses; provided a practice environment that is professionally rewarding to registered nurses, thereby increasing job satisfaction and retention; and gave purpose, direction, and organization to the nursing department.

Hinton-Walker and Raborn (1989) described the implementation of the Neuman Systems Model at Jefferson Davis Memorial Hospital in Mississippi. They developed a patient classification system based on the Neuman Systems Model client system variables. The Patient Classification Worksheet is used to determine patient needs, staffing mix, and costs of nursing services.

Dunn and Trépanier (1989) described the implementation of the Neuman Systems Model as a guide for a community-based educational program for perinatal clients in Ontario, Canada. Their Maternal/Fetal Assessment Tool permits viewing the pregnant woman and her fetus as a single client system made up of two overlapping individuals. The tool focuses on assessment of sources of stressors, within the context of all Neuman Systems Model client system variables. A similar Neonatal/Family Assessment Tool focuses on assessment of sources of stressors for the neonate and the family. Later, Trépanier, Dunn, and Sprague (1995) described the development of the Perinatal Risk-Grading Tool, which facilitates systematic identification, differentiation, and prioritizing of perinatal risks. This tool was derived from the Neuman Systems Model lines of defense and resistance and the client system variables. Risks are graded as A (client system is steady and within the usual wellness state), B (moderate risk), or C (great risk), and standardized care plans are available for each level of risk.

Murphy (1990) used the Neuman Systems Model to organize an integrative review of literature about breast-feeding successes and failures. The literature review led to development of a preliminary screening tool to identify women at risk for early weaning.

Fulbrook (1991) described implementation of the Neuman Systems Model as a guide for nursing practice with clients in an intensive care unit. Fulbrook's Assessment Tool facilitates assessment of client system variables, as well as information about the family. Each client system variable is cross-tabulated with major systems in the body (e.g., respiratory), to enable identification of many specific details. The Care Plan allows the nurse to select relevant common primary and secondary prevention interventions for a 24-hour period and to add individualized prevention interventions.

Cotten (1993) used the Neuman Systems Model to develop the Interdisciplinary High Risk Assessment Tool for Rehabilitation Inpatient Falls. This tool permits evaluation of patient risks for falling at rehabilitation centers.

Schlentz (1993) described use of the Neuman Systems Model in a long-term care facility. She developed the Minimum Data Set Format, which identifies 18 common client system problems (e.g., delirium, cognitive loss) in relation to primary, secondary, and tertiary prevention interventions.

McGee (1995) described use of the Neuman Systems Model as a guide for occupational health nursing practice. In this setting, nursing practice focuses on reduction of stressors that might have noxious effects on populations of workers. The Decision Matrix for Nursing Intervention tool focuses on primary prevention interventions associated with various stressors, within the context of client system variables. The Format for Evaluation permits documentation of evaluation of the outcomes of primary prevention interventions.

Felix and colleagues (1995) described the application of the Neuman Systems Model to nursing practice in a chronic care facility. The Nursing Health Assessment Tool and Nursing Care Plan Tool focuses on tertiary prevention interventions, within the context of client system variables, and emphasizes functional activities and activities of daily living.

Carrigg and Weber (1997) recently developed and tested the psychometric properties of the first tool that focuses on a specific client system variable. The Spiritual Care Scale (SCS) is a 30-item scale that encompasses three spiritual dimensions—faith, empowerment, and meaningfulness. The SCS measures spiritual care for clients and distinguishes spiritual care from psychosocial care. The internal consistency reliability was excellent, with a Cronbach's alpha coefficient of .94.

Some clinical tools have been developed by nurse educators to facilitate students' use of the Neuman Systems Model as a guide for nursing practice. Johnson and colleagues (1982) described a group of clinical tools developed for master's students at Texas Woman's University (TWU). The Grid for Stressor Identification guides assessment of types and sources of stressors encountered by clients. The Guide for Assessment of the Structural Components of a System permits documentation of the status of the basic structure, and the lines of defense and resistance across client system variables for individuals, groups, families, or communities. The Guide for Data Synthesis to Derive Nursing Diagnosis permits documentation of clients' responses to stressors and the etiology of each stressor. The Guide for Planning Theoretically Derived Nursing Practice permits documentation of nursing diagnoses; the theoretically derived nursing plan, goals, and intervention; and the expected outcomes and evaluation. The Format for Evaluation of Theoretically Derived Nursing Practice permits documentation of the evaluation of expected and actual outcomes in relation to each nursing diagnosis, goal, and intervention.

Ziegler (1982) extended the work of her TWU faculty colleagues by developing the Neuman Systems Model Nursing Diagnosis Taxonomy. The taxonomy of nursing diagnoses is directly derived from the Neuman Systems Model. Ziegler organized the taxonomy in relation to (1) the client system (individual, family, group, community), (2) the level of response (primary, secondary, tertiary), (3) the client subsystem responding to the stressor (physiological, psychological, sociocultural), (4) the source of the stressor (intrasystem, intersystem, extrasystem), and (5) the type of stressor (physiological, psychological, sociocultural). Diana Newman (personal communication, June 15, 2000) has extended the taxonomy by adding the developmental and spiritual variables.

McHolm and Geib (1998) described the application of the Neuman Systems Model to teaching health assessment and the nursing process. Their Assessment and Analysis Guideline Tool facilitates students' assessment of the client's health status and their formulation of nursing diagnoses.

The Neuman Systems Model also has been used to guide development of protocols for clinical practice. Baker (1982) developed the Protocol of Potential Interventions for the Psychological Needs of the Patient with COPD. She focused on the psychological crisis that can occur following onset of chronic obstructive pulmonary disease, when the client begins to realize the extent of disease-imposed limitations. The protocol emphasizes the fear, anxiety, lowered self-esteem, and depression experienced by the client and the prevention interventions required to strengthen the lines of defense.

Cardona (1982) developed the Nursing Protocol for Management of Immobilization. The protocol was designed for clients who are immobilized due to hip fracture. The protocol focuses on identification of intrapersonal, interpersonal, and extrapersonal stressors; assessment of the lines of defense and resistance; identification of priorities, expectations, and support systems within the context of the three types of stressors and the client system variables; and selection of prevention interventions.

Cardona (1982) also developed the Nursing Protocol for Management of Mental Confusion. This protocol encompasses a list of goals and associated interventions, rationale, and outcomes for clients who are mentally confused.

Cunningham (1982) derived the Protocol for Pain from the Neuman Systems Model. This protocol includes a list of prevention interventions, with associated rationale and outcomes, for reduction of pain experienced by clients who do not request pain relief due to attitudes toward pain relief measures and cultural group affiliation.

The Neuman model is an effective model for use with individuals as clients and with patient populations. Through the use of the many and varied adaptations over time and by many nurses, the model also has proven to be flexible and beneficial. During two decades of use, it has been established that the model can organize care for any client in any setting and guide nurses to provide a higher quality of care.

CLIENT AS FAMILY

Neuman (1989, 1995) provided a case example to demonstrate the use of her Assessment and Intervention Tool when the family is the client system. The family case example features assessment of the family's major stressors; documentation of the family's perception of their condition and the caregiver's perception of the family's condition; the statement of a nursing diagnosis based on the family's variance from wellness; and prevention interventions to stabilize the family.

Reed (1982) developed the first specific Neuman Systems Model–based clinical tool for use with the family as the client system. The Guide for Family Assessment, which is a modification of Neuman's (1974) original Assessment and Intervention Tool, permits assessment of the family's lines of defense, resistance, and stressors; statement of a nursing diagnosis and goals; identification of appropriate prevention interventions; and evaluation of the outcomes of the prevention interventions.

Mischke-Berkey, Warner, and Hanson (1989) developed the Family Systems Stressor–Strength Inventory. This Likert-type clinical tool includes three parts: general family system stressors assessment (e.g., family member feels unappreciated, has insufficient "me" time), specific family system stressors assessment (e.g., a family member identifies a particular problem, such as time for family after work), and an assessment of family strengths (e.g., communicate and listen to each other, affirm and support one another). Each family member completes the Inventory, and the results of the family members' scores are correlated. The Inventory facilitates identification of family stressors and focuses attention on family strengths. Mischke-Berkey and Hanson (1991) went on to develop a pocket guide for family assessment and intervention that is brief and practical. The pocket guide includes separate family and clinician forms of the Family Systems Stressor–Strength Inventory.

Flannery (1991) developed the FAMLI-RESCUE tool, which guides collection and evaluation of data about family functioning. The tool was designed for use by neuroscience nurses working in acute care settings. Flannery noted that she wanted to focus the nurse's attention on the family of the hospitalized client, because she believes that their inclusion would enhance the client's recovery and strengthen the bond between client and family. The FAMLI-RESCUE tool permits identification of specific weaknesses in family functioning that interfere with the ability of family members to communicate and interact, needs for change, and family resources that might facilitate the client's recovery.

CLIENT AS COMMUNITY

Benedict and Sproles (1982) introduced use of the Neuman Systems Model as a guide for nursing practice with the community as the client system. Their Community Assessment Guide focuses on intracommunity, intercommunity, and extracommunity factors, and incorporates both the community's and the health planner's perceptions of stressors.

Beddome (1989, 1995) described the application of the Neuman Systems Model to the geopolitical community or an aggregate community. She defined a *geopolitical community* as a broader community involving beliefs, laws, and resources that affect the larger system. In contrast, an *aggregate community* is one that involves only the immediate caregiving system (both client and care providers). The Community-as-Client Assessment Guide focuses on intrasystem, intersystem and extrasystem factors. Although many aspects of assessment are the same for geopolitical and aggregate communities, some aspects are different. For example, within the sociocultural intersystem, aggregate community data include ethnic composition of personnel, languages spoken, and membership in associations. In contrast, geopolitical community data include the cultural composition of the population and languages spoken, guiding values, positions and roles, associations and clubs, services to strengthen families (e.g., senior day care), and services for special groups (e.g., handicapped people and new immigrants). Beddome pointed out that home health care nurses would typically focus on aggregate communities, whereas public health nurses would typically focus on geopolitical communities.

CLIENT AS ORGANIZATION

Bowman (1982) reported the earliest application of the Neuman Systems Model to an organization. She developed the Systems-Based Assessment Tool for Child Day-Care Centers. Bowman focused attention on what she called intracenter factors, intercenter factors, and extracenter factors in relation to stressors and resources. The tool guides assessment of the stressors and resources and facilitates determination of the best method to manage the stressors and maintain or increase the resources.

Kelley, Sanders, and Pierce (1989, 1995) focused attention on the nurse administrator at the personal, department, and organizational levels. Their Neuman Systems-Management Tool for Nursing and Organizational Systems permits the nurse administrator to assess, resolve, prevent, and evaluate stressors in any type of administrative setting, and measures the total system response to an environmental stressor. The tool facilitates identification of the nursing administrator's stressors and personal factors for all client system variables, identification of problems across various administration levels (e.g., middle management), development of goals and an action plan, and formulation of outcome statements.

CONCLUSION

The Neuman Systems Model clinical tools are practical and effectively guide wholistic assessment and prevention interventions for individual, family, community, and organization client systems (Table 4-1). Collectively, the tools guide clinical practice with a wide array of client systems in diverse health care settings.

The review of the clinical tools presented in this chapter provides direction for future work. First, the validity and reliability of the existing clinical tools need to be determined, so that users can determine when and under what conditions each tool is most effectively used. Next, many tools have been developed for use with individuals, but many more are needed for use with families, communities, and organizations. Finally, clinical tools that focus on portions of the content of the Neuman Systems Model are needed. For example, a tool is needed for assessment of individuals' internal, external, and created environments. Given the broad scope of the Neuman Systems Model, the creation of new clinical tools is limitless. Commitment to the task is all that is required.

REFERENCES

Baker, N. A. (1982). Use of the Neuman Model in planning for the psychological needs of the respiratory disease patient. In B. Neuman (Ed.), *The Neuman Systems Model: Application to nursing education and practice* (pp. 241–51). Norwalk, CT: Appleton-Century-Crofts.

Beckman, S. J., Boxley-Harges, S., Bruick-Sorge, C., & Eichenauer, J. (1998). Evaluation modalities for assessing student and program outcomes. In L. Lowry (Ed.), *The Neuman Systems Model and nursing education: Teaching strategies and outcomes* (pp. 149–60). Indianapolis: Sigma Theta Tau International Center Nursing Press.

Beddome, G. (1989). Application of the Neuman systems model to the assessment of community-as-client. In B. Neuman (Ed.), *The Neuman Systems Model* (2nd ed., pp. 363–74). Norwalk, CT: Appleton & Lange.

Beddome, G. (1995). Community-as-client: A Neuman-based guide for education and practice. In B. Neuman (Ed.), *The Neuman Systems Model* (3rd ed., pp. 567–79). Norwalk, CT: Appleton & Lange.

Beitler, B., Tkachuck, B., & Aamodt, D. (1980). The Neuman model applied to mental health, community health, and medical–surgical nursing. In J. P. Riehl & C. Roy (Eds.), *Conceptual models for nursing practice* (2nd ed., pp. 170–78). Norwalk, CT: Appleton-Century-Crofts.

Benedict, M. B., & Sproles, J. B. (1982). Application of the Neuman model to public health nursing practice. In B. Neuman (Ed.), *The Neuman Systems Model: Application to nursing education and practice* (pp. 223–40). Norwalk, CT: Appleton-Century-Crofts.

Bowman, G. E. (1982). The Neuman assessment tool adapted for child day-care centers. In B. Neuman (Ed.), *The Neuman Systems Model: Application to nursing education and practice* (pp. 324–34). Norwalk, CT: Appleton-Century-Crofts.

Breckenridge, D. M. (1982). Adaptation of the Neuman Systems Model for the renal client. In B. Neuman (Ed.), *The Neuman Systems Model: Application to nursing education and practice* (pp. 267–77). Norwalk, CT: Appleton-Century-Crofts.

Breckenridge, D. M., Cupit, M. C., & Raimondo, J. M. (1982). Systematic nursing assessment tool for the CAPD client. *Nephrology Nurse,* January/February, 24, 26–27, 30–31.

Burke, M. E., Sr., Caper, C. F., O'Connell, R. K., Quinn, R. M., & Sinnott, M. (1989). In B. Neuman (Ed.), *The Neuman Systems Model* (2nd ed., pp. 423–44). Norwalk, CT: Appleton & Lange.

Cardona, V. D. (1982). Client rehabilitation and the Neuman model. In B. Neuman (Ed.), *The Neuman Systems Model: Application to nursing education and practice* (pp. 278–90). Norwalk, CT: Appleton-Century-Crofts.

Carrigg, K. C., & Weber, R. (1997). Development of the Spiritual Care Scale. *Image: Journal of Nursing Scholarship, 29,* 293.

Clark, F. (1982). The Neuman Systems Model: A clinical application for psychiatric nurse practitioners. In B. Neuman (Ed.), *The Neuman Systems Model: Application to nursing education and practice* (pp. 335–53). Norwalk, CT: Appleton-Century-Crofts.

Cotten, N. C. (1993). An interdisciplinary high risk assessment tool for rehabilitation inpatient falls. *Master's Abstracts International, 31,* 1732.

Cunningham, S. G. (1982). The Neuman model applied to an acute care setting: Pain. In B. Neuman (Ed.), *The Neuman Systems Model: Application to nursing education and practice* (pp. 291–96). Norwalk, CT: Appleton-Century-Crofts.

Dunbar, S. B. (1982). Critical care and the Neuman model. In B. Neuman (Ed.), *The Neuman Systems Model: Application to nursing education and practice* (pp. 297–307). Norwalk, CT: Appleton-Century-Crofts.

Dunn, S. I., & Trépanier, M. J. (1989). Application of the Neuman model to perinatal nursing. In B. Neuman (Ed.), *The Neuman Systems Model* (2nd ed., pp. 407–22). Norwalk, CT: Appleton & Lange.

Felix, M., Hinds, C., Wolfe, S. C., & Martin, A. (1995). The Neuman Systems Model in a chronic care facility: A Canadian experience. In B. Neuman (Ed.), *The Neuman Systems Model* (3rd ed., pp. 549–65). Norwalk, CT: Appleton & Lange.

Flannery, J. (1991). FAMLI-RESCUE: A family assessment tool for use by neuroscience nurses in the acute care setting. *Journal of Neuroscience Nursing, 23,* 111–15.

Fulbrook, P. R. (1991). The application of the Neuman Systems Model to intensive care. *Intensive Care Nursing, 7,* 28–39.

Gunter, L. M. (1982). Application of the Neuman Systems Model to gerontic nursing. In B. Neuman (Ed.), *The Neuman Systems Model: Application to nursing education and practice* (pp. 196–210). Norwalk, CT: Appleton-Century-Crofts.

Hinton-Walker, P., & Raborn, M. (1989). Application of the Neuman Model in nursing administration and practice. In B. Henry, C. Arndt, M. DiVincenti, & A. Marriner-Tomey (Eds.), *Dimensions of nursing administration: Theory, research, and practice.* Boston: Black Scientific Publications.

Johnson, M. N., Vaughn-Wrobel, B., Ziegler, S., et al. (1982). Use of the Neuman health-care systems model in the master's curriculum: Texas Woman's University. In B. Neuman (Ed.), *The Neuman Systems Model: Application to nursing education and practice* (pp. 130–52). Norwalk, CT: Appleton-Century-Crofts.

Kelley, J. A., & Sanders, N. F. (1995). A systems approach to the health of nursing and health care organizations. In B. Neuman (Ed.), *The Neuman Systems Model* (3rd ed. pp. 347–64). Norwalk, CT: Appleton & Lange.

Kelley, J. A., Sanders, N. F., & Pierce, J. D. (1989). A systems approach to the role of the nurse administrator in education and practice. In B. Neuman (Ed.), *The Neuman Systems Model* (2nd ed., pp. 115–38). Norwalk, CT: Appleton & Lange.

McGee, M. (1995). Implications for use of the Neuman Systems Model in occupational health nursing. In B. Neuman (Ed.), *The Neuman Systems Model* (3rd ed., pp. 657–67). Norwalk, CT: Appleton & Lange.

McHolm, F. A., & Geib, K. M. (1998). Application of the Neuman Systems Model to teaching health assessment and nursing process. *Nursing Diagnosis: The Journal of Nursing Language and Classification, 9,* 23–33.

McInerney, K. A. (1982). The Neuman Systems Model applied to critical care nursing of cardiac surgery clients. In B. Neuman (Ed.), *The Neuman Systems Model: Application to nursing education and practice* (pp. 308–15). Norwalk, CT: Appleton-Century-Crofts.

Mirenda, R. M. (1986). The Neuman model in practice. *Senior Nurse, 5*(3), 26–27.

Mischke-Berkey, K., & Hanson, S. M. H. (1991). *Pocket guide to family assessment and intervention.* St. Louis: Mosby–Year Book.

Mischke-Berkey, K., Warner, P., & Hanson, S. (1989). Family health assessment and intervention. In P. J. Bomar (Ed.), *Nurses and family health promotion: Concepts, assessment, and interventions* (pp. 115–54). Baltimore: Williams & Wilkins.

Murphy, N. G. (1990). Factors associated with breastfeeding success and failure: A systematic integrative review. *Master's Abstract International, 28,* 275.

Neuman, B. (1974). The Betty Neuman health-care systems model: A total person approach to patient problems. In J. P. Riehl & C. Roy (Eds.), *Conceptual models for nursing practice* (pp. 99–114). New York: Appleton-Century-Crofts.

Neuman, B. (1982). *The Neuman Systems Model: Application to nursing education and practice.* Norwalk, CT: Appleton-Century-Crofts.

Neuman, B. (1989). *The Neuman Systems Model* (2nd ed.). Norwalk, CT: Appleton & Lange.

Neuman, B. (1995). *The Neuman Systems Model* (3rd ed.). Norwalk, CT: Appleton & Lange.

Neuman, B., & Young, R. J. (1972). A model for teaching total person approach to patient problems. *Nursing Research, 21,* 264–69.

Reed, K. (1982). The Neuman Systems Model: A basis for family psychosocial assessment. In B. Neuman (Ed.), *The Neuman Systems Model: Application to nursing education and practice* (pp. 188–95). Norwalk, CT: Appleton-Century-Crofts.

Schlentz, M. D. (1993). The minimum data set and the levels of prevention in the long-term care facility. *Geriatric Nursing, 14,* 79–83.

Trépanier, M. J., Dunn, S. I., & Sprague, A. E. (1995). Application of the Neuman Systems Model to perinatal nursing. In B. Neuman (Ed.), *The Neuman Systems Model* (3rd ed., pp. 309–20). Norwalk, CT: Appleton & Lange.

Ziegler, S. M. (1982). Taxonomy for nursing diagnosis derived from the Neuman Systems Model. In B. Neuman (Ed.), *The Neuman Systems Model: Application to nursing education and practice* (pp. 55–68). Norwalk, CT: Appleton-Century-Crofts.

Using the Neuman Systems Model to Guide Nursing Practice in the United States: Nursing Prevention Interventions for Postpartum Mood Disorders

Diane Fashinpaur

Postpartum mood disorders (PPMDs) strike without warning and can potentially shatter the lives of affected women and their families. At a time when family members anticipated joy, they find themselves grappling with the effects of an unexpected illness that robs the new mother, and consequently other family members, of happiness.

PPMDs pose tremendous stressors that threaten the very system cores of the identified patient and her family. The threat is magnified when PPMDs go unrecognized and untreated. Despite the existence of a considerable body of literature addressing mood disorders that begin after childbirth, development of services that specifically meet the needs of affected women and their families remains a relatively neglected area of health care. This care gap is due in part to the fact that PPMDs often go undetected by primary health care providers (Gruen, 1990; Seeley, Murray, & Cooper, 1996). Informed nurses who regularly interact with childbearing families are uniquely positioned to create innovative strategies for promoting the mental health of childbearing women and their families. The Neuman Systems Model provides a framework on which to base primary, secondary, and tertiary nursing prevention interventions that focus on retaining, attaining, and maintaining the mental health and system stability of women and families potentially or actually affected by PPMDs (Fashinpaur & Spisak, 1995; Fashinpaur, 1997).

The purpose of this chapter is to facilitate nurses' recognition of PPMDs and the subsequent development of nursing diagnoses and appropriate prevention interventions. The chapter begins with a discussion of PPMDs viewed within the context of the Neuman Systems Model and includes brief descriptions of currently recognized PPMD syndromes. Next, several PPMD assessment tools, followed by a list of potential intrapersonal, interpersonal, and extrapersonal PPMD stressors and client reactions are provided to assist in the development of nursing diagnoses. The chapter concludes with recommendations for primary, secondary, and tertiary prevention interventions to help childbearing families affected by PPMDs to retain, attain, and maintain optimal mental well-being.

POSTPARTUM MOOD DISORDERS AND THE NEUMAN SYSTEMS MODEL

Expansion of knowledge about the presentation of and appropriate treatment for PPMDs has occurred over the past 15 years. The health care community at large, however, has been slow to develop a clear understanding of these disorders. Consequently, affected women and their families often struggle to avail themselves of timely and appropriate treatment. Nurses caring for childbearing families must ensure that their knowledge about PPMD presentation, associated potential stressors, and appropriate prevention interventions is current and comprehensive. The Neuman Systems Model offers a method of viewing clients and their families wholistically and multidimensionally within a system perspective. Conceptualization of PPMDs within the Neuman Systems Model framework will assist nurses to devise appropriate interventions to best shield families from the impact of stressors associated with these disorders.

According to the Neuman Systems Model, each individual family member, and the family unit collectively, is a system with a basic structure or core. The basic structure of each client system, whether considered individually or collectively as a family unit, has life-giving energy resources that are protected by a flexible line of defense, a normal line of defense, and lines of resistance. When considering PPMDs in the context of the Neuman Systems Model, *client* refers to the mother as the patient of record and/or her entire family as a unit.

When internal or external stressors threaten or break through an individual family member system's lines of defense and resistance, each other family member, as well as the collective family system, are affected. Consequently, acute PPMD stressors that threaten or invade a new mother's flexible and normal lines of defense can potentially result in reactions that will undoubtedly cause some degree of instability within the systems of her infant, partner, and any other children, and on the family system as a whole (Harberger, Berchtold, & Honikman, 1992; Martell, 1990).

Experts devoting considerable time to the study of PPMDs recognize at least four distinct diagnoses in this category: postpartum major depression, postpartum panic disorder, postpartum obsessive–compulsive disorder, and postpartum psychosis (Cohen et al., 1994; Hamilton, 1989; Hamilton & Sichel, 1992; Kendall-Tackett, 1993). The course and duration of PPMDs are variable, but left untreated, episodes may last from months to years (Hamilton & Harberger, 1992). An overview of each PPMD is presented here; a comprehensive differential description and definition of each PPMD syndrome is beyond the scope of this chapter.

Postpartum major depression, which Wisner (1991) states affects 10 to 15 percent of women who give birth, is difficult to accurately characterize due to its insidious onset and atypical presentation. Most cases begin within the first week to three months after delivery. Although the typical course and duration are not well established, for some women postpartum major depression has been known to last a year or more (Wisner, 1991). Case illustrations of postpartum major depression often reflect the symptoms of major depression as defined in the fourth edition of the *Diagnostic and Statistical Manual of Mental Disorders* (DSM-IV) (American Psychiatric Association, 1994). Symptoms may include depressed mood, diminished interest or pleasure in activities (anhedonia), appetite disturbance, sleep disturbance, psychomotor agitation or retardation, fatigue, feelings of worthlessness, excessive guilt, decreased concentration, and recurrent thoughts of death or suicidal ideation. Many affected mothers commonly complain of experiencing fuzzy or muddled thinking, and they are bothered by serious doubts about their ability to care for their infants.

Postpartum panic disorder commonly presents as a first lifetime episode in the postpartum period (Cohen et al., 1994). Because panic disorder has not been widely studied as it relates to childbearing, information is not clearly established about incidence and onset in the postpartum. Some women with pregravid panic disorder are at risk for an escalation of symptoms following childbirth (Fernandez, 1992). Panic disorder is commonly characterized by recurrent unexpected panic attacks that may or may not be accompanied by frequent avoidance of activities, places, or situations (agoraphobia) perceived by the client to be instrumental in the onset of an attack. Symptoms of panic may include palpitations, sweating, trembling, sensations of smothering or choking, chest pain, nausea, dizziness, derealization (feelings of unreality), and fear of losing control or dying (DSM-IV). Medical conditions that can mimic panic symptoms include asthma, cardiac arrhythmias, electrolyte imbalances, hyperthyroidism, hypothyroidism, mitral valve prolapse, and true vertigo. Therefore, a thorough history and physical examination including appropriate laboratory testing is essential (Fernandez, 1992).

Sichel, Cohen, and Dimmock (1993) have studied women with new-onset postpartum obsessive–compulsive disorder (OCD). They report clinical features that include rapidly escalating obsessions to harm (e.g., by drowning or stabbing) the newborn, increased generalized anxiety, and disrupted mother–infant relationships. The study mothers did not experience psychotic symptoms nor were any of their obsessive thoughts ever acted out. Since obsessional thought is often confused with psychotic thought (Wisner, 1991), making the distinction is important. In fact, new mothers with OCD find their obsessions most upsetting and unwanted and often will distance themselves from their infants due to the fear that they may harm their babies. As with postpartum panic disorder, the incidence and onset of postpartum OCD have not been established.

The fortunately rare postpartum psychosis occurs in about 2 per 1,000 deliveries and usually begins within the first month, most often the first week, after delivery (Wisner, 1991). Wisner described the typical presentation of an episode of postpartum psychosis as follows:

> After several days of normal functioning, the woman experiences one or two nights of falling and staying asleep and an increase in irritability. The symptoms then progress rapidly and can include disorganization, bizarre behavior, elation, and rapid mood changes,

distractibility, hallucinations and increased activity levels. The confused, disorganized presentation has been observed and recorded throughout history. (p. 7)

Postpartum psychosis carries an increased risk of maternal suicide and infanticide. Commonly exhibited symptoms are guilt of delusional proportions involving the infant or spouse, guilt feelings over infanticidal thoughts, and bizarre beliefs that the infant is possessed by the devil (Wisner, 1991). An episode of postpartum psychosis, because of its florid presentation, is generally recognized early and treated quickly.

It is crucial to recognize that PPMDs are distinctly different from the more commonly recognized "baby blues," which are experienced by 50 to 80 percent of new mothers, beginning two to five days after delivery and resolving spontaneously within a week or so (Stowe & Nemeroff, 1995). Mothers who experience "baby blues" may exhibit any combination of the following symptoms: brief episodes of sadness, crying, irritability, anxiety, elation, headache, insomnia, confusion, forgetfulness, and ambivalent thoughts about the baby (Wisner, 1991). Caregivers who confuse the less severe PPMD syndromes with "baby blues" will unintentionally thwart affected mothers' attempts to get timely help. In contrast to the early treatment generally afforded a woman experiencing a postpartum psychosis, a new mother in the throes of postpartum depression, postpartum panic disorder, or postpartum OCD may have her help-seeking behaviors met with trivialization and discouragement by others, including uninformed health care providers. A sense of shame or failure and fear of stigmatization pose additional barriers to a woman's search for appropriate help (Harberger, Berchtold, & Honikman, 1992). Because early recognition, diagnosis, and treatment of PPMDs may result in a shorter recovery time (Fernandez, 1992), early case finding and referral are of utmost importance.

NURSING ASSESSMENT AND DIAGNOSIS

Given the need for improvement in early identification of PPMDs by care providers, nurses who work with childbearing families must sharpen their assessment and diagnostic skills in this area. By becoming familiar with appropriate PPMD assessment tools and developing a working knowledge of the stressors commonly found to be associated with PPMDs, nurses who care for childbearing families will be well prepared to advocate appropriately and develop interventions for PPMD clients.

Several screening tools are available for assessment of a new mother's psychosocial status in the postpartum period. One PPMD assessment tool is the Neuman Postpartum Mood Questionnaire (NPMQ), which was designed by the author within the context of the Neuman Systems Model. Other available PPMD assessment measures, which are not based on the Neuman Systems Model, include the Edinburgh Postnatal Depression Scale (EPDS) (Cox, Holden, & Sagovsky, 1987) and the Postpartum Depression Checklist (PDC) (Beck, 1995).

The NPMQ is a PPMD assessment tool intended for use in initiating dialogue between the nurse and new mother about her postpartum emotional status that will provide data for the development of a nursing diagnosis. Like Clark's (1982) Depression Symptom Checklist, the NPMQ consists of assessment items categorized by variable domain. Eighteen questions assess for potential reactions to PPMD stressors in the physiological, psychological, sociocultural, and spiritual variable domains. Three additional questions assess for potential stressors in the developmental variable domain. Sample

NPMQ questions from each variable domain are provided in Table 5-1. Suggestions for use of the NPMQ include asking the mother to complete the questionnaire prior to mutual discussion with the nurse or having the nurse use the tool to guide her interview. The NPMQ is not designed to be scored; rather, this tool is meant to facilitate mutually collaborative exploration of each item on the list. If discussion of the items reveals that the mother is experiencing significant distress, referral to a mental health specialist for further evaluation and possible treatment may be indicated. For example, immediate referral for psychiatric intervention and measures to keep mother, infant, and other family members safe are indicated if suicidal or homicidal intent is elicited. Even if a mother is not significantly distressed, administering the NPMQ will prompt discussion of possible areas in which the mother is experiencing minor stressors for which the nurse may offer prevention interventions that will strengthen the lines of defense and resistance.

The EPDS is a brief, 10-item, self-report scale (Cox, Holden, & Sagovsky, 1987). Women who score 10 or higher on the EPDS might well benefit from further assessment and treatment. A possible drawback of the EPDS is that it does not allow mothers to elaborate on or clarify their perceptions of their distress (Beck, 1995). However, mutual discussion between client and caregiver about client responses to the individual EPDS items and the total test score can help clarify caregiver and client perceptions about any identified client reactions to PPMD stressors.

Beck's (1995) PDC is intended to be administered by the health care provider in the context of an interview and allows for exploration of the woman's feelings and presence of symptoms. A list of 11 symptoms based on themes that emerged in Beck's (1992) phenomenological study of postpartum depressed women, the PDC allows the caregiver to identify which symptoms are experienced by a particular patient. The PDC is not scored, nor is it meant to establish a diagnosis. Rather, like the NPMQ, the PDC promotes discourse between a new mother and a nurse that will be most helpful in determining need for further evaluation of a new mother's mental status.

TABLE 5-1. Sample Items from the Neuman Postpartum Mood Questionnaire (NPMQ)

Physiological:
1. Have you experienced sleep disturbance, particularly difficulty sleeping even when the baby is asleep?   Yes _____   No _____
2. Have you experienced any disturbance in appetite?   Yes _____   No _____

Psychological/Cognitive:
1. Have you been feeling unusually sad?   Yes _____   No _____
2. Are you experiencing anxious or frightened feelings?   Yes _____   No _____

Sociocultural:
1. Have you felt as though you are a "bad mother"?   Yes _____   No _____
2. Do you feel distanced from your baby or husband?   Yes _____   No _____

Spiritual:
1. Do you feel you have lost the person you used to be?   Yes _____   No _____
2. Have you been feeling hopeless?   Yes _____   No _____

Developmental:
1. Have you experienced depression or anxiety in the past?   Yes _____   No _____
2. Have family members experienced anxiety or depression?   Yes _____   No _____

Assessment of a new mother's psychosocial status in the months following birth should be routine. Nurses working in obstetric or pediatric practices should ask new mothers to complete brief assessment tools at the time of regularly scheduled six-week and three-month postpartum checkups or at selected pediatric/well child clinic visits during the infant's first year. By explaining that completion of the tool/questionnaire is requested of *all* new mothers in a particular provider's practice, nurses will allay mothers' fears that they have been singled out or suspected of experiencing difficulty. Completing a PPMD inventory gives a mother the opportunity and "permission" to share concerns that she might otherwise not have disclosed. Collaborative review of the assessment tool is crucial in that it allows the client and nurse to mutually examine any client reactions to potential PPMD stressors. Thus, as uniquely prescribed in the Neuman Systems Model Nursing Process Format, both client and caregiver perceptions are determined for relevant goal setting. Subsequent to clarification of client and caregiver perceptions about potential and actual reactions to PPMD stressors, client prevention intervention goals can be mutually determined.

An assessment that reveals a mother's reactions to PPMD stressors signals the need for attention to the psychosocial status of all family members, given the potential impact of PPMD stressors on an entire family unit. Although no tool specifically designed to assess families affected by PPMDs currently exists, the Neuman Family Assessment Measure (NFAM) (K. Reed, personal communication, March 31, 2000), is an instrument based on the Neuman Systems Model that would be a suitable assessment tool for the family as a system. The instrument allows each family member to identify his or her top 10 stressors from a list of 24 common family life stressors. In addition, the NFAM includes 10 to 12 items addressing various aspects of each of the family's five variable domains. Each family member has the opportunity to respond to each item, and the accompanying clinician forms and scoring guidelines allow the interviewer to tabulate and compare family members' responses. Affected family members may find interpersonal sharing about their reactions to intrapersonal, interpersonal, and extrapersonal PPMD stressors difficult without facilitation by an objective caregiver. Thus, collaborative review among family members and caregiver of individual family responses to the NFAM provides a method to foster open communication leading to clarification about individual family member perceptions of and reactions to PPMD stressors.

Nurses directly involved in the care of women diagnosed with PPMDs could supply patients with enough copies of the NFAM for all family members capable of completing the tool. After the individually completed instruments have been returned and tabulated, an appointment can be made with a mental health nurse clinician for the family as a unit to review individual family member responses and subsequently clarify client and caregiver perceptions about family member reactions to stressors. Mutually identified problem areas can be discussed and prioritized for goal setting and prevention intervention planning that will strengthen family system lines of resistance and promoting wellness.

Use of the assessment tools, as well as developing a working knowledge of the intrapersonal, interpersonal, and extrapersonal stressors commonly associated with PPMDs will assist in the development of nursing diagnoses. Specific causative stressors at the root of PPMDs have not been absolutely established, and experts in the field continue to explore possible biological and/or psychosocial contributory factors. Women most likely at risk are those who have experienced prior postpartum-onset depression or anxiety or episodes of mood disorder at other times. A family history of affective disorders also increases a woman's risk. Other contributory stressors include a crisis or major stress during pregnancy, problematic delivery, social isolation following childbirth, lack of help from close family members, childhood abuse, and trauma (Gruen, 1990; Hamilton & Harberger, 1992; Sebastian, 1998).

The manner in which the client system copes with the stressors imposed by a postpartum mood disorder is determined to a great degree by the strengths or weaknesses of the client system's lines of resistance for each of five interacting variable domains: physiological, sociocultural, developmental, psychological, and spiritual. How an affected mother reacts to the stressors impinging on her individual system within the context of each of these variable domains will determine the degree to which the entire family system and individual family members' systems are altered. Conversely, the responses of the individual family members to the mother's stress reactions will affect the course of her illness, as well as the degree to which the PPMD affects remaining family members systems. Whether the family members' responses have a positive or negative effect on a mother's condition will depend on strengths or weaknesses inherent in the lines of resistance of the patient/family systems. Nursing prevention interventions that focus on augmenting the strengths of the family system's lines of resistance will help to strengthen the family's defenses against impinging stressors. An examination of intrapersonal, interpersonal, and extrapersonal stressors and potential reactions commonly experienced by clients struggling with PPMDs will serve as a guide in the development of appropriate nursing interventions for this population.

As all families are unique, the following discussion of stressors and potential reactions associated with PPMDs is not exhaustive. However, the intrapersonal, interpersonal, and extrapersonal stressors and reactions identified and discussed here are commonly experienced by many affected family units.

Potential Intrapersonal PPMD Stressors

Common intrapersonal PPMD stressors include:

- Previous personal or family history of depression/anxiety
- Mother's altered hormonal environment
- Physiological changes resulting from childbirth
- Knowledge deficit about existence and manifestation of PPMDs
- Difficult pregnancy/delivery
- Sleep deprivation due to altered schedule
- Demands related to care of an infant
- Role alterations
- Mother's past history of physical or sexual abuse

When PPMD stressors invade a new mother's normal line of defense, she and each other family member will uniquely experience the impact intrapersonally. Affected mothers are typically shocked to find that they are experiencing such unexpected feelings. For example, overwhelming sadness, confusion, anxiety, and distorted thought processes cause mothers to feel frightened, ashamed, guilty, and doubtful of their abilities to parent and successfully nurture their infants. They may take on the formidable task of pretending that all is well due to fear of disapproval and rejection from friends and husbands. While attempting to "put on a happy face," their condition can steadily deteriorate (Harberger, Berchtold, & Honikman, 1992).

Partners of women with a PPMD also experience reactions to intrapersonal stressors and are at risk of experiencing a mental disorder (Ballard et al., 1994; Lovestone & Kumar, 1993). Fathers often express anger, fear, or frustration, which they disguise as anger, when their partner exhibits symptoms of a PPMD. In their examination of the father's experience, Meighan and colleagues (1999) found that men experience confusion, a sense of loss of control, and helplessness at being unable to help their spouses overcome their mental conditions.

Children in an affected family also have been found to exhibit reactions to intrapersonal stressors. Cogill and colleagues (1986) found that young children of depressed mothers may subsequently perform poorer cognitively. Additionally, Gross and colleagues (1994) pointed out that preschool children of depressed mothers may experience lower social competence and more behavior problems than children whose mothers are not depressed. Furthermore, a mother's affective illness may adversely affect her relationship with her infant (Stein et al., 1991).

The vulnerability of family systems is demonstrated by the effects of intrapersonal PPMD stressors on individual family members. Because of the interdependence of family members, PPMD stressors experienced intrapersonally will inevitably result in reactions that affect interpersonal relationships within the family system.

Potential Interpersonal PPMD Stressors

Common interpersonal PPMD stressors include:

- Roles altered by addition of a family member
- Knowledge deficit about existence and presentation of PPMDs
- Increased demands and responsibilities related to parenting an infant
- Marital distress
- Difficult or compromised infant
- Unsupportive or absent partner
- Recent stressful family life events

Interpersonal stressors for family members affected by PPMDs are those that occur externally to each individual member system, as well as between or among individual member systems. For example, alterations in the role expectations and communication patterns of mothers, their partners, and the children in affected families will affect the interpersonal relationships of all members of the family unit and threaten the stability of the family system.

A mother's temporary inability to function at the level to which she and her family are accustomed may result in instability of the couple relationship (Dimitrovsky, Perez-Hirshberg, & Itskowitz, 1983; Meighan et al., 1999; Zuckerman & Beardslee, 1987). Reactions to PPMD stressors may threaten even the strongest of marital bonds. Furthermore, affected mothers' distress may be magnified as a result of the absence of a partner or by having a partner who must work long hours or who is limited in the ability to offer behavioral and emotional support (Morse, 1993). In addition, fathers identify sadness over loss of intimacy and loss of how things used to be (Meighan et al., 1999).

Other serious interpersonal consequences of PPMD include child abuse and neglect (Hanford, 1985).

Potential Extrapersonal PPMD Stressors

The potential intrapersonal and interpersonal stressors associated with PPMDs clearly take a toll on family systems. Beyond the stressors perceived within and between individual family members, extrapersonal stressors related to PPMDs render further insult on the affected family units. Common extrapersonal PPMD stressors are:

- Health care providers' knowledge deficits regarding PPMDs
- Trivialization of PPMDs by health care providers and the general public
- General cultural stigmatization around issues of mental health
- Distancing from affected family unit by family/friends
- Geographic isolation from extended family members

Extrapersonal stressors are external and at a distance from the boundaries of both the individual family member and the family unit systems. Extrapersonal PPMD stressors can be levied on families by outside persons and institutions or society at large.

Gaps in the knowledge of health care providers about the presentation and appropriate treatment for PPMDs can thwart an affected family's search for adequate help. Adequate information about PPMDs is curiously absent in the obstetric and gynecologic texts (Sebastian, 1998). Furthermore, minimization of PPMD symptoms by those whom the family considers to be "the experts" may cause the family to discontinue help-seeking behaviors and result in further deterioration of their situation.

The health care system places major emphasis on the period of pregnancy and childbirth. Information abounds concerning protocols to ensure well-being of the woman and baby throughout pregnancy and delivery. In contrast, little, if any, attention is given to the psychosocial needs of the new family following the arrival of a baby.

The stigma that surrounds psychiatric disorders in the United States is magnified in the case of PPMDs due to a culture that fosters projection of the predominantly positive aspects of new motherhood in the media and popular literature. A new mother's inability to live up to societal expectation may result in the distancing of her friends and criticism from members of the extended family. Negative reactions of family and friends decrease the base of extrafamilial support so important to the development of any young family. A lack of extrafamilial support will be even more acutely felt by the young family experiencing a PPMD due to the difficulty commonly experienced in accessing outside resources of assistance.

In many cases, geographic distance, not the absence of extended family emotional support, will be the cause of increased hardship for a family battling a PPMD. Over the past several decades, it has become increasingly common for young families to move farther away from families of origin, making it difficult to garner help from close relatives in the early weeks following childbirth. A first-time mother may have little or no experience with child care, particularly if her family of origin is small (Sebastian, 1998). A first-time mother experiencing a PPMD far away from her extended family will be left to cope by relying on her own already depleted resources.

The examples of intrapersonal, interpersonal, and extrapersonal stressors and potential reactions given here support the contention that PPMDs are the cause of much personal suffering, place increased demands on health care systems for services, and, in fortunately rare instances, can result in the demise of family systems as a result of irreversible marital conflict, infanticide, or maternal suicide.

Considering the seriousness of possible outcomes of PPMDs, nurses who regularly interact with childbearing families must focus attention on the development of prevention interventions that will augment the mother's and family system's lines of defense and resistance toward an optimal functional level.

PREVENTION INTERVENTIONS

Childbirth educators; nurses working in neonatal intensive care units, obstetricians' offices, and pediatricians' offices; nurse counselors; nurse practitioners; nurse midwives; lactation consultants; and visiting nurses are well positioned to lessen the toll that PPMDs can take on young families. Nursing prevention interventions addressing PPMDs will serve to increase the breadth of knowledge about these conditions among health care providers and lay persons and also will also help to decrease the stigma surrounding these illnesses.

Primary Prevention Interventions

Primary prevention interventions are those intended to reduce the possibility of the client's encounter with stressors and are meant to strengthen the client system's flexible line of defense. The childbearing family's flexible line of defense will be strengthened by learning about the nature of PPMDs and possible factors that put women at risk. A strong flexible line of defense will promote the young family's retention of optimal system stability. Thus, education and awareness-raising around the issues of PPMDs are primary prevention interventions of critical importance.

First and foremost, nurses must increase their own knowledge about PPMDs so that they may serve as educators for their patients and colleagues. The literature is replete with information about the presentation and treatment of PPMDs, and several resources speak directly and comprehensively to the role nurses play in assisting families to cope with PPMDs (Beck, 1999; Comitz, Comitz, & Semprevivo, 1990; Kendall-Tackett, 1993). Unfortunately, some nurses and other health care providers continue to hold on to the belief that if they question clients about mood disorders, they will plant a seed that will ultimately blossom into the actual experience of such an illness. This myth must be dispelled, freeing nurses who care for young families to openly share information that will assist in strengthening their clients' flexible lines of defense. There are a number of mechanisms by which informed nurses can impart knowledge about PPMDs. These educational efforts include:

- Provision of in-service education programs about PPMDs for colleagues and co-workers
- Including material on PPMDs in maternal and child nursing curricula
- Sharing information in childbirth preparation classes (Comitz, Comitz, & Semprevivo, 1990) about the nature of PPMDs as well as factors that may put women at risk
- Increasing the availability of information about PPMDs in obstetricians' and pediatricians' offices

- Developing informational brochures about PPMDs and including these in the discharge materials provided to new mothers on postpartum units
- Targeting information about PPMDs to underserved populations who may have even greater difficulty accessing pertinent information regarding these conditions
- Writing professional articles about PPMDs for magazines popular with women and young families
- Delivering presentations about the relationship between childbearing and mental health to young mother and parent groups
- Ensuring that educational materials about PPMDs are available in local public libraries and at women's resource centers within the community

By implementing these prevention interventions and by creating other ways to share information, nurses will strengthen the flexible defense lines of the systems of the women and families with whom they work, thus preventing PPMD experiences. Primary prevention intervention will reduce or eliminate the impact of PPMD stressors on the normal defense lines and lines of resistance of childbearing client systems.

Secondary Prevention Interventions

Secondary prevention interventions are those nursing actions that help to protect the basic/core structures of the mother's and family's systems once the normal lines of defense have been invaded by PPMD stressors. Timely assessment, early case finding, and accessing appropriate treatment for PPMDs are important secondary prevention interventions. Nursing assessment resulting in a PPMD diagnosis indicates that stressors have invaded the mother's and family system's normal lines of defense and steps must be taken to augment client systems' lines of resistance within the five variable domains, to protect the client systems' basic cores. Nursing prevention interventions to consider include:

- Helping affected families to mobilize usual support systems
- Teaching appropriate anger expression
- Encouraging the appropriate expression of anger
- Assisting family to arrange for uninterrupted sleep (Martell, 1990)

In most cases of PPMD, it is crucial that nurses offer early referral for appropriate treatment.

The treatment of postpartum psychiatric illness depends on the particular syndrome identified, as well as the level of its severity. Treatment options include supportive psychotherapy, psychotropic medication, and group support (Fernandez, 1992; Wisner, 1992).

Cognitive therapy and interpersonal therapy are methods of psychotherapy commonly used in the treatment of PPMDs (Sebastian, 1998). Cognitive therapy is a collaborative approach in which the therapist guides the client to discover how the quality of thoughts may negatively affect emotions and behaviors (Freeman et al., 1990). A client and therapist engaged in interpersonal psychotherapy focus on the possible connections between a presenting mood disorder and the client's current interpersonal relationships (Engler & Coleman, 1992; Stuart & O'Hara, 1995). Psychotherapy should be supportive, focus on the here and now, and explore possible social factors when the woman's symptoms have diminished (Fernandez, 1992). In-depth psychotherapy may not be necessary for all patients. However, psychotherapy is strongly suggested for patients with a history of traumatic childhood, including incest, physical abuse, and foster care placements; current domestic violence; and unsatisfactory and dysfunctional relationships with partner and family (Wisner, 1992).

It is recommended that nurses working with childbearing families compile and maintain a readily available list of local advanced practice nurse therapists, psychologists, and social workers experienced in both providing psychotherapy and in working with women with PPMDs and their families. Mental health specialists who are familiar with PPMDs and consequent patient/family reactions to these disorders are best suited to assist this population with their restabilization efforts. In mild PPMD cases, psychotherapy alone may prove sufficient for adequately addressing signs and symptoms; however, when there is no improvement, psychotropic medications are commonly added to the treatment regimens.

Medications most often used to treat PPMDs include selective serotonin reuptake inhibitors (SSRIs) or tricyclic antidepressants (TCAs). Prior to the commencement of pharmacological treatment, a thorough medical diagnostic assessment must be performed, including history, physical, and laboratory evaluations, including a thorough thyroid screen (Fernandez, 1992; Wisner, 1992). The clinical picture dictates the duration of treatment. When treatment is begun early in the illness, and when symptoms are mild, shorter periods of treatment up to four months are usually sufficient. When treatment is begun late in the course of illness, if affective symptoms are severe, or a significant obsessive component is present, longer periods of medication may be required. Treatment lasting from six months to a year after delivery is common (Fernandez, 1992). In view of the fact that earlier treatment onset may shorten the course of postpartum mental illness, the importance of nurses adopting improved methods of wholistic assessment and case finding needs to be underscored.

Community support plays an important adjunctive role in helping affected families to attain optimal wellness. Partly in response to the all-too-common trivialization of the signs and symptoms of postpartum psychiatric illness, a network of mutual aid, self-help, and volunteer support services has stretched across the United States and Canada during the past 15 years. Depression After Delivery (DAD) and Postpartum Support International (PSI) are two organizations dedicated to providing assistance to women and families affected by PPMDs (Table 5-2). These organizations offer education, advocacy, and access to appropriate referral resources (Harberger, Berchtold, & Honikman, 1992). Depending on location, support group services may vary to include telephone support or regularly scheduled group meetings. In some areas, groups are available for both mothers and fathers. Participation in a support group is valuable to clients as it offers a safe arena in which to share experiences, thereby alleviating guilt, shame, and sense of aloneness. Nurses need to become familiar with available community support services. Where little or no such support services exist, nurses might consider initiating support group activities. Formal or informal PPMD support group meetings can be held in a variety of places, such as meeting rooms at hospitals, clinics, local churches, or public libraries. Both DAD and PSI, as well as colleagues experienced in work with groups, can provide guidance and information on support group development.

Adequate assessment for and timely case finding of PPMDs, followed by early referral to appropriate psychotherapeutic and psychobiological treatments augmented by community group support, will provide affected clients the best chance for attaining

TABLE 5-2. Resources for Postpartum Mood Disorders

Support Groups

United States

Depression After Delivery (DAD)
1-888-440-PPMD
www.behavenet.com/dadinc/

Postpartum Support International (PSI)
805-967-7636
www.postpartum.net

Canada

PASS-CAN (Postpartum Adjustment Support Services–Canada)
905-844-9009
passcan@vdnetmmp.net

Pacific Post Partum Support Society
(PPPSS)
604-255-7999

Professional Organization

Marcé Society
North American representative:
Michael O'Hara, PhD (319)-335-2452
Department of Psychology
University of Iowa
Iowa City, IA 52242

Helpful Books for Parents

Placksin, S. (1994). *Mothering the new mother.* New York: New Market Press.
Kleiman, K. R., & Raskin, V. D. (1994). *This isn't what I expected.* New York: Bantam.
Sebastian, L. (1998). *Overcoming postpartum depression and anxiety.* Omaha, NE: Addicus Books.
Roan, S. (1997). *Every woman's guide to diagnosis, treatment, & prevention.* Holbrook, MA: Adams Media Corporation.

wellness and preserving life-sustaining energy through secondary prevention interventions. Attention must then turn to maintaining gains achieved through the application of secondary prevention interventions.

Tertiary Prevention Interventions

Tertiary prevention interventions are those nursing interventions designed to maintain wellness once a client system has regained stability achieved through secondary prevention interventions. Tertiary prevention interventions for PPMDs include:

- Continued community group support
- Use of measures to prevent reoccurrence of a PPMD following subsequent childbirth

The healing process often continues long after signs and symptoms have resolved for women who have recovered from PPMDs. Continued group support involvement, in the form of lending assistance to others affected by PPMDs, may help some recovered clients to sustain gains made in the process of attaining system stability. Indeed, the DAD and PSI support groups are organized and facilitated predominantly by individuals who have successfully recovered from PPMDs.

Women who have experienced a PPMD once are at significant risk of reoccurrence after subsequent deliveries (Hamilton & Sichel, 1992). Nurses must keep abreast of continuing advancements in the prevention and treatment of PPMDs in order to share this information with recovered clients who plan to have more children. By utilizing the knowledge and self-awareness gained through participation in their own secondary prevention interventions, and by learning about current prevention and treatment methods, recovered clients will be in a good position to successfully cope with stressors after subsequent childbirth. Thus, tertiary prevention nursing interventions, such as continued support and education about prevention of PPMDs, proceed full circle to become primary prevention interventions that strengthen client systems' flexible lines of defense in the event of future pregnancy.

CONCLUSION

The recognition and timely treatment of PPMDs is a relatively neglected area of health care in which nurses can make a measurable difference. Kendall-Tackett (1993) has recognized that nurses who work with young families play a vital and often heroic role. Guided by the Neuman Systems Model, nurses who regularly provide care to childbearing families can develop and implement primary, secondary, and tertiary prevention interventions that will greatly reduce stressors of families experiencing PPMDs. This chapter is offered as a primary prevention intervention that acts as a springboard for colleagues in their development of interventions to help young families retain, attain, and maintain optimal wellness and family system integrity around psychosocial issues related to childbearing.

REFERENCES

American Psychiatric Association. (1994). *Diagnostic and statistical manual of mental disorders* (4th ed.). Washington, DC: Author.

Ballard, C. G., Davis, R., Cullen, P. C., Mohan, R. N., & Dean, C. (1994). Prevalence of postnatal psychiatric morbidity in mothers and fathers. *British Journal of Psychiatry, 164,* 782–88.

Beck, C. T. (1992). The lived experience of postpartum depression: A phenomenological study. *Nursing Research, 41,* 166–70.

Beck, C. T. (1995). Screening methods for postpartum depression. *Journal of Obstetrical, Gynecological, and Neonatal Nursing, 24,* 308–12.

Beck, C. T. (1999). Postpartum depression: Stopping the thief that steals motherhood. *AWONNN Lifelines, 3*(4), 41–44.

Clark, F. (1982). The Neuman Systems Model: A clinical application for psychiatric nurse practitioners. In B. Neuman (Ed.), *The Neuman Systems Model: Application to nursing education and practice* (pp. 335–53). Norwalk, CT: Appleton-Century-Crofts.

Cogill, S. R., Caplan, H. L., Alexandra, H., Robson, K. M., & Kumar, R. (1986). Impact of maternal postnatal depression on cognitive development of young children. *British Medical Journal, 292,* 1165–66.

Cohen, L. S., Sichel, D. A., Dimmock, J. A., & Rosenbaum, J. F. (1994). Postpartum course in women with preexisting panic disorder. *Journal of Clinical Psychiatry, 55,* 289–92.

Comitz, S., Comitz, G., & Semprevivo, D. (1990). Postpartum psychosis: A family's perspective. In S. Flagler & D. M. Semprevivo (Eds.), *NAACOG's Clinical issues in perinatal and women's health nursing* (pp. 410–18). Philadelphia: Lippincott.

Cox, J., Holden, J., & Sagovsky, R. (1987). Detection of postnatal depression: Development of the 10-item Edinburgh Postnatal Depression Scale. *British Journal of Psychiatry, 150,* 782–86.

Dimitrovsky, L., Perez-Hirshberg, M. , & Itskowitz, R. (1983). Depression during and following pregnancy: Quality of family relationships. *Journal of Psychology, 121,* 213–18.

Engler, J., & Coleman, D. (1992). *The consumer's guide to psychotherapy.* New York: Fireside Books.

Fashinpaur, D. (1997, March). Application of Neuman's System Model: Nursing interventions for families affected by postpartum mood disorders. Paper presented at the Sixth Biennial International Neuman Systems Model Symposium, Boston, MA.

Fashinpaur, D., & Spisak, D. (1995, November). Postpartum mood disorders: Interventions through an academic nurse managed center. Paper presented at the Thirteenth Annual National Conference of the Society for Education and Research in Psychiatric–Mental Health Nursing, Nashville, TN.

Fernandez, R. J. (1992). Recent clinical management experience. In J. A. Hamilton & P. N. Harberger (Eds.), *Postpartum psychiatric illness: A picture puzzle* (pp. 78–89). Philadelphia: University of Pennsylvania Press.

Freeman, A., Pretzer, B., Fleming, B., & Simon, K. (1990). *Clinical applications of cognitive therapy.* New York: Plenum.

Gross, D., Conrad, D., Fogg, L., & Wothke, W. (1994). A longitudinal model of maternal self-efficacy, depression, and difficult temperament during toddlerhood. *Research in Nursing and Health, 17,* 207–15.

Gruen, D. (1990). Postpartum depression: A debilitating yet often unassessed problem. *Health and Social Work, 15,* 261–70.

Hamilton, J. A. (1989). Postpartum psychiatric syndromes. In B. L. Parry (Ed.), *Women's disorders: The psychiatric clinics of North America* (pp. 67–82). Philadelphia: Saunders.

Hamilton, J. A., & Harberger, P. N. (Eds.). (1992). *Postpartum psychiatric illness: A picture puzzle.* Philadelphia: University of Pennsylvania Press.

Hamilton, J. A., & Sichel, D. A. (1992). Prophylactic measures. In J. A. Hamilton & P. N. Harberger (Eds.), *Postpartum psychiatric illness: A picture puzzle* (pp. 219–34). Philadelphia: University of Pennsylvania Press.

Hanford, P. (1985). Postpartum depression: What it is. What helps? *Canadian Nurse, 81*(1), 30–33.

Harberger, P. N., Berchtold, N. G., & Honikman, J. I. (1992). In J. A. Hamilton & P. N. Harberger (Eds.), *Postpartum psychiatric illness: A picture puzzle* (pp. 41–60). Philadelphia: University of Pennsylvania Press.

Kendall-Tackett, K. (1993). *Postpartum depression: A comprehensive approach for nurses.* Newbury Park, CA: Sage.

Lovestone, S., & Kumar, R. (1993). Postnatal psychiatric illness: The impact on partners. *British Journal of Psychiatry, 163,* 210–16.

Martell, L. (1990). Postpartum depression as a family problem. *Maternal and Child Nursing, 15,* 90–93.

Meighan, M., Davis, M. W., Thomas, S. P., & Droppleman, P. G. (1999). Living with postpartum depression: The father's experience. *American Journal of Maternal and Child Nursing, 24,* 202–208.

Morse, C. (1993). Psychosocial influences in postnatal depression. *Australian Journal of Advanced Nursing, 10,* 26–31.

Sebastian, L. (1998). *Overcoming postpartum anxiety and depression.* Omaha, NE: Addicus Books.

Seeley, S., Murray, L., & Cooper, P. (1996). The outcome for mothers and babies of health visitor interventions. *Health Visitor, 69,* 135–38.

Sichel, D. A., Cohen, L. S., & Dimmock, J. A. (1993). Postpartum obsessive–compulsive disorder: A case series. *Journal of Clinical Psychiatry, 54,* 156–59.

Stein, A., Gath, D. H., Bucher, J., et al. (1991). The relationship between postnatal depression and mother–child interaction. *British Journal of Psychiatry, 158,* 46–52.

Stowe, Z., & Nemeroff, C. (1995). Women at risk for postpartum-onset major depression. *American Journal of Obstetrics and Gynecology, 173,* 639–45.

Stuart, S., & O'Hara, M. (1995) Interpersonal psychotherapy for postpartum depression. *Journal of Psychotherapy Practice and Research, 4*(1), 18–29.

Wisner, K. L. (1991). Postpartum disorders: Identification of postpartum psychiatric illness. *North Carolina Family Physician, 42*(4), 6–8.

Wisner, K. L. (1992). Treatment of postpartum psychiatric illness. *North Carolina Family Physician, 43*(2), 18–20.

Zuckerman, B., & Beardslee, W. (1987). Maternal depression: A concern for pediatricians. *Pediatrics, 79,* 110–17.

six

Using the Neuman Systems Model to Guide Nursing Practice in Canada

John A. Crawford, Michael A. Tarko

The purpose of this chapter is to document the utilization of the Neuman Systems Model for psychiatric nursing practice from a Canadian perspective. In this chapter, narratives from practicing Canadian psychiatric–mental health nurses are presented to illustrate how their psychiatric nursing practice has been influenced by the Neuman Systems Model. The narratives explicate the use of the Neuman Systems Model with diverse client populations and clinical practice contexts.

THE DOUGLAS COLLEGE ADVANCED DIPLOMA PROGRAM IN PSYCHIATRIC NURSING

Over the past 11 years, Douglas College, Faculty of Health Sciences, Department of Psychiatric Nursing, has offered a clinically focused Advanced Diploma Program in Psychiatric Nursing (ADPN) comprised of 30 credit hours of study using a distance education delivery model. The Neuman Systems Model was selected as the conceptual model of nursing to guide psychiatric nursing curriculum development in the program. Psychiatric nurses enrolled in the ADPN at Douglas College are educated to focus on the wellness of the client system regarding environmental stressors and reactions to stressors. The client system is viewed as an individual, family, group, or community, and is a composite of the five Neuman Systems Model interrelated client system variables—physiological, psychological, sociocultural, developmental, and spiritual. The wholistic view of the Neuman Systems Model provides a comprehensive framework that guides the practice of the over 500 registered psychiatric nurses (RPNs) and registered nurses (RNs) who have enrolled in the program since 1989, including 97 graduates (Leah Ponting, personal communication, September 25, 2000).

THE NEUMAN SYSTEMS MODEL AND NURSING PRACTICE

Fawcett (1998) asserted that conceptual models of nursing provide the foundation for advanced psychiatric nursing practice. She pointed out that psychiatric nurses demonstrate an advanced level of psychiatric nursing practice when using the Neuman Systems Model conjointly with one or more therapeutic modalities. Psychiatric nurses who use the Neuman Systems Model to analyze and synthesize client assessment data and frame their psychiatric nursing interventions within the prevention-as-intervention process of primary, secondary, and tertiary care, striving collaboratively with clients for client system stability, provide evidence of theory-based psychiatric nursing care (August-Brady, 2000, Fawcett, 1998; Neuman, 1995). The use of the Neuman Systems Model prevention interventions are central to health promotion activities with diverse client populations in mental health environments.

Neuman, Newman, and Holder (2000) asserted that the concepts of leadership and scholarship associated with the Neuman Systems Model are requisite for a conceptual model of nursing necessary for twenty-first century scientific nursing practice. They posited that the very nature of the Neuman Systems Model conceptual breadth, flexibility, and systemic properties provide benchmarks for the integration of leadership and scholarly professional nursing practice suitable for the changing commission of health care as the profession of nursing embarks on a new century. They espouse that the new century requires new styles and patterns of delivering health care services. Additionally, they proposed that the Neuman Systems Model provides a systematic framework for organizing and supporting the diversity of future health care roles and functions. Neuman and colleagues pointed out that the Neuman Systems Model facilitates Sigma Theta Tau International's 1996 Arista II proposals for preferred nursing activities "because it provides the right directives for future role definition, care activities, and evaluation of [w]holistic care outcomes. The model becomes a useful research tool for interim as well as outcome evaluation" (Neuman, Newman, & Holder, 2000, p. 61).

August-Brady (2000) asserted that the research associated with the Neuman Systems Model prediction of health outcomes in the context of prevention as intervention is limited, and that further inquiry is required with concepts such as the flexible and normal lines of defense, the created environment, and the interrelatedness of core client system variables to foster increased clarity with the theory of prevention as intervention in the new century.

Neuman (1998) posited that the Neuman Systems Model provides a broad conceptual umbrella for nursing practice and pointed out that the model can be used to complement the Omaha System for patient classification, thus providing practitioners with an organizing nursing model and a set of specific tools that facilitate a partnership with client populations supported by evidenced-based nursing practice. Neuman maintained that the complementary nature of the Neuman Systems Model and the Omaha System can be utilized to promote health and wellness by members of the interdisciplinary team within a cross-cultural and international context of interdisciplinary health care practice.

The utility of the Neuman Systems Model for professional nursing practice in general and psychiatric nursing practice in particular is documented in the nursing literature, which reflects an international context of nursing practice (Beynon et al., 1997; Craig & Morris-Coulter, 1995; Fawcett, 1997; Gigliotti, 1998; Knight, 1990; Moore & Munro, 1990; Neuman, 1989, 1995, 1996, 1998; Neuman, Newman, & Holder, 2000; Owens, 1995; Reed, 1993; Smith, 1989; Stuart & Wright, 1995).

The Individual as Client System

Psychiatric nurses studying in the ADPN program at Douglas College are educated to view the client/client system as a composite of five interrelated variables—physiological, psychological, sociocultural, developmental, and spiritual (Neuman, 1995). Assessment of the client/client system comprises an in-depth wholistic health assessment of each variable and focuses on client wellness and strengths related to environmental stressors and reactions to stressors, in accordance with Neuman's conceptualization of the individual as client (Crawford & Gunderson, 1997; Gunderson, 1997).

The Neuman Systems Model has developed credibility among the nursing community for its utility in diverse practice settings. McHolm and Geib (1998) published a guideline tool (Malone College Department of Nursing Assessment and Analysis Tool) as an example of the application of the Neuman Systems Model to health assessment and nursing diagnosis, illustrating the utility of the Neuman Systems Model and links to the North American Nursing Diagnosis Association taxonomy in planning nursing care. Gigliotti (1998) illustrated the integration of the Neuman Systems Model with the theory of nursing diagnosis in postpartum nursing through a systematic case study analysis, which Lunney (as cited in Gigliotti, 1998) asserted is a significant contribution to knowledge development on the topic. Other nurses have described application of the Neuman Systems Model to nursing practice through the use of case illustrations with an elderly client admitted to hospital with a diagnosis of myocardial infarction complicated by congestive heart failure and pulmonary edema (Smith, 1989); clients diagnosed with multiple sclerosis in which the author has adapted the Neuman Systems Model for use in an acute care medical context (Knight, 1990); and planning care for a 26-year-old woman with Down's syndrome (Owens, 1995). Moreover, Moore and Munro (1990) applied the Neuman Systems Model to mental health nursing of older adults, asserting that it is imperative to focus on the total person who is interacting with the environment, with the goal of system stability achieved by assisting the client to attain and maintain the maximal level of functioning irrespective of any compromised physical or mental state.

The Group as Client System

Nurses enrolled in the Douglas College ADPN program who study group counseling examine the theoretical foundations of group counseling for psychiatric nursing practice (Crawford, 1999). Theoretical frameworks of selected group counseling approaches are introduced, including goals, key concepts, therapeutic processes, basic techniques, group leader role and functions, member role and functions, and strengths and limitations for group counseling practice. The key elements of group structure and process from a systems perspective are delineated for psychiatric nursing practice. The utility of the theoretical frameworks regarding group structure and stages of group work in working with selected diverse client populations are explicated. Key concepts associated with group work are discussed and the 10 theoretical approaches to group work described by Corey (2000) are delineated. Nurses demonstrate integration and synthesis of group concepts through planning, conducting, analyzing, and evaluating a group using the Neuman Systems Model and group theory. The Neuman Systems Model applied to group as client enables psychiatric nurses to practice at an advanced level of psychiatric nursing when combining the Neuman Systems Model with one or more therapeutic modalities (Fawcett, 1998).

Psychiatric nurses studying group theory and process in the ADPN program develop a group proposal and conduct a group in a health care setting to demonstrate application of systems theory concepts to group process and group structure. Analysis of the group examines the intra-, inter-, and extrasystem stressors for the group leaders and each group member. The group as a whole can be analyzed by way of identification of intra-, inter-, and extragroup stressors. Mossing (as cited in Crawford, 1999) asserted that the flexible line of defense is envisioned as being similar to that of individuals and includes environmental noises, esthetics of the room, and room temperature, which may affect the buffering potential for the group. Further, she stated that the normal line of defense is envisioned as being identified when the group has developed cohesion and establishes a way of working within the group. The internal lines of resistance are envisioned by Mossing as the degree of trust experienced between group members and the leader as well as strengths of the support for one another and the depth of commitment to learning from each other in the group. The central core of the group is envisioned by Mossing as the common values and beliefs that hold the group together.

The Family as Client System

The Neuman Systems Model adapted to family health assessment and intervention is documented in the nursing literature (Hanson & Mischke, 1996; Reed, 1982, 1989, 1993). Reed (1982, 1989) discussed the Neuman Systems Model structures and concepts in terms of family theory and delineates family process and structure concepts related to the Neuman Systems Model, thus providing direction for family assessment and intervention (Reed, 1993). Nurses enrolled in the Douglas College ADPN program who study family assessment in psychiatric nursing are guided primarily by Reed's contribution in linking family theory process and structure concepts to the Neuman Systems Model using the Family Assessment Guide developed by Mossing and Westwood (1999). The family assessment guide provides direction for data collection and analysis using the Neuman Systems Model. Nurses collect data pertaining to general information about the family system such as composite of the family, relationship in family, age, marital status, highest level of education obtained, occupations, and reasons for referral. Data are collected using a screening level assessment for each member of the family system using Neuman's five client system variables. Those five variables are compressed into four areas to assess the family system as client: (1) psychosocial and cultural relationship characteristics; (2) physical status; (3) family developmental characteristics; and (4) spiritual influences (Mossing & Westwood, 1999). Using the Neuman Systems Model nursing process format of nursing diagnosis, nursing goals, and nursing outcomes enables the psychiatric nurse to plan collaboratively with the family system to achieve optimal family system stability (Mossing & Westwood, 1999).

According to Hanson and Mischke (1996), the Neuman Systems Model concepts modified for client as family system use include "client, basic structure; flexible line of defense; normal line of defense; lines of resistance; stressors; degree of reaction; primary, secondary, and tertiary prevention; reconstitution; and intrapersonal, interfamily, and extrafamily factors" (pp. 169–70). The three-step Neuman Systems Model nursing process (nursing diagnosis, nursing goals, and nursing outcomes) helps the psychiatric nurse to plan for optimal family system stability.

Reed (1989) delineated elements of family theory as factors influencing the family's flexible line of defense as follows: role enactment; rule implementation; decision-making mechanisms; task allocation processes; and bonding patterns. Reed posited that the factors influencing the family's normal line of defense include communication patterns, problem-solving mechanisms; mechanisms for meeting family members' needs for intimacy and affection; and ways of dealing with loss and change. Further, Reed asserted that factors influencing the family's lines of resistance include interrelatedness, interdependence, values, and beliefs. Reed explicated examples of primary prevention strategies as career counseling, parenting classes, and premarital counseling. Secondary prevention strategies include family crisis intervention, grief work, and marital counseling. Tertiary prevention strategies include family therapy, rehabilitative courses, and use of support groups. Reed (1989) maintained that use of the Neuman Systems Model Nursing Process Format (Appendix C, Table C-1) enables novice nurses to begin to understand family theory using the nursing process to care for clients, thus rendering the Neuman Systems Model "a positive impetus for family intervention, the final goal being maintenance of family stability" (p. 195).

The Community as Client System

Beddome (1995) developed the Community-as-Client Assessment Guide, which is an adaptation of the Neuman Systems Model that guides data collection for geopolitical and aggregate needs from the perspectives of clients and health care providers. Beddome delineated eight subsystems associated with the inter- and extrasystems of geopolitical and aggregate clients—health and safety, sociocultural, education, communication and transportation, recreation, economics, law and politics, and religion.

Nurses enrolled in the Douglas College ADPN program who study community concepts examine concepts related to community and community mental health for psychiatric nursing practice (Gunderson, 1999). Moreover, nurses are introduced to definitions of community and social and cultural considerations in community mental health. Further, examination of community mental health from a historical perspective, methods for assessing community, use of the Neuman Systems Model envisioned by way of the Community-as-Partner Model developed by Anderson and McFarlane (as cited in Gunderson, 1999), and approaches to community intervention are delineated (Gunderson, 1999). Using the Neuman Systems Model, Anderson and McFarlane explicated eight subsystems that affect residents of a community—physical environment, safety and transportation, education, politics and government, health and social services, communication, economics, and recreation, with the core and the subsystems comprising the assessment wheel.

In the Douglas College ADPN program, nurses enrolled in the PNUR 720: Clinical Focus Concepts for Clinical Practice and the PNUR 730: Clinical Focus Course for Psychiatric Nursing Practice, the concept of community is expanded to include the health care delivery system for selected clients/client systems (Advanced Diploma Working Group, 2000a,b). For example, nurses conduct a service system assessment in which they assess and analyze community variables to identify strengths, duplication, gaps, and limitations associated with services available to meet client system needs. Based on the analysis, they formulate a nursing diagnosis and identify strategies to strengthen the services available to enhance client system stability. Further, a change proposal is developed to address system stressors based on relevant nursing diagnoses.

PSYCHIATRIC–MENTAL HEALTH NURSES' PERSPECTIVES

RPNs and RNs who use the Neuman Systems Model consistently indicate the model has enhanced their professional identity and self-confidence in working within the interdisciplinary health care team. Psychiatric nurses find that the Neuman Systems Model provides them with the conceptual framework and rationale needed to provide wholistic, competent, and high-quality mental health care to their clients. In addition, the practitioners indicate that the model facilitates critical thinking and clinical judgment, thereby enhancing their clinical practice through expanded role(s) and scope of psychiatric mental health nursing practice.

PSYCHIATRIC–MENTAL HEALTH NURSES' PERSPECTIVES

The Nurses as Contributors

Twenty psychiatric/mental health nurses (RPNs, RNs) who already graduated from or currently are enrolled in courses in the ADPN program at Douglas College were invited to submit a narrative describing how their practice has been influenced through use of the Neuman Systems Model. All of the nurses are registered/licensed to practice by their respective provincial professional association/college and are engaged in active clinical practice. Sixteen of the 20 nurses are graduates of diploma psychiatric programs, and 4 are graduates of diploma general nursing programs; one nurse has diplomas in both general nursing and mental/psychiatric nursing. One nurse has completed a bachelor's degree in psychiatric nursing, 8 nurses have completed the ADPN program, 12 currently are enrolled in courses. In addition, two nurses have certificates in psychiatric–mental health nursing. The group included 10 staff nurses, 1 home care nurse, 1 unit coordinator, 1 nurse clinician, 1 psychiatric behavior consultant, 1 mobile response nurse–Car 87, 1 community mental health nurse, 1 mental health counselor, 1 day hospital coordinator, 1 program director, and 1 instructor/coordinator. Two nurses work in an acute psychiatric unit in a general hospital, two in a provincial psychiatric hospital, and one each in a day hospital, a public school system, a college system, a short-term assessment unit/long-term care facility, a personal care home, a home care agency, a community mental health agency, a community agency, a forensic/psychiatric hospital, youth forensic services, child and adolescent services, a crisis stabilization unit, mental health emergency services–Car 87/urgent emergent services–mobile response, consulting services, counseling services, and a critical care/community hospice. Four nurses work with children and adolescents; 11 with adults; and 3 with the elderly. Two other nurses provide psychiatric nursing services to clients across the life span.

Managing the Narratives

The nurses who submitted narratives completed a consent form granting permission to use their narratives and to identify each contributor by name. The rich text of each narrative was read thoroughly, and open coding was used to identify key ideas and concepts. Further exploration and analysis facilitated identification of higher-order themes/organizers. Fawcett's (2000) version of the rules for Neuman Systems Model–based nursing practice, as well as the diagram of the Neuman Systems Model (Chapter 1, Figure 1-3), the Neuman Systems Model Nursing Process Format (Appendix C, Table C-1), and the Neuman Systems Model Assessment and Intervention Tool: Format for Prevention as Intervention (Appendix C, Table C-6) were used to guide the analysis and organize key concepts and themes explicated in the nurses' narratives. The key concepts and themes are interwoven in the narratives of the nurses and illustrate the use of various Neuman Systems Model concepts in the nurses' practice. Further clarification and refinement of the narratives was facilitated by using constant comparative analysis (Glaser & Strauss, 1967; Strauss & Corbin, 1990). Trustworthiness and rigor, including auditability, credibility, and fittingness were considered using criteria identified by Denzin and Lincoln (1994) and Lincoln and Guba (1985). Credibility was considered paramount and was achieved by staying close to the nurses' words and using quotations whenever possible.

Three major themes emerged from the narratives related to how the Neuman Systems Model has influenced the nurses' practice: Enhancing Psychiatric Nursing Practice, Expanding Scope of Practice, and Adapting the Neuman Systems Model to Enhance Client System Wellness. Subthemes related to Enhancing Psychiatric Nursing Practice include: Viewing the Professional Self Differently, Viewing the Client System Differently—Having a Framework and Focusing on Wholism, and Viewing the Client System Differently—Focusing on Strengths and Wellness. Working with Client Systems emerged as a subtheme related to Expanding Scope of Practice. Subthemes related to Adapting the Neuman Systems Model to Enhance Client Wellness include: Working with the Client Differently—Focusing on Prevention as Intervention, Focusing on Nursing Process Differently, Focusing on Individual Systems, Focusing on Group as Client System, Focusing on Family as Client System, Focusing on Community and Aggregates as Client Systems, Focusing on Students as Client System, Focusing on the Interdisciplinary Team as Client System, and Using the Concentric Rings in Working with Client Systems—Drawing the Circle and Standing in the Circle. The subthemes address specific Neuman Systems Model concepts and principally address one of the three major themes, though they mirror all three themes to some degree. Subthemes associated with the nurses' quotations highlight the themes and subthemes.

Enhancing Psychiatric Nursing Practice

Most of the nurses commented on how the Neuman Systems Model has had a positive impact on and changed how they view their practice and on how they view their clients. The nurses perceive that the Neuman Systems Model provides them with a conceptual framework and rationale that assists them to provide systematic, wholistic, competent, and high-quality mental health care to their clients. In addition, the nurses indicated that the model facilitates critical thinking and clinical judgment, thereby enhancing their clinical practice through expanded role(s) and scope of psychiatric–mental health nursing practice. As Claire stated, "The Neuman Systems Model has sharpened my critical thinking skills and clinical judgments so I formulate individualized and wholistic care plans for clients."

Viewing the Professional Self Differently. RPNs and RNs consistently indicated the Neuman Systems Model has enhanced their professional identity and self-confidence in working collaboratively within the interdisciplinary health care team.

Viewing the Client Differently—Having a Framework and Focusing on Wholism. Most of the nurses commented on how the Neuman Systems Model provides them with a framework to look at client systems in a systematic and wholistic manner. In addition to wholism, Lorraine indicated that the model enables her to focus on health and stressors. Lorraine stated:

> The Neuman Systems Model helps me to view my clients in a more wholistic way: I now take into consideration all factors which have affected or may affect my client's health (e.g., environmental factors). I more readily identify actual and potential stressors in my clients' lives and I am able to structure my nursing actions around those identified stressors. This increases the likelihood that my clients will deal with those stressors more effectively.

For Tracey and Tara, system stability, interrelationships among systems and stressors are important. Tracey wrote:

> The NSM affords me a pathway to adapt a systematic way of delivering quality and comprehensive health care. System balance for clients . . . is the goal of my health care delivery. It is important in my nursing practice to explore all areas of my client's system to identify that all areas are working in harmony. . . . I can understand how my client functions with other systems like family and the community. I am able to identify stressors that may affect my client's well-being. With all of this I am able to provide a complete, dynamic, and diverse level of health care for my clients.

Tara added:

> Neuman's Systems Model has impacted my nursing practice by allowing me to attain a greater sense of wholistic nursing care. In my current practice within the geriatric community, I have grown to view individual aspects of the client's life as subparts of the system. In order to have wellness within the client system, all parts need to work harmoniously. As a practitioner, it is my goal to carefully consider the interrelationship of all these working parts in the total health of my clients.

Viewing the Client Differently—Focusing on Strengths and Wellness. Some of the nurses commented on how their thinking has changed and how they appreciate the Neuman Systems Model because it enables them to focus on strengths and wellness in contrast to focusing on illness. Theresa talked about focusing on wellness and assessment in the context of her practice and said:

By no means do I consider myself an expert with the NSM. I feel its use can be modified slightly to better fit a particular situation as long as the major components of the model remain intact. In my use [of the model] at Forward House, which is a place where people with mental illnesses that live in the community can go for support, socializing, and activities, among other things, I have come to see the NSM as a tool for motivation. Because the NSM focuses on wellness rather than illness, I tend to use it as a measure of growth and successes for the client. It is easy to see how far some of them have come in a specific amount of time. Also, although we do not gather lengthy histories on clients, I have the knowledge of the five variables in the back of my mind and what each entails. Knowing this assists me in assessing whether or not someone is decompensating. This is how my practice has changed by becoming more aware of all the facets of the people I assist and trying to be more thorough in assessing any problems.

Marg, who works with children and adolescents, indicated that the Neuman Systems Model "offers an opportunity to explore this population using a broader, strength-focused framework of reference . . . a change in focus from the usual 'what they did not accomplish' paradigm to a way of thinking which focused on strengths and protective factors." Marg used the framework "to develop a questionnaire, which examined quality of life issues for adolescents who had been given the diagnosis of either pervasive developmental disorder or Asperger's syndrome and received treatment at MATC in Winnipeg." Marg added:

Because of the focus on wellness and strength, it gave me the concepts and structure to shift my thinking away from a more traditional "deficit" mindset. The variables . . . broadened the focus to take into account areas which not only allowed me to change my conceptualization around this grouping of adolescents but also helped me present this "new way" of thinking to the "kids" as well. The focus on strengths and the ability of the client[s] to reconceptualize themselves using the Neuman model was particularly helpful for this population. Often, this group's special/ idiosyncratic interests are viewed as "odd" or maladaptive. Taking strengths into account, even though they may not fit the norm, were seen to be means to reinforce the normal line of defense. The use of this model allowed for a shift in focus from seeing things, which could be defined as pathological in the traditional sense to being reconceptualized as a means of preserving and strengthening lines of defense and ultimately the core of the individual. The practical application of these concepts enabled an alternate view of the client to be presented, not only from a clinical perspective, but also from the perspective of individuals relating to each other as unique beings and partners in their relationship.

Expanding Scope of Practice

Expanding the scope of their psychiatric nursing practice emerged as a second major theme from the nurses' narratives, including one subtheme related to working with client systems. As with the first major theme, key Neuman Systems Model concepts and components are interwoven into the nurses' narratives and both themes to some extent. A number of nurses articulated the impact the model has had on expanding the scope of their psychiatric nursing practice. In addition to emphasizing wholism, Leslie Ann,

Claire, Shelley, and Terry talked about how their roles have changed in working with different client systems.

Working with Client Systems. The model has enabled these nurses to expand their focus of care from individuals to include families, groups, and community. Leslie Ann wrote:

> The Neuman Systems Model has provided me with the framework for a comprehensive wholistic approach that I can apply to individuals, families, and the community. It is important for nurses to expand their thinking to include a systems approach to allow for more flexibility and creativity in our roles as nurses.

In talking about changes in her role within the mental health system, Claire stated:

> My risk assessments have developed . . . to a more wholistic approach, which assesses not just the client's current presentation but further identifies the client's strengths, stressors, premorbid levels of function, coping mechanisms, support systems, and availability of resources. In addition, the systems approach has given me valuable insights into recognizing my own role as a nurse within the mental health system. I recognize the importance of sharing knowledge, beliefs, and ideas amongst mental health professionals and agencies, and the value of partnerships with police and other agencies to improve the community as a whole.

Debbie wrote about how she promotes Neuman Systems Model concepts in her role of unit coordinator. She stated:

> The Neuman Systems Model enabled me to change my view of the person from a specific, medical disease process, to one of a wholistic comprehensive view. Neuman assisted me in viewing the client as a unique, multidimensional being, and . . . I promote these concepts and assist the staff with applying this approach to client care, as well as in assisting the physicians with their focused interviews.

Shelley, who works primarily with elderly clients in home care, identified the importance of community resources and family in working with this client population. As Shelly put it:

> The Neuman Systems Model has influenced my scope of practice as a registered psychiatric nurse working in home care. A large population of our clientele [is] the elderly. The Neuman Systems Model has a way of helping me focus on the client as a whole. In home care, the client becomes more dependent on the community resources available to them in order to maintain the optimal level of wellness and functioning at home for as long as possible. The Neuman Systems Model also helps me focus on the family of the client, as many family members care for their loved ones and the health and stability of them are extremely important to the overall wellness of the client and the family.

Terry added that the Neuman Systems Model has provided her with a framework reflecting her own personal style of nursing with clients and her involvement in community development. She stated:

It has resulted in my ability to care more wholistically—in a way that respects the true needs of the person. It honors where the person has come from, where the person is presently, and where the person needs and desires to go in his or her continuum of the wellness journey. It also honors the family, the group, and the community in their search for health. I am learning in my newest role in community development that the Neuman systems model also supports the development of a healthy organization whose goal is to serve a community of people.

Adapting the Model to Enhance Client System Wellness

The third major theme that emerged from the nurses' narratives reflect their use of key concepts and components of the Neuman Systems Model in adapting the model for use with various client systems, including service system providers/agencies. As with the first two major themes, key model concepts and components are interwoven into the nurses' narratives and both subthemes to some extent.

Working with the Client Differently—Focusing on Prevention as Intervention. A number of the nurses made specific reference to use of the prevention-as-intervention component of the model. Jesse wrote that she appreciates "the inclusion of the individual client's strengths at all three levels of prevention as intervention [as she] can validate the client's abilities rather than focus primarily on his/her disabilities." Sherry commented:

> Since I have incorporated the Neuman Systems Model into my psychiatric nursing practice, I focus more on primary prevention and the client's level of wellness rather than on client illness. I have also become more aware of client environmental stressors and their effects on client health and system stability. My assessments are more comprehensive and multidimensional; this in turn has helped me create more specific, individualized, and effective care plans.

Leslie Ann highlighted the importance of health promotion and empowerment as roles for nurses in assisting client systems to work toward wellness. Leslie Ann expanded on this by saying:

> I believe in the importance of health promotion and illness and this model also supports that. Neuman believes that the healthier the system, the lower the reaction to stress and the faster one can rebound from stress. Importance is placed on strengthening the coping skills of individuals, families, and communities, and empowering people and their communities to find ways to attain, retain, and maintain their goals. Keeping in mind the threefold responsibility of this approach, it allows the nurse to take on many roles to foster resiliency in our clients and our communities. The end result of our efforts will be healthier and stronger individuals, families, and communities.

Sandra articulated the utility of the prevention-as-intervention components of the model to assist her in developing programs and services for clients with dual diagnoses. As she stated:

> Betty Neuman's statement [of] the purpose of the model is to help nurses organize the nursing field within a broad systems perspective as a logical way of dealing with its grow-

ing complexity encouraged me to organized the systems to provide primary, secondary, and tertiary prevention for the dual-diagnosis client. My next project is to coordinate a family support group, for families who have a family member in the Inpatient Unit or Day Hospital/Programs. Leaders will be from the Day Hospital/Program and Mental Health with a volunteer from the community family group attending every two weeks encouraging membership in the community group. Families from the community group may return to the group if their family member returns to programming. Our system has been enriched with the shared care and even though we are rural and remote, a lot of the isolation was self-imposed.

Furthermore, as Terry put it, in addressing stressors, the variables, empowerment, and prevention as intervention:

With the knowledge of what these stressors are, it becomes crystal clear what level of intervention is required. As a nurse, one may ask "Is this a gap or need that requires primary preventative intervention, safeguarding the integrity of the individual before the stressor has challenged or affected the inner reserves of wellness of the person, or is it in a secondary preventative mode, which will lessen the impact that the stressor has already placed on the core of wellness?" I am confident that the model facilitates what it is that the client needs, not what I have imagined his or her need to be or where I think they need to be in their journey of wellness. I believe that this kind of caring empowers the individual to grow towards their vision of wellness.

Viewing Clients Differently—Focusing on Nursing Process. Several nurses discussed how the Neuman Systems Model Nursing Process Format facilitated their work with clients. Pamela, who works on a short-term assessment unit in a long-term care facility and jokingly acknowledges "admitting the whole family" when a client is admitted, wrote:

Wow!!! A model that connected the issues of family support; identified strengths as well as weaknesses; allows for primary, secondary, and tertiary intervention; and dares to include psychological, physiological, spiritual, developmental, and sociocultural dimensions. I needed to involve the informal systems and the environment for the client's benefit. The interactions and the networks were not part of the assessments or the interventions previously. [The] NSM model assesses the degree of reaction and interactions to develop wholistic patient care plans. The model allows for in-depth assessments and interventions. I use it for patient care and staff development. When a patient is admitted, I assess the whole person, the supports, the physical dimensions of the previous living environment, the stressors affecting the system, spiritual level of being, previous level of functioning, and present level of coping. This model helps organize large amounts of information on the five dimensions or variables for a wholistic assessment. Short-term goals and long-term goals are more inclusive, describing education for the client as well as the informal support. It documents psychological stressors that affect the physical body; poor motivation and low self-esteem do have an effect on the client's ability to function and poor coping skills need to be in the care program. Finally, a model that includes the spiritual variable. Feelings that affect a client's ability to respond to stress sometimes open the door to alternate interventions. The power of prayer and power of

faith have been the needed intervention for rehabilitation and reconciliation for many patients. The patients are able to place value on the interventions and the nurse is the facilitator.

Scott indicated that the model provides a systematic perspective in using the first
step of the Neuman Systems Model Nursing Process Format, including the client's environment, in assisting clients to achieve wellness. According to Scott:

> The Neuman Systems Model has influenced my practice as a psychiatric nurse in a posi-
> tive way. It provides me with a guideline, or framework so to speak, in which to collect,
> organize, and synthesize client data in a systematic, wholistic, and logical manner. By in-
> corporating a systems perspective and by viewing the client in his/her/its entire environ-
> ment (both internal and external), the Neuman Systems Model has enabled me to better
> serve my client population, assisting each to attain, retain, and maintain the highest pos-
> sible level of wellness.

For Mary, the model enables her to provide therapeutic care as an outcome of nursing actions for individuals with unique needs. As Mary stated:

> Utilizing the Neuman Systems Model (NSM) has been a rewarding and enlightening ex-
> perience for me, both personally and professionally. Since applying the model to my nurs-
> ing practice, I have clearly acquired a more organized and purposeful approach to nurs-
> ing. Adopting the NSM framework has strengthened my level of nursing practice by
> guiding and directing me in a logical and practical manner so I provide efficient therapeu-
> tic care. Moreover, NSM has helped me to focus on each patient in a holistic manner and
> as an individual with unique needs, which is essential to the provision of quality psychi-
> atric care.

Focusing on Individual as Client System. Jesse commented on how focusing on the individual as client system and use of the nursing process is reflected in her practice, and
Terry focuses on the use of the lines of defense to assist in understanding the client's perception of stressors affecting the client system. Jesse stated:

> This model fits so nicely with psychiatric nursing. The five variables (physiological, psy-
> chological, sociocultural, developmental, and spiritual) very much address the different
> parts that comprise a person. The explicit addition of the spiritual variable is especially
> refreshing given that this is what gives us meaning and essence of life. Assessment of
> these variables gives me a complete picture of the client. This comprehensive data set pro-
> vides clear direction whereon to base my psychiatric nursing interventions. By using this
> model, I've gone beyond the usual assessment of physical and psychological components.
> [The model] leaves open for a broad range of interventions to take place that could si-
> multaneously impact the multidimensions of a person.

Terry reflected on how, when working in a hospice, she was able to identify the interrelationship among individual as client and church as family. She wrote:

> I was asked to support a young mother who came to the office in her grief following the
> death of her son who had died suddenly. Surprisingly, she spoke over and over, not of

the grief at the loss of her child, but of her husband's abandonment and her own siblings who she always felt never really cared for her and as she described, "always put me down." As I stood with her in the lines of defense within the Neuman [Systems] Model, appreciating her strong faith, her boisterous and very vocal ways that had served her well in the past, it dawned on me what it was that she was mourning at this moment. She was mourning the loss of her supports—her family core. She was also mourning over her lack of self-esteem, an important component of an individual's inner core. What she was looking for when she came to us was a way to build herself up, to replenish her inner core. By strengthening her inner core, the next, perhaps most hardest step, being the grief work from her child's death could then be done. The initial means to her goal for moving towards wellness was for someone to show caring and for a sense of family. She was able to find that caring and the family atmosphere within a new church who cared and appreciated her just as she was and provided her with the needed spiritual support.

Focusing on Group as Client System. Terry also talked about her work in developing and conducting bereavement groups, including the role of facilitator. She stated:

I was new to facilitating adult groups, having spent time mostly with children in bereavement workshops. I learned that structure was an important feature for adults at the onset of the group's time together in order to create safe boundaries to explore their grief, as was the child's. Once trust could be established, and each person sensed some inclusion and made a decision to be part of the structure, then there was a sense of cohesion. The work for what each person came to do in his or her grief journey could then begin. I began to understand my role in standing in the lines of defense with a new group—that the only structure that is present is the one the facilitator creates. And how important this structure is! Unlike families, the group core has not yet been established. The core must first be formed before it can perform as a unit. I learned that the environmental structure that the facilitator creates must be strong enough for members to feel safe in, yet flexible enough to be relinquished once each member comes together to form a unit, bringing their own rules and boundaries and direction for growth. The facilitator becomes the structure and foundation only until such time as the group decides to commit to one another from the sharing of commonalities, values, and goals. The group will then perform like family in their structure, function, and development.

Focusing on Family as Client System. Both Jesse and Terry asserted how the model has broadened their perspectives in viewing family as client. For Jesse:

Viewing the family as a unit of care from a system's theory perspective, as in the NSM, has helped me understand the interrelatedness of the parts—the individual family members, and how they affect the whole—the family unit. As a front-line psychiatric nurse I work with individual clients, yet I do consider the family to be integral in the planning of care of the individual client. The health/wellness promotion aspect of this model is a positive force towards helping families reach levels of wellness they may have thought were not possible. This provides the family with a proactive stance towards their health rather than being reactive towards illness.

Terry, using the analogy of a fortress, wrote about her experience in working with families experiencing loss. She said:

> I learned to appreciate the beauty of the family and how it performs in order to maintain, attain, and retain the family's wellness by assuming a structure that protects its core from the stresses and strains of living. Certain necessary defenses need to be in place. These lines encircle the family core, ensuring its survival. They are like the walls of protection that encircle the family fortress, and include those duties and tasks that will protect the fortress. The walls represent the structure needed and the duties represent the functions that help to uphold the structures surrounding the core. The concepts that lie closest to the family, ensuring its survival, are the values—beliefs, interrelatedness, and interdependence of each of its physical, cultural, social developmental, and spiritual variables. Combined together, it creates the strongest glue and identifies to the world a unique family structure.

Focusing on Community and Aggregates as Client System.   Several nurses submitted narratives related to the use of the model with community/aggregates as client system. Della wrote:

> My area of practice is as a mental health worker for a private agency. I travel to First Nations communities to provide therapy to adults and children. One area I do a great deal of work in is debriefing after a crisis on the reserve. I found the Neuman Systems Model very helpful in my work area. This model is an asset for assisting me to organize my thinking in planning a community intervention. It is important in the midst of a traumatic event to systematically look at individual problem areas and their impact on each other. I am able to take the community as a whole and identify the strengths and weaknesses. Then, using the model, I am able to strengthen the lines of defense around the weaker area to protect it from further trauma. Since learning of the model, I now carry a copy with me and use it when I am involved in a community intervention. It is a valuable tool [that] is a reminder to be aware of the whole community and the many interrelated areas. By using this method, I am able to problem-solve with the crisis team to ensure all trauma areas are covered.

Sandra wrote about developing health care services for a client population through community development and partnerships. She noted:

> Rural and remote nursing is isolating, limiting, and a challenge when developing follow-up care for your clients, especially dual-diagnosis or concurrent-disorder patients/clients. I was so focused on my patient/client and caught up in my narrow scope I failed to look up and spend even a moment on our system or the person as a system, until I started to read about the Betty Neuman's Systems Model (1995). Traditionally, our system focused on the person's persistent mental illness, and the ongoing alcohol and drug abuse was seen as a symptom or form of self-medicating. Often, patients/clients were referred to Alcohol and Drug Services and told they could be re-referred after they had addressed the alcohol/drug issue. The Mental Health System spoke very little to the Alcohol and Drug System here in our region over issues that current staff didn't know about or understand. We were all busy providing care, so the situation became static. After thinking about Betty Neuman's Systems Model and talking about the alcohol and drug abuse among our

patients/clients the next step for me was to advocate for a treatment program for concurrent disordered patients/clients. I approached Alcohol and Drug Services with the problems of concurrent-disorder patients, hoping they would provide the expertise and treatment for this group of patients and I could relax about this issue and get back to my routine. The issue of who would do the treatment was not resolved, as they didn't have the expertise in mental health, but they agreed to support and be a partner in a dual-diagnosis program. An interested staff member from Alcohol and Drug phoned, and the problems and possible solutions were discussed after our literature search. We decided that patients/clients lacked knowledge about concurrent-disorder issues. Working together, we developed a training manual with 12 lessons. We also developed an ongoing support group with leaders from Alcohol and Drug Services and Mental Health. These staff members represented Day Hospital/Programs, Mental Health, and Alcohol and Drug Services. The one system that was missing was peer counselors and someone who was interested in developing a Dual Diagnosis Anonymous Group. The BC Schizophrenia Society was approached, and a consumer who completed the Bridges program and has an AA background has taken up the challenge. To the consumer, the flow of the groups was natural and seamless.

Focusing on Students as Client System.
Jane and Cynthia work in the education system with special needs students. Jane teaches employment preparation in a college setting to young adults with developmental disabilities, and Cynthia works with children with special needs in the public school system. For Jane:

> Every student . . . comes from a different background and is at a different level of functioning academically, socially, emotionally, and developmentally from their peers . . . [and] face many stressors when living away from home for the first time. For the instructors . . . integrating Neuman's five variables . . . offers a natural framework on which to base individual and class course content and provides guidelines for the appropriate placement of each student in work experiences. Accurate assessment of each variable on an ongoing basis provides students and instructors with valuable information on the level of wellness that individual students are experiencing. Knowledge of the stressors in one variable affecting all the other variables and the student's overall performance provides instructors with guidelines to modify individual programs. Students may be referred to appropriate professionals, may change their schedules or be encouraged to access counseling to assist them to cope with stressors. Following the Neuman Systems Model has proven to increase retention in the program and contributes greatly to the success of the special needs population in this college environment.

Focusing on the Interdisciplinary Team as Client System.
Several nurses talked about the utility of the Neuman Systems Model in the context of the interdisciplinary team. Debbie wrote, "The format of our multidisciplinary meetings now follow the five variables, allowing the whole team to utilize the Neuman concepts. The comprehensive care plans used on the unit have been adapted to ensure all aspects of the person are considered."

Using the Concentric Rings in Working with Client Systems.
Two nurses working in very diverse practice settings described how their use of the Neuman Systems Model concentric rings assists them in working with client systems.

Drawing the Circles. Cynthia wrote that working in the public school system with various members of the interdisciplinary team can be very challenging and that in team meetings:

> Every member brings their own concerns and information about the student, as well as their own desired goals. By physically drawing the circle that represents the basic structure of the student's being I can effectively demonstrate the known, the unknown, and universal stressors that are impacting this student. Everyone's input can be shown on the diagram, and I can demonstrate the importance of the lines of defense and resistance as well as the uniqueness of this student. The impact of [the] team actually seeing recognizable stressors and strengths around the student's basic structure has a significant importance on how they, in turn, view the student. I often hear my colleagues comment, "I never looked at it that way before," or "That didn't occur to me." Many of our meetings deal with students' coping methods and resources, and the NSM shows the significance of their assessment and evaluation.

Cynthia added that in working with First Nations children and their caregivers, "The use of a circle to depict the basic core and surrounding circular lines of defense and resistance is also significant . . . the circle is very important in their own life teachings, and as such carries more meaning, interpretation, and acceptance."

Standing in the Circles. Terry, reflecting on her attending the 1999 Neuman Systems Model Symposium in Vancouver and the words shared by Dr. Neuman, wrote:

> Dr. Neuman said something like this: "We must always remember the wellness each client has within when we are standing with our clients in our time with them. We must remember to look up and outward with them, not down and inward." Dr. Neuman's words, combined with her systems model taught through the advanced psychiatric nursing diploma at Douglas College has been the change agent for the way that I now show caring. Each time I am with an individual, a family, a group, or a community, I have pictured in my mind standing in that circular Neuman Systems Model with them, in whatever the lines of defense they are in, looking outward and seeing with them their vision for wellness, as well as viewing with them all the ways that they have attempted wellness in the face of many challenges of adversity.

Jewel summarized the utility of the Neuman Systems Model succinctly by stating, "In clinical applications, the Neuman Systems Model provides a comprehensive conceptual framework which offers depth and breadth to psychiatric nursing practice."

CONCLUSION

The nurses' narratives indicate how their practice has changed by using the Neuman Systems Model, viewing their practice wholistically. They apply the model through a shift to include wellness as well as variances from wellness. Explicit in their narratives are the use of components of the model, including the individual's being comprised of five variables, and the individual's being influenced by and reacting to stressors, which is analyzed in the context of the lines of defense and resistance. The psychiatric nurses recognize their role in assisting clients to retain, attain, and maintain, and retain optimal client system wellness by focusing on client strengths using the Neuman Systems Model Nursing Process Format. The three levels of prevention as intervention are considered in planning collaborative psychiatric nursing care with diverse client populations, as indicated in the themes and subthemes that emerged from the narratives.

Several components of the model were not explicitly addressed by the nurses in their narratives. The nurses appear to be less able to articulate several components of the model and struggle with such components as the created environment and the process of reconstitution.

Canadian psychiatric nurses currently employed in diverse mental health settings are being challenged. In the midst of a global psychiatric nursing shortage and declining national and provincial health care resources and services, strategic short-term and long-term psychiatric nursing human resource planning is needed to meet current and future demands and challenges and to begin to address quality of life issues. Documentation from the literature and the nurses' narratives further supports the utility of the Neuman Systems Model for theory-based psychiatric nursing practice in Canada, to enhance and strengthen the mental health system and services to client systems.

The Neuman Systems Model and its utility with client populations enables psychiatric nurses to provide comprehensive, wholistic psychiatric nursing care, working as an integral part of the interdisciplinary health care team. The notion of advanced psychiatric nursing practice is realized when psychiatric nurses base their practice on a conceptual model of nursing and further expand their practice by way of incorporating one or more modalities (e.g., family and group theory and constructs) as a component of their psychiatric nursing care (Fawcett, 1998). Stuart and Wright (1995) asserted that psychiatric nurses "need to evaluate the client's functional status, quality of life and satisfaction with care received. Wholistic psychiatric nursing care must focus on the integrated experience of individuals in their internal and external environment and not merely target symptomatic relief" (p. 271). Psychiatric nurses have opportunities to employ primary, secondary, and tertiary prevention strategies in their work across diverse practice settings with individuals, groups, families, and communities. Psychiatric nursing practice–based research is needed regarding client system outcomes of Neuman Systems Model–based care to provide evidence-based practice, enhance psychiatric nursing care, and further the development of the model in the twenty-first century, as well as psychiatric nursing as a profession.

ACKNOWLEDGMENT

The authors gratefully acknowledge the following psychiatric–mental health nurses (RPNs and RNs) for the insightful, inspiring, and significant contributions made to this chapter by sharing how the Neuman Systems Model has influenced their psychiatric–mental health nursing practice. Your narratives explicate the utility of the Neuman Systems Model in working with diverse client populations, in diverse contexts of practice, and in urban and rural geographic regions of Canada. Your narratives reflect theory-based psychiatric–mental health nursing practice and contribute both to client wellness and to the growth and development of the profession of psychiatric nursing and mental health nursing in Canada. Thank you!

Theresa Baldwin, RPN, Forward House, Parksville, British Columbia

Cynthia Booton, RPN, Psychiatric Nurse, Public School System, Rural British Columbia

Tracey Eklund, RPN, Psychiatric Behavior Consultant, Michener Services, Red Deer, Alberta

Scott Gaucher, RPN, ADPN, Nurse 1, Riverview Hospital, Port Coquitlam, British Columbia

Pam Gulay-Lester, RPN, Staff Psychiatric Nurse, Short Term Assessment Unit/Long Term Care, Capital Care Norwood, Edmonton, Alberta

Jane Hillary, RPN, ADPN, Olds College, Olds, Alberta

Jewel Jasmins, RMN, RN, Nurse Clinician, Psychiatry Program, Surrey Memorial Hospital, Surrey, British Columbia

Tara Kerr, RPN, BHSc(PN), Staff Psychiatric Nurse, Rock Lake Personal Care Home, Pilot Mound, Manitoba

Shelley Kluk, RPN, Geriatric Home Care Psychiatric Nurse, Yorkton, Saskatchewan

Leslie Ann Langdon, RN, CPMHN(C), Mental Health Nurse, Health and Community Services–Central, Lewisporte, Newfoundland

Della Mansoff, RPN, ADPN, Mental Health Counsellor, Foster Counselling, Brandon, Manitoba

Mary Perkovic, RN, CPMHN(C), Forensic Unit, Lakehead Psychiatric Hospital, Thunder Bay, Ontario

Sandra Ramsay, RPN, ADPN, Coordinator, Day Hospital, Northern Interior Health Board, Prince George Regional Hospital, Prince George, British Columbia

Marg Synyshyn, RPN, ADPN, Program Director, MATC & Child and Adolescent Mental Health Services, Winnipeg Regional Health Authority, Winnipeg, Manitoba

Jesse Spencer, RPN, Staff Psychiatric Nurse, Short Stay Assessment Unit (2-East), St. Paul's Hospital, Vancouver, British Columbia

Debbie Wait, RN, ADPN, Unit Coordinator, Crisis Stabilization Unit, Quesnel, British Columbia

Lorraine Waring, RPN, ADPN, Nurse 1, Riverview Hospital, Port Coquitlam, British Columbia

Terry Webber, RN, Critical Care, Community Hospice & Family Care Givers, Surrey, British Columbia

Claire Winson-Jones, RPN, Mental Health Emergency Services/Car 87, Surrey Central Mental Health Team, Urgent Emergent Services/Mobile Response Nurse, Surrey, British Columbia

Sherry Zeer, RPN, Youth Forensic Psychiatric Services, Burnaby, British Columbia

REFERENCES

Advanced Diploma Working Group (2000a). *PNUR 720: Clinical focus concepts for psychiatric nursing practice* (6th ed.). New Westminster, BC: Douglas College.

Advanced Diploma Working Group (2000b). *PNUR 730: Application of clinical focus concepts for psychiatric nursing practice* (6th ed.). New Westminster, BC: Douglas College.

August-Brady, M. (2000). Prevention as intervention. *Journal of Advanced Nursing, 31,* 1304–1308.

Beddome, G. (1995). Community-as-client assessment: A Neuman-based guide for education and practice. In B. Neuman (Ed.), *The Neuman Systems Model.* (3rd ed., pp. 567–75). Norwalk, CT: Appleton & Lange.

Beynon, C. E., Chadwick, P. L., Chang, N. J., et al. (1997). The Neuman Systems Model: Reflections and projections. *Nursing Science Quarterly, 10,* 18–21.

Corey, G. (2000). *Theory and practice of group counseling* (5th ed.). Belmont, CA: Wadsworth/Thomson Learning.

Craig, D. M., & Morris-Coulter, C. (1995). Neuman implementation in a Canadian psychiatric facility. In B. Neuman (Ed.), *The Neuman Systems Model.* (3rd ed., pp. 397–406). Norwalk, CT: Appleton & Lange.

Crawford, J. A. (1999). *PNUR 704: Group counseling for psychiatric nursing practice* (4th ed.). New Westminster, BC: Douglas College.

Crawford, J. A., & Gunderson, J. (1997). *PNUR 707: Health assessment: The psychological, sociocultural, developmental and spiritual variables.* New Westminster, BC: Douglas College.

Denzin, N., & Lincoln, Y. (Eds.). (1994). *Handbook of qualitative research.* Thousand Oaks, CA: Sage.

Fawcett, J. (1997). Conceptual models as guides for psychiatric nursing practice. In A. W. Burgess (Ed.), *Psychiatric nursing: Promoting mental health* (pp. 627–42). Stamford, CT: Appleton & Lange.

Fawcett, J. (1998). Conceptual models and therapeutic modalities in advanced psychiatric nursing practice. In A. W. Burgess (Ed.), *Advanced practice psychiatric nursing* (pp. 41–52). Stamford, CT: Appleton & Lange.

Fawcett, J. (2000). *Analysis and evaluation of contemporary nursing knowledge: Nursing models and theories.* Philadelphia: Davis.

Gigliotti, E. (1998). You make the diagnosis—Case study: Integration of the Neuman Systems Model with the theory of nursing diagnosis in postpartum nursing. *Nursing Diagnosis: Journal of Language and Classification, 9,* 14, 34–38.

Glaser, B., & Strauss, A. (1967). *The discovery of grounded theory.* Chicago: Aldine.

Gunderson, J. (1997). *PNUR 705: Health assessment: The physiological variable.* New Westminster, BC: Douglas College.

Gunderson, J. (1999). *PNUR 702: Community concepts* (5th ed.). New Westminster, BC: Douglas College.

Hanson, S. M. H., & Mischke, K. B. (1996). Family assessment and intervention. In P. Bomar (Ed.), *Nurses and family health promotion: Concepts, assessment, and interventions* (2nd ed., pp. 165–87). Philadelphia: Saunders.

Knight, J. B. (1990). The Betty Neuman Systems Model applied to practice: A client with multiple sclerosis. *Journal of Advanced Nursing, 15,* 447–55.

Lincoln, Y., & Guba, E. (1985). *Naturalistic inquiry.* Beverly Hills, CA: Sage.

McHolm, F. A., & Geib, K. G. (1998). Application of the Neuman Systems Model to teaching health assessment and nursing process. *Nursing Diagnosis: Journal of Language and Classification, 9,* 23–33.

Moore, S. L., & Munro, M. F. (1990). The Neuman System Model applied to mental health nursing of older adults. *Journal of Advanced Nursing, 15,* 293–99.

Mossing, J., & Westwood, A. (1999). *PNUR 708: Family assessment in psychiatric nursing practice* (4th ed.). New Westminster, BC: Douglas College.

Neuman, B. (1989). The Neuman Systems Model. In B. Neuman (Ed.), *The Neuman Systems Model* (2nd ed., pp. 3–63). Norwalk, CT: Appleton & Lange.

Neuman, B. (1995). *The Neuman Systems Model* (3rd ed.). Norwalk, CT: Appleton & Lange.

Neuman, B. (1996). The Neuman Systems Model in research and practice. *Nursing Science Quarterly, 9,* 67–70.

Neuman, B. (1998). Neuman Systems Model and the Omaha system. *Image: Journal of Nursing Scholarship, 30,* 8.

Neuman, B., Newman, M. L., & Holder, P. (2000). Leadership–scholarship integration: Using the Neuman Systems Model for the 21st century professional nursing practice. *Nursing Science Quarterly, 13,* 60–63.

Owens, M. (1995). Care of a woman with Down's syndrome using the Neuman Systems Model. *British Journal of Nursing, 4,* 752–58.

Reed, K. S. (1982). The Neuman Systems Model: A basis for family psychosocial assessment. In B. Neuman (Ed.), *The Neuman Systems Model: Application to nursing education and practice* (pp. 188–95). Norwalk, CT: Appleton-Century-Crofts.

Reed, K. S. (1989). Family theory related to the Neuman Systems Model. In B. Neuman (Ed.), *The Neuman Systems Model* (2nd ed., pp. 385–96). Norwalk, CT: Appleton & Lange.

Reed, K. S. (1993). Adapting the Neuman Systems Model for family nursing. *Nursing Science Quarterly, 6,* 93–97.

Smith, M. C. (1989). Neuman's model in practice. *Nursing Science Quarterly, 2,* 116–17.

Strauss, A., & Corbin, J. (1990). *Basics of qualitative research: Grounded theory procedures and techniques.* Newbury Park, CA: Sage.

Stuart, G. W., & Wright, L. K. (1995). Applying the Neuman Systems Model to psychiatric nursing practice. In B. Neuman (Ed.), *The Neuman Systems Model* (3rd ed., pp. 263–73). Norwalk, CT: Appleton & Lange.

PART III

THE NEUMAN SYSTEMS MODEL AND NURSING RESEARCH

seven

Guidelines for Neuman Systems Model–Based Nursing Research

Margaret Louis, Betty Neuman, Jacqueline Fawcett

The Neuman Systems Model was initially envisioned as an organizing schema for clinical courses (Neuman & Young, 1972). Within just a few years, however, the model was being used as a guide for nursing research. When used as a guide for nursing research, the focus of the four nursing metaparadigm concepts must be modified. *Person* becomes each research participant or subject, as well as the researcher, and *environment* becomes the setting in which the research takes place or the situation that is required for a prevention intervention. *Health* becomes the wellness or illness state of the research participants. *Nursing* becomes the research procedure(s) employed in the resolution of the problem under study, which results in the data collected and analyzed to answer the study questions or test the study hypotheses.

This chapter identifies guidelines for Neuman Systems Model–based research. These guidelines are applicable to Neuman Systems Model–based research conducted by one or more members of any health care discipline. The chapter includes an explanation of each guideline, as well as a discussion of issues surrounding the conduct of interdisciplinary research.

THE NEUMAN SYSTEMS MODEL RESEARCH GUIDELINES

Rudimentary guidelines for Neuman Systems Model–based nursing research were extracted from the content of the model several years ago (Fawcett, 1989) and were refined over time (Fawcett, 1995a, 2000). The refinements were stimulated by a conversation among the Neuman Systems Model trustees (personal communication, April 24, 1993) and discussions of Neuman Systems Model–based research found in the literature (Gigliotti, 1997; Grant, Kinney, & Davis, 1993; Neuman, 1996). The most recent refinements, which are the result of dialogue among the three authors of this chapter, are presented in Table 7-1. Although the guidelines initially were targeted to nursing, our interest in the multidisciplinary use of the Neuman Systems Model called for their extrapolation to other disciplines concerned with studying the health of individuals, families, and communities. Consequently, the guidelines listed in Table 7-1 have been written for researchers in all health care disciplines.

The first guideline stipulates that one purpose of Neuman Systems Model–based research is to predict the effectiveness of primary, secondary, and tertiary prevention inter-

TABLE 7-1. Guidelines for Neuman Systems Model–Based Research

1. Purpose of the Research	One purpose of Neuman Systems Model–based research is to predict the effects of primary, secondary, and tertiary prevention interventions on retention, attainment, and maintenance of client system stability. Another purpose of Neuman Systems Model–based research is to determine the cost, benefit, and utility of prevention interventions.
2. Phenomena of Interest	The phenomena of interest encompass the physiological, psychological, sociocultural, developmental, and spiritual variables; the properties of the central core of the client/client system; the properties of the flexible and normal lines of defense and the lines of resistance; the characteristics of the internal, external, and created environments; the characteristics of intrapersonal, interpersonal, and extrapersonal stressors; and the elements of primary, secondary, and tertiary prevention interventions.
3. Problems to Be Studied	The precise problems to be studied are those dealing with the impact of stressors on client system stability with regard to physiological, psychological, sociocultural, developmental, and spiritual variables, as well as the lines of defense and resistance.
4. Research Methods	Research designs encompass both inductive and deductive research using qualitative and quantitative approaches and associated instrumentation. Data encompass both the client system's and the investigator's perceptions, and may be collected in inpatient, ambulatory, home, and community settings.
5. Study Participants	Study participants can be the client systems of individuals, families, groups, communities, organizations, or collaborative relationships between two or more individuals. The investigator also is a study participant.
6. Data Analysis	Data analysis techniques associated with both qualitative and quantitative methodologies are appropriate. Quantitative methods of data analysis should consider the flexible line of defense as a moderator variable and the lines of resistance as a mediator variable.
7. Contributions to Knowledge Development	Neuman Systems Model–based research findings advance understanding of the influence of prevention interventions on the relation between stressors and client system stability.
8. Research and Clinical Practice	Research is linked to clinical practice through the use of research findings to direct practice. In turn, problems encountered in clinical practice give rise to new research questions

ventions on retention, attainment, and maintenance of client system stability. This means that the ultimate focus of the research is to determine whether prevention interventions are effective ways to retain, attain, or maintain the stability of a client system. This aspect of the first guideline must be understood within the context of the progression of research necessary for building the knowledge base of a discipline. In particular, it is important to understand that tests of prevention interventions must not be conducted prior to adequate descriptions and explanations of relevant phenomena. In other words, descriptive and correlational research must be done prior to the quasi-experimental or experimental research that will test the effectiveness of prevention interventions (Fawcett, 1999).

Another purpose of Neuman Systems Model–based research is to determine the cost, benefit, and utility of prevention interventions. This aspect of the first guideline means that attention must be given to the efficiency of prevention interventions. Efficiency is perhaps best viewed within an economic context. Fawcett and Russell (2001) explained that "The economic principle of efficiency demands that the services produced by a society have the highest attainable total value, given limited resources and technology" (p. 111). Both production efficiency and allocative efficiency must be considered. Production efficiency refers to producing or delivering effective prevention interventions at the lowest possible cost, focuses attention on the costs of delivering particular prevention interventions and associated Neuman Systems Model practice processes, and is determined by cost-effectiveness analysis. This type of economic analysis involves the systematic study of the effects and costs of alternative methods or programs for achieving the same objective. In the case of Neuman Systems Model–based research, the objective is optimal client system stability. In contrast, allocative efficiency refers to maximizing population health given existing constraints; focuses attention on the level of personnel, technology, and expenditures that produce the maximum effect, as well as on the frequency and dose of prevention interventions that produce the maximum effect; and is determined by cost–benefit analysis. This type of economic analysis involves study of one or more methods or programs for achieving a given objective and measurement of both benefits and costs in monetary units. Once again, the objective for Neuman Systems Model–based research is optimal client system stability.

The second guideline stipulates that the phenomena to be studied encompass the concepts of the Neuman Systems Model—physiological, psychological, sociocultural, developmental, and spiritual variables; the central core of the client system; the flexible and normal lines of defense and the lines of resistance; the internal, external, and created environments; intrapersonal, interpersonal, and extrapersonal stressors; and primary, secondary, and tertiary prevention interventions. Although the most comprehensive studies would incorporate all of those concepts, any one study may involve just one, two, or a few of the concepts. Accordingly, a description of types of stressors or an explanation of the relation between a particular type of stressor and a physiological stressor reaction, for example, is appropriate subject matter for Neuman Systems Model–based research.

The third guideline stipulates that the precise problems to be studied are those dealing with the impact of stressors on client system stability with regard to physiological, psychological, sociocultural, developmental, and spiritual variables, as well as the flexible and normal lines of defense and the line of resistance. This guideline should not be interpreted to mean that descriptive and correlational studies cannot be conducted. Rather, the guideline directs the researcher to always consider how, for example, a descriptive study of types of stressors encountered by a person, a family, or a community might be used in future research that is designed to examine the impact of those stressors on one of the lines of defense, the lines of resistance, and/or one or more of the client system variables.

The fourth guideline addresses research methods. It stipulates that research designs encompass both inductive and deductive research using qualitative and quantitative approaches and associated instrumentation. To date, no specific research methods have been derived from the Neuman Systems Model. Consequently, any qualitative or quantitative approach that is logically compatible with the Neuman Systems Model may be used. Here, it is important to recognize the need to uncouple particular methods or approaches from the frames of reference from which they were derived. For example, the grounded theory approach was developed within the context of a sociological conceptual frame of reference that encompasses a basic social problem, a social process, and a trajectory (Glaser & Strauss, 1967). If an investigator wished to use the grounded theory approach to study Neuman Systems Model phenomena, the techniques of grounded theory, such as theoretical sampling and constant comparative analysis, would have to be uncoupled or separated from the original sociological conceptual frame of reference. If a particular research technique cannot be separated from its original conceptual frame of reference, it would not be appropriate for use with the Neuman Systems Model. Furthermore, the approach selected must take into account another aspect of this guideline, namely, that data encompass both the client system's and the investigator's perceptions. This portion of the fourth guideline is a direct derivative of the Neuman Systems Model Process Format, which takes into account both the client system's and the caregiver's perceptions when formulating a diagnosis, goals, and outcomes. Still another aspect of the fourth guideline stipulates that data may be collected in inpatient, ambulatory, home, and community settings. This portion of the guideline is a direct derivative of the sites considered appropriate for Neuman Systems Model–based clinical practice.

The fifth guideline stipulates that study participants can be the client systems of individuals, families, groups, communities, or organizations. This means that the legitimate participants in Neuman Systems Model–based research encompass all client systems of interest in the Neuman Systems Model. Care must be taken to clearly identify the client system of interest. For example, if families are to be the study participants, then each family is considered the unit of analysis, rather than the individuals who comprise the family. Feetham (1991) and Sullivan and Fawcett (1991) pointed out that the responses of individuals who are members of particular families should not be considered family data; rather, they refer to those responses as family-related or individual-level data. In contrast, family or relational data are the responses of the family unit as a whole or the conversion of data from two or more members of each family into a single score. Similarly, if the client system is a group or a community, the entire group or community must be considered the unit of analysis, rather than the individuals who happen to be members of the group or community. In addition, the fifth guideline stipulates that the investigator also is a study participant. This portion of the guideline follows from the fourth guideline, which stipulates that both client systems' and investigators' perceptions be taken into account. Accordingly, the investigator must be a participant in the study. Although investigators participate in all studies by virtue of their selection of the research questions and methodology, the Neuman Systems Model requires investigators to document their perceptions of the study participants' responses to the questions posed. For example, if a study focuses on study participants' level of anxiety about an extrapersonal stressor, such as a laboratory test, the investigator must record the study participants' responses to an instrument that measures anxiety, as well as his or her own perception of each participant's level of anxiety.

The sixth guideline stipulates that data analysis techniques associated with both qualitative and quantitative methodologies are appropriate. This guideline requires that care must be taken to select the data analysis technique that is logically compatible with the particular research method used and also with the Neuman Systems Model. As noted in the discussion of the fourth guideline, it is important to uncouple the data analysis technique from its parent conceptual frame of reference. Furthermore, in keeping with the fifth guideline, data analysis techniques must permit comparisons of study participants' and investigators' perceptions. The sixth guideline also stipulates that quantitative methods of data analysis should consider the flexible line of defense as a moderator variable and the lines of resistance as a mediator variable. (The use of the term *variable* here is not to be confused with the five client system variables. Here, *variable* is used in the research sense of empirical data. For example, the flexible line of defense might be represented in a study by the number of hours of sleep in the past 24 hours experienced by each individual in a study. The research variable in this example would be "number of hours of sleep in the past 24 hours." The "number of hours of sleep in the past 24 hours" then would be treated as a moderator variable in the data analysis.)

Gigliotti (1997) pointed out that inasmuch as the flexible line of defense is a cushion or buffer that is activated in response to a stressor, any variable representing this line of defense should be regarded as a moderator variable, which specifies "the conditions under which effects will hold" (p. 139). Similarly, inasmuch as the lines of resistance are viewed as coming between a stressor and the central core, or blocking the stressor from entering the central core, any variable representing these lines should be regarded as a mediator variable, which enhances understanding of "why certain effects occur" (p. 141). In particular, a mediator specifies the following linear path: x (the stressor) $\rightarrow$ m (the lines of resistance) $\rightarrow$ y (the central core).

The seventh guideline stipulates that Neuman Systems Model–based research findings advance understanding of the influence of prevention interventions on the relation between stressors and client system stability. Such an understanding is the ultimate goal of Neuman Systems Model–based research. It must not be forgotten, however, that each of the many steps required to attain understanding of the influence of prevention interventions contribute in their own equally valuable ways to knowledge development. That is, the findings of descriptive and correlational research are as valuable in terms of knowledge development as are the findings of quasi-experimental and experimental research.

The eighth guideline stipulates that research is linked to clinical practice through the use of research findings to direct practice, and that, in turn, problems encountered in clinical practice give rise to new research questions. This guideline means that the findings of Neuman Systems Model–based studies can be used to formulate recommendations regarding use of particular prevention interventions in clinical practice (Fawcett, 1995b; Louis, 1995). Furthermore, clinical practice problems can serve as a catalyst for new research questions.

ISSUES IN THE APPLICATION OF THE NEUMAN SYSTEMS MODEL–BASED RESEARCH GUIDELINES

The Neuman Systems Model is a conceptual frame of reference that is appropriate for use by members of all health care disciplines; it is truly a multidisciplinary perspective that fosters interdisciplinary collaboration in clinical practice and research. Accordingly, the research guidelines presented in this chapter have been written in such a way that they are applicable to all health care disciplines.

The Neuman Systems Model multidisciplinary perspective is in keeping with the promotion of multidisciplinary and interdisciplinary approaches in contemporary clinical practice. McCloskey and Maas (1998) pointed out, "Interdisciplinary teams are being promoted in health care as the means to find solutions to costs and quality problems" (p. 157). The Neuman Systems Model is an ideal conceptual model for those purposes. But McCloskey and Maas (1998) also pointed out the danger of interdisciplinary approaches. They stated:

> Nurses who always have wanted to be an equal partner on a health care team are eagerly participating in and promoting the team approach. . . . [However,] some nurses are abandoning discipline-specific successes because they have been led to believe that a disciplinary focus is not consistent with an interdisciplinary approach. We believe that real danger for the profession of nursing exists if this happens and that patient care will suffer from the loss of the nursing perspective and the accountability of nurses for their interventions. (p. 157)

Although the Neuman Systems Model research guidelines certainly can and should be used to study the outcomes of interdisciplinary practice, it is important that the members of each discipline tailor the research guidelines to their discipline, in order to identify the distinctive outcomes of their distinctive prevention interventions. For example, the first guideline directs all health researchers to focus on the costs, benefits, and utility of prevention interventions. This guideline can be tailored by nurse researchers to their special interest in identifying nurse-sensitive outcomes and documenting those as outcomes of *nursing* practice, in order to justify the utility of and payment for *nursing* services. Thus, the guideline can be considered a mandate for nurse researchers to design studies that include the collection and analysis of data related to the costs and benefits of *nursing* prevention interventions for individuals, families, and communities.

The ideal Neuman Systems Model–based study would clearly reflect all eight Neuman Systems Model research guidelines and would be conducted by a multidisciplinary research team. Such a study would consider all five client system variables, the three types of stressors, the lines of defense and resistance, the central core, and one or more types of prevention interventions. In addition, such a study would include the perceptions of both the study participants and the investigators.

CONCLUSION

Application of the guidelines for Neuman Systems Model–based research that were presented in this chapter is evident in Chapters 10 and 11. An integrated review of the published reports of Neuman Systems Model research is the subject matter of Chapter 8.

The research tools that have been used to measure concepts of the Neuman Systems Model are identified and discussed in Chapter 9.

REFERENCES

Fawcett, J. (1989). *Analysis and evaluation of conceptual models of nursing* (2nd ed.). Philadelphia: Davis.

Fawcett, J. (1995a). *Analysis and evaluation of conceptual models of nursing* (3rd ed.). Philadelphia: Davis.

Fawcett, J. (1995b). Constructing conceptual–theoretical–empirical structures for research. In B. Neuman (Ed.), *The Neuman Systems Model* (3rd ed., pp. 459–71). Norwalk, CT: Appleton & Lange.

Fawcett, J. (1999). *The relationship of theory and research* (3rd ed.). Philadelphia: Davis

Fawcett, J. (2000). *Analysis and evaluation of contemporary nursing knowledge: Nursing models and theories.* Philadelphia: Davis.

Fawcett, J., & Russell, G. A conceptual model of nursing and health policy. *Policy, Politics, and Nursing Practice, 2,* 108–116.

Feetham, S. L. (1991). Conceptual and methodological issues in research of families. In A. L. Whall & J. Fawcett (Eds.), *Family theory development in nursing: State of the science and art* (pp. 55–68). Philadelphia: Davis.

Gigliotti, E. (1997). Use of Neuman's lines of defense and resistance in nursing research: Conceptual and empirical considerations. *Nursing Science Quarterly, 10,* 136–43.

Glaser, B., & Strauss, A. (1967). *The discovery of grounded theory.* Chicago: Aldine.

Grant, J. S., Kinney, M. R., & Davis, L. L. (1993). Using conceptual frameworks or models to guide nursing research. *Journal of Neuroscience Nursing, 25,* 52–56.

Louis, M. (1995). The Neuman model in nursing research: An update. In B. Neuman (Ed.), *The Neuman Systems Model* (3rd ed., pp. 473–80). Norwalk, CT: Appleton & Lange.

McCloskey, J. C., & Maas, M. (1998). Interdisciplinary team: The nursing perspective is essential. *Nursing Outlook, 46,* 157–63.

Neuman, B. (1996). The Neuman Systems Model in research and practice. *Nursing Science Quarterly, 9,* 67–70.

Neuman, B., & Young, R. J. (1972). A model for teaching total person approach to patient problems. *Nursing Research, 21,* 264–69.

Sullivan, J., & Fawcett, J. (1991). The measurement of family phenomena. In A. L. Whall & J. Fawcett (Eds.), *Family theory development in nursing: State of the science and art* (pp. 69–84). Philadelphia: Davis.

eight

The Neuman Systems Model and Research: An Integrative Review

Jacqueline Fawcett, Sandra K. Giangrande

T he purpose of the chapter is to describe a project that was designed to integrate the publicly available Neuman Systems Model–based research literature.[1,2] The Neuman Systems Model, like other conceptual models of nursing, guides research by stating the purpose of the research, the phenomena making up the domain of inquiry, the problems to be investigated, the methodological directives about how the domain is to be investigated, and the contributions that the research makes to the advancement of nursing knowledge.

REVIEWS OF NEUMAN SYSTEMS MODEL–BASED RESEARCH

Four other reviews of Neuman Systems Model–based research have been published. Louis and Koertvelyessy (1989) identified 44 studies by means of a survey of schools of nursing in the United States, Canada, and Europe and classified the studies according to research design and the Neuman Systems Model phenomena studied. Several of the studies were unpublished and no information, even in abstract form, was given by Louis and Koertvelyessy. A major limitation of Louis and Koertvelyessy's review was their failure to conduct a search of the literature to identify all of the Neuman Systems Model–based studies that had been published.

Louis (1995) later identified 84 additional Neuman Systems Model–based studies from a computer-assisted literature search, along with a personal contact list made available by Betty Neuman. Many of the studies were listed as "in process" theses or dissertations or papers presented at the biennial Neuman Systems Model symposia. The research review focused on how various studies reflected the Neuman Systems Model research rules, or guidelines.

Gigliotti's (2001) integrative review focused on an analysis of nine Neuman Systems Model–based studies. The purpose of her review was to determine the extent of support for propositions that link various concepts of the Neuman Systems Model. Gigliotti reported her difficulty with interpreting the results of the studies, due primarily to the investigators' failure to include all relevant Neuman Systems Model concepts in their research designs.

Fawcett and Giangrande's (2001) earlier integrative review was limited to the 62 Neuman Systems Model–based research reports that were published as journal articles or book chapters. This chapter extends the review by adding data from doctoral dissertations and master's theses. More specifically, the integrative review presented in this chapter sought to extend the existing reviews by identifying and reviewing all published Neuman Systems Model–based research through 1997, to add a quantitative component to the previous narrative reviews, to identify and classify existing programs of Neuman Systems Model–based research, and to delineate directions for future programmatic research. The review was conducted with the Neuman Systems Model research guidelines (see Chapter 7) in mind, because those guidelines convey the widely known content and focus of the Neuman Systems Model. The long-range goal of the project is to use the integrative review as a catalyst for the establishment of networks of researchers who are interested in filling in gaps and extending knowledge of the phenomena encompassed by the Neuman Systems Model.

METHOD FOR THE INTEGRATIVE REVIEW

The project was guided by Cooper's (1989) method of integrating research. The five stages of Cooper's method are: problem formulation, data collection, data evaluation, analysis and interpretation, and public presentation.

Stage 1: Problem Formulation

The problem as formulated was to: (1) identify all published Neuman Systems Model–based research reports, including journal articles, book chapters, master's theses, and doctoral dissertations; (2) classify each research report according to type of research, Neuman Systems Model phenomena studied, extent of Neuman Systems Model usage evident, findings, and scientific merit; and (3) draw conclusions regarding evidence of programs of Neuman Systems Model–based research and directions for future programmatic research.

Stage 2: Data Collection

The sample for the project encompassed research reports published through 1997 that were explicitly based on the Neuman Systems Model. The literature included in the project analysis was limited to the end date of 1997 due to available funding, the time required for retrieval and analysis of the literature and preparation of the report, and a lack of confidence that literature searches conducted in 1998 through mid-2000 yielded a comprehensive list of publications for those years, due to the time lag for indexing in computerized databases. Hand searches of several journals in the private collection of the first author were done. All issues through 1997 of *Advances in Nursing Science, Image: Journal of Nursing Scholarship, Nursing Science Quarterly, Research in Nursing and Health,* and *Western Journal of Nursing Research* were examined, as were all issues from 1967 through 1997 of *Nursing Research.* Hand searches of all three editions of *The Neuman Systems Model* (Neuman, 1982, 1989, 1995) also were done. In addition, computer-assisted searches were done through June 1999, using the CD-ROM and then the online versions of *Index Medicus* (Medline); *International Nursing Index* (INI; available online as part of Medline); *Cumulative Index to Nursing and Allied Health Literature* (CINAHL), which includes citations for selected doctoral dissertations; and *Dissertation Abstracts International* (DAI), which includes both doctoral dissertations and master's theses (master's abstracts are published in *Master's Abstracts International,* which is a component of the DAI computer database). Moreover, the first author had done hand searches of all volumes of the printed versions of INI, CINAHL, and DAI from the mid-1970s through the early 1990s, prior to the widespread availability of the CD-ROM and online versions of those databases. Only those publications in which the Neuman Systems Model was explicitly cited as the basis for the study were included in the sample. Citations for all research reports included in the sample are listed in the chapter bibliography.

Although the authors of integrative reviews of research typically attempt to locate the "fugitive" unpublished literature, a decision was made to limit the current project to published reports of research. The rationale for that decision was partly empirical and partly pragmatic. The empirical rationale was based on the knowledge that the "file draw problem" (Rosenthal, 1979) is not a major one in nursing because nursing journals tend to publish reports of studies with statistically significant and nonsignificant findings. Furthermore, integrative research reviews that included a comparison of the results of more versus less flawed studies (the more flawed studies are less likely, of course, to be published) have found no difference in the strength of theoretical relations (e.g., Smith & Glass, 1977) or have found evidence of stronger relations in the better studies (e.g., Devine & Cook, 1983; Wampler, 1982). Moreover, Heater, Becker, and Olson (1988) found no evidence of a statistically significant difference in effect size for published and unpublished studies. The pragmatic rationale was based on the understanding that there is no systematic way to identify the unpublished research, and that it is exceedingly difficult to obtain full reports of such studies. In addition, lists of unpublished Neuman Systems Model–based research (Louis, 1995; Louis & Koertvelyessy, 1989) revealed that they are in the form of papers presented at conferences—which are available only in abstract form in proceedings or have been subsequently published in journals or book chapters—or in progress dissertations and master's theses—which eventually would be available from University Microfilms.

The various search strategies yielded 200 research reports. The reports encompassed 59 journal articles; 2 abstracts published in journals, one of which was published only as an abstract, and the other only as an abstract in English (the full report was published in Chinese); 3 book chapters; 81 master's theses; and 55 doctoral dissertations. A photocopy of each journal article, book chapter, and journal abstract was made. The full reports of all dissertations were either already in the private collection of the first author or were purchased from University Microfilms. The abstracts of all master's theses were printed from the online databases.

Stage 3: Data Evaluation

The research reports were evaluated using a code book developed by the first author.[3] The code book contained 9 general information elements, 19 scientific merit elements, and 19 Neuman Systems Model elements (Table 8-1). The Neuman Systems Model elements reflected the content of the Neuman Systems Model (see Chapter 1 and Appendix A) and the Neuman Systems Model research guidelines (see Chapter 7). Intrarater reliability was established at 92 percent in one round, using 10 randomly selected research reports. Interrater reliability was established at 80 percent between two independent coders in two rounds, using the same 10 randomly selected research reports.

TABLE 8-1. Coding Elements

General Information—9 Coding Elements

Study code number
Year of publication
Type of publication
Study focus
Other phenomenon (not part of Neuman Systems Model) studied
Other framework (not Neuman Systems Model) also used
School (for master's theses and doctoral dissertations)
Secondary analysis
Publication of theses or doctoral dissertation in journal or book

Scientific Merit—19 Coding Elements

Statement of study purpose given
Hypotheses specified
Theoretical significance and clinical significance of study evident
Study variables defined
Type of research
Sample size justified
Actual sample size
Specific client system identified
Gender of client system identified
General clinical condition specified
Specific clinical condition specified
Setting for data collection given
Evidence of validity of instruments given
Evidence of reliability of instruments given
Procedure explained
Type of data analysis
Data analysis techniques appropriate
Results given for each research question/hypothesis
Statistical significance of results reported

Neuman Systems Model—19 Coding Elements

Overview of Neuman Systems Model
Client system of interest

(continues)

TABLE 8-1. Coding Elements *(continued)*

Neuman Systems Model—19 Coding Elements *(continued)*
Client system and/or nurse preceptions of interest
Types of stressors of interest
Environment of interest
Which lines of defense/resistance of interest
Central core/basic structure of interest
Variables of interest
Physiological variables of interest
Psychological variables of interest
Sociocultural variables of interest
Developmental variables of interest
Spiritual variables of interest
Type(s) of prevention intervention of interest
Study variables linked to Neuman Systems Model concepts
Empirical indicators linked to Neuman Systems Model concepts or to study variables
Propositions about study variables linked to Neuman Systems Model relational propositions
Conclusions regarding Neuman Systems Model stated
Major Neuman Systems Model focus of study

Stage 4: Analysis and Interpretation

Analysis.   This chapter includes comprehensive analyses of the 117 research reports published as journal articles ($n = 59$), book chapters ($n = 3$), and dissertations ($n = 55$). The chapter also includes less comprehensive analyses of the abstracts of the 81 master's theses and the 2 abstracts published in journals.

Three-quarters (75 percent) of all 200 studies focused on clinical nursing topics. Slightly more than one-eighth (14 percent) of the studies focused on nursing administration, just under one-tenth (9 percent) focused on nursing education, and a few (2 percent) focused on continuing nursing education. Slightly more than one-third (34 percent) of the studies were experimental, one-quarter (25 percent) were correlational, and almost two-fifths (37 percent) were descriptive. The remaining few (4 percent) studies were designed to develop and/or test instruments. One of the studies published as a journal article was a secondary analysis of data, as were four dissertations and one master's thesis.

Just over one-third (34 percent) of all 200 studies focused on development or testing of Neuman Systems Model–derived prevention interventions. Almost one-quarter (24 percent) focused on perception of stressors and slightly less than one-tenth (8 percent) focused on reactions to stressors. Almost one-tenth (9 percent) focused on one or more of the five Neuman Systems Model client system variables. A few studies focused on the lines of defense and/or resistance (5 percent) or the central core (1 percent). Other studies focused on various client system perceptions (3 percent), coping (2 percent), or the environment (2 percent). Still others focused on the Neuman Systems Model nursing process (2 percent) or development and testing of instruments derived from the Neuman Systems Model (2 percent). Some other studies focused on evaluation of Neuman Systems Model–based nursing education programs (5 percent) or clinical agencies in which the Neuman Systems Model was used to guide practice (2 percent). The focus of the remaining studies (1 percent) could not be determined from the content of the research report.

More specific analyses were done according to type of publication—journal articles and book chapters, doctoral dissertations, and abstracts of master's theses and abstracts published in journals. The results of the analysis of the journal articles and book chapters are presented in Table 8-2, and the results of the analysis of the doctoral dissertations are presented in Table 8-3. The results of the analysis of the abstracts of master's theses are presented in Table 8-4.

Six (10 percent) of the 59 journal articles were based on master's theses; another four (7 percent), on doctoral dissertations. These research reports were included in the analysis of the journal articles and book chapters (Table 8-2), as well as in the analysis of the doctoral dissertations (Table 8-3) or the master's theses (Table 8-4). There is, then, some overlap in the data presented in the various tables, although that overlap is minimal.

The findings of six other doctoral dissertations were published as journal articles, but the Neuman Systems Model was not cited in those articles; therefore, the articles are not included in any analyses reported in this chapter nor are they listed in the journal articles section of the bibliography. These journal articles were located by means of online searches using the name of the author of each dissertation.

Journal Articles and Book Chapters. The first known Neuman Systems Model–based study published as a journal article or book chapter appeared in 1983 (Ziemer, 1983); the article reports Ziemer's (1982) dissertation research. As can be seen in Table 8-2, almost three-quarters (72 percent, $n = 44$) of the 62 research reports published as journal articles or book chapters focused on clinical topics, and almost one-half (45 percent, $n = 28$) were designed as experiments. Slightly more than one-third (37 percent, $n = 23$) of the studies investigated the effects of Neuman Systems Model prevention interventions. Additional analysis indicated that 6 (26 percent) of those 23 studies focused solely on primary prevention interventions, and 1 (5 percent), on tertiary prevention interventions; no studies focused solely on secondary prevention interventions. Ten (44 percent) of the 23 studies focused on some combination of primary, secondary, and tertiary prevention interventions. Six (26 percent) of the 23 reports did not specify the type of prevention intervention(s) studied.

Almost two-thirds (61 percent, $n = 38$) of the reports included an overview of the Neuman Systems Model that was sufficient for understanding the linkage between the model and the study purposes. However, only one-half ($n = 31$) of the reports included explicit linkages between particular Neuman Systems Model concepts and all study variables. Moreover, just one-fifth (21 percent, $n = 13$) of the reports included explicit linkages between Neuman Systems Model relational propositions and at least some of the propositions about the study variables.

Conclusions regarding the utility of the Neuman Systems Model for the study conducted or the implications of the study findings for the credibility of the Neuman Systems Model were evident in just two-fifths (39 percent, $n = 24$) of the 62 reports. The issue of credibility is particularly critical in that almost one-third (30 percent, $n = 3$) of the 10 correlational studies and slightly more than one-eighth (14 percent, $n = 4$) of the 28 experimental studies yielded results that were not statistically significant. Furthermore, another 30 percent ($n = 3$) of the 10 correlational studies and 54 percent ($n = 15$) of the

TABLE 8-2. Analysis of Neuman Systems Model–Based Research Reports Published as Journal Articles and Book Chapters ($n = 62$)

	n	%
Study Focus		
Clinical	44	72%
Administrative	9	14%
Educational	7	11%
Continuing education	2	3%
Type of Research		
Instrument development	2	3%
Descriptive	22	36%
Correlational	10	16%
Experimental	28	45%
Neuman Systems Model Primary Study Focus		
Prevention interventions	23	37%
Perception of stressors	12	19%
Stressor reaction	6	10%
One or more of the Neuman Systems Model variables	3	5%
Lines of defense/resistance	3	5%
Neuman Systems Model nursing process	3	5%
Client system perceptions	2	3%
Development of research instrument/clinical tool	2	3%
Environment	2	3%
Nursing curriculum	2	3%
Nursing in a clinical agency	2	3%
Client system coping	1	2%
Basic structure/central core	1	2%
Overview of the Neuman Systems Model		
Neuman Systems Model only named	7	11%
Brief overview given	14	23%
Overview sufficient to understand relation of Neuman Systems Model to study	38	61%
Comprehensive overview but not fully tied to study	3	5%
Neuman Systems Model Concept Linkages		
All study variables linked to Neuman Systems Model concepts	31	50%
Some study variables linked to Neuman Systems Model concepts	21	34%
No study variables linked to Neuman Systems Model concepts	10	16%
Empirical Indicators		
All Neuman Systems Model concepts or study variables linked to empirical indicators	55	89%
Some Neuman Systems Model concepts or study variables linked to empirical indicators	3	5%
No Neuman Systems Model concepts or study variables linked to empirical indicators	4	6%

TABLE 8-2. Analysis of Neuman Systems Model–Based Research Reports Published as Journal Articles and Book Chapters (*n* = 62) *(continued)*

Neuman Systems Model Relational Propositions

Relational propositions not required	19	31%
Neuman Systems Model relational propositions not stated	23	37%
Neuman Systems Model relational propositions stated but not linked to any propositions about study variables	7	11%
Neuman Systems Model relational propositions stated and linked to some propositions about study variables	3	5%
Neuman Systems Model relational propositions stated and linked to all propositions about study variables	10	16%

Conclusions Regarding Neuman Systems Model

Conclusions regarding utility or credibility of Neuman Systems Model *not* stated	38	61%
Conclusions regarding utility and/or credibility of Neuman Systems Model stated explicitly	24	39%

Sample Size

Sample size justified	5	8%

Instruments

Validity data given	25	40%
Reliability data given	29	47%

Research Findings: All Studies (*n* = 62)

Not statistically significant	7	11%
Statistically significant	10	16%
Mixed	19	31%
Statistical significance not reported	5	8%
Statistical significance not relevant	21	34%

Research Findings: Correlational Studies (*n* = 10)

Not statistically significant	3	30%
Statistically significant	3	30%
Mixed	3	30%
Statistical significance not reported	1	10%

Research Findings: Experimental Studies (*n* = 28)

Not statistically significant	4	14%
Statistically significant	6	21%
Mixed	15	54%
Statistical significance not reported	3	11%

TABLE 8-3. Analysis of Neuman Systems Model–Based Doctoral Dissertations ($n = 55$)

	n	%*
Study Focus		
Clinical	41	75%
Administrative	4	7%
Educational	9	16%
Continuing education	1	2%
Type of Research		
Instrument development	1	2%
Descriptive	16	29%
Correlational	22	40%
Experimental	16	29%
Neuman Systems Model Primary Study Focus		
Prevention interventions	13	24%
Perception of stressors	11	20%
Stressor reaction	3	5%
One or more of the Neuman Systems Model variables	9	16%
Lines of defense/resistance	6	11%
Client system perceptions	1	2%
Development of research instrument/clinical tool	1	2%
Environment	2	4%
Nursing curriculum	8	14%
Nursing in a clinical agency	1	2%
Overview of the Neuman Systems Model		
Brief overview given	6	11%
Overview sufficient to understand relation of Neuman Systems Model to study	44	80%
Comprehensive overview but not fully tied to study	5	9%
Neuman Systems Model Concept Linkages		
All study variables linked to Neuman Systems Model concepts	36	65%
Some study variables linked to Neuman Systems Model concepts	14	26%
No study variables linked to Neuman Systems Model concepts	5	9%
Empirical Indicators		
All Neuman Systems Model concepts or study variables linked to empirical indicators	51	93%
No Neuman Systems Model concepts or study variables linked to empirical indicators	4	7%
Neuman Systems Model Relational Propositions		
No relational propositions stated	1	2%
Relational propositions not required	14	25%
Neuman Systems Model relational propositions not stated	14	25%

TABLE 8-3. Analysis of Neuman Systems Model–Based Doctoral Dissertations (*n* = 55) *(continued)*

Neuman Systems Model Relational Propositions *(continued)*

Neuman Systems Model relational propositions stated but not linked to any propositions about study variables	6	11%
Neuman Systems Model relational propositions stated and linked to some propositions about study variables	3	5%
Neuman Systems Model relational propositions stated and linked to all propositions about study variables	17	31%

Conclusions Regarding Neuman Systems Model

Conclusions regarding utility or credibility of Neuman Systems Model *not* stated	5	9%
Conclusions regarding utility and/or credibility of Neuman Systems Model stated explicitly	50	91%

Sample Size

Sample size justified	24	44%

Instruments

Validity data given	36	66%
Reliability data given	44	80%

Research Findings: All Studies (*n* = 55)

Not statistically significant	1	2%
Statistically significant	8	14%
Mixed	33	60%
Statistical significance not relevant	13	24%

Research Findings: Correlational Studies (*n* = 22)

Statistically significant	5	23%
Mixed	17	77%

Research Findings: Experimental Studies (*n* = 16)

Not statistically significant	1	6%
Statistically significant	2	13%
Mixed	13	81%

Totals may not equal 100% due to rounding.

28 experimental studies yielded a combination of statistically significant and nonsignificant results.

Relatively few reports included mention of specific Neuman Systems Model phenomena. Indeed, further analysis of the 62 reports revealed that 95 percent (*n* = 59) were not explicit with regard to the type of environment (internal, external, created) considered, 92 percent (*n* = 57) did not specify whether the central core was of interest, and 84 percent (*n* = 52) did not explicate the type of variables (physiological, psychological, sociocultural, developmental, spiritual) studied. Furthermore, 69 percent (*n* = 43) of the 62 reports did not indicate which lines (flexible and normal lines of defense, lines of resist-

TABLE 8-4. Analysis of Neuman Systems Model–Based Abstracts of Master's Theses ($n = 81$)

	n	%
Study Focus		
Clinical	62	77%
Administrative	17	21%
Educational	1	1%
Continuing education	1	1%
Type of Research		
Instrument development	4	5%
Descriptive	36	44%
Correlational	16	20%
Experimental	25	31%
Neuman Systems Model Primary Study Focus		
Prevention interventions	32	39%
Perception of stressors	23	28%
Stressor reaction	7	8%
One or more of the Neuman Systems Model variables	5	6%
Lines of defense/resistance	2	3%
Neuman Systems Model nursing process	1	1%
Client system perceptions	2	3%
Development of research instrument/clinical tool	2	3%
Environment	1	1%
Nursing curriculum	1	1%
Nursing in a clinical agency	2	3%
Client system coping	2	3%
Could not be determined	1	1%
Conclusions Regarding Neuman Systems Model		
Conclusions regarding utility or credibility of Neuman Systems Model *not* stated	74	91%
Conclusions regarding utility and/or credibility of Neuman Systems Model stated explicitly	7	9%
Research Findings: All Studies ($n = 81$)		
Not statistically significant	19	23%
Statistically significant	15	18%
Mixed	11	14%
Statistical significance not reported	12	15%
Statistical significance not relevant	24	30%
Research Findings: Correlational Studies ($n = 16$)		
Not statistically significant	4	25%
Statistically significant	7	44%
Mixed	2	12%
Statistical significance not reported	3	19%
Research Findings: Experimental Studies ($n = 25$)		
Not statistically significant	12	48%
Statistically significant	5	20%
Mixed	3	12%
Statistical significance not reported	5	20%

ance) were relevant, and 50 percent ($n = 31$) did not specify the type(s) of stressors (intrapersonal, interpersonal, extrapersonal) considered. Almost three-quarters of the studies (74 percent, $n = 46$) were designed to examine only the perceptions of the study participant, despite the Neuman Systems Model emphasis on both client system (study participant) and caregiver (researcher) perceptions.

The scientific merit of the studies varied. The stated purpose of the study was sufficient for understanding in the vast majority (94 percent, $n = 58$) of the 62 reports, as was the explanation of study procedures (89 percent, $n = 55$). The theoretical significance and/or the clinical significance of the study were explained in all but two (3 percent) of the reports. In addition, the data analysis procedures were appropriate for the research questions in most (89 percent, $n = 55$) studies. However, slightly more than two-fifths (42 percent, $n = 26$) of the studies that employed inferential statistical procedures did not explicitly state the hypotheses that were tested.

Sample size ranged from 1 to 864 participants. In general, the size of the sample was adequate for the study purpose and the research design, but very few investigators (8 percent, $n = 5$) mentioned any justification for the number of participants, either in the narrative or as a power analysis. The modal study participant was an individual (in 82 percent [$n = 51$] of the 62 studies) adult (21 percent, $n = 13$) client system with a clinical condition that required surgery (31 percent, $n = 19$). Nurses were the study participants in almost one-fifth (19 percent, $n = 12$) of the 62 studies. Data were collected most frequently in inpatient facilities (31 percent [$n = 19$] of the studies) or the community (13 percent, $n = 8$).

Many reports did not include psychometric data for the instruments used (Table 8-2). Moreover, just one-fifth (19 percent, $n = 12$) of the reports included information regarding the appropriateness of the instruments for the population from which the sample was drawn, and even fewer (16 percent, $n = 10$) included reliability data for the particular study sample.

Doctoral Dissertations. The first known Neuman Systems Model–based doctoral dissertations were published in *Dissertation Abstracts International* in 1982 (Dunbar, 1982; Ziemer, 1982). Neuman Systems Model–based dissertations have been conducted by students enrolled in the doctoral programs at 17 different universities (Table 8-5); the majority were conducted by doctoral students at the University of Alabama at Birmingham (56 percent, $n = 31$).

As can be seen in Table 8-3, three-quarters (75 percent, $n = 41$) of the 55 dissertations focused on clinical topics, and more than one-quarter (29 percent, $n = 16$) were designed as experiments. Almost one-quarter (24 percent, $n = 24$) of the studies investigated the effects of Neuman Systems Model prevention interventions. Further analysis revealed that 12 (50 percent) of those 24 studies focused solely on primary prevention interventions, and one (4 percent), on tertiary prevention interventions; no studies focused solely on secondary prevention interventions. Five (21 percent) of the 24 studies focused on some combination of primary, secondary, and tertiary prevention interventions. One (4 percent) of the 24 reports did not specify the type of prevention intervention(s) studied.

The vast majority (80 percent, $n = 44$) of the reports included an overview of the Neuman Systems Model that was sufficient for understanding the linkage between the model and the study purposes. However, only two-thirds (65 percent, $n = 36$) of the re-

TABLE 8-5. Colleges and Universities at Which Neuman Systems Model–Based Doctoral Dissertations and Master's Theses Were Conducted

College or University	n	%*
Doctoral Dissertations (n = 55)		
University of Alabama at Birmingham	31	56%
University of Pennsylvania	4	7%
Catholic University	2	4%
University of California, Los Angeles	2	4%
University of Pittsburgh	2	4%
University of South Carolina	2	4%
University of Texas at Austin	2	4%
Case Western Reserve University	1	2%
Clark University	1	2%
Oregon Health Sciences University	1	2%
University of Georgia at Athens	1	2%
University of Massachusetts at Amherst	1	2%
University of Miami	1	2%
University of Michigan	1	2%
University of Utah	1	2%
Wayne State University	1	2%
Widener University	1	2%
Master's Theses (n = 81)		
D'Youville College	34	42%
University of Nevada, Las Vegas	10	12%
Medical College of Ohio at Toledo	8	10%
Grand Valley State University	6	7%
California State University, Dominguez Hills	5	6%
Madonna University	2	3%
University of Alaska Anchorage	2	3%
University of Mississippi Medical Center	2	3%
California State University, Fresno	1	1%
San Diego State University	1	1%
San Jose State University	1	1%
Southern Connecticut State University	1	1%
Texas Woman's University, Denton	1	1%
Uniformed Services University of the Health Sciences	1	1%
University of Alabama in Huntsville	1	1%
University of Louisville	1	1%
University of Lowell	1	1%
University of Manitoba (Canada)	1	1%
University of New Mexico	1	1%
University of Northern Colorado	1	1%

Totals may not equal 100% due to rounding.

ports included explicit linkages between particular Neuman Systems Model concepts and all study variables. Moreover, just one-third (36 percent, $n = 20$) of the reports included explicit linkages between Neuman Systems Model relational propositions and at least some of the propositions about the study variables.

Conclusions regarding the utility of the Neuman Systems Model for the study conducted or the implications of the study findings for the credibility of the Neuman Systems Model were evident in 50 (91 percent) of the 55 dissertations. The issue of credibility is particularly critical in that more than three-quarters (77 percent, $n = 17$) of the 22 correlational studies and more than four-fifths (81 percent, $n = 13$) of the 16 experimental studies yielded a combination of statistically significant and nonsignificant results.

Few dissertations included specification of the particular Neuman Systems Model phenomena studied. Indeed, further analysis of the 55 dissertations revealed that 85 percent ($n = 47$) of the dissertations were not explicit with regard to the type of environment (internal, external, created) considered, 82 percent ($n = 45$) did not specify whether the central core was of interest, and 62 percent ($n = 34$) did not explicate the type of variables (physiological, psychological, sociocultural, developmental, spiritual) studied. Furthermore, 64 percent ($n = 35$) of the 55 dissertations did not indicate which lines (flexible and normal lines of defense, lines of resistance) were relevant, and 42 percent ($n = 23$) did not specify the type(s) of stressors (intrapersonal, interpersonal, extrapersonal) considered. Almost three-quarters of the studies (73 percent, $n = 40$) were designed to examine only the perceptions of the study participant, despite the Neuman Systems Model emphasis on both client system (study participant) and caregiver (researcher) perceptions.

The scientific merit of the dissertations was adequate but not outstanding. The stated purpose of the study was sufficient for understanding in almost all (98 percent, $n = 54$) 55 dissertations, as was the explanation of study procedures (96 percent, $n = 53$). The theoretical significance and the clinical significance of the study were explained 48 (87 percent) dissertations; only theoretical significance was explained in another six (11 percent) dissertations, and only clinical significance was explained in the remaining one (2 percent) dissertation. In addition, the data analysis procedures were appropriate for the research questions in the vast majority (98 percent, $n = 54$) of the dissertations. However, almost one-fifth (18 percent, $n = 10$) of the studies that employed inferential statistical procedures did not explicitly state the hypotheses that were tested.

Sample size ranged from 1 to 9,068 participants; the study with the largest number of participants was a secondary analysis of existing data. In general, the size of the sample was adequate for the study purpose and the research design, but less than one-half (44 percent, $n = 24$) of the dissertations included any justification for the number of participants, either in the narrative or as a power analysis. The modal study participant was an individual (in 85 percent [$n = 47$] of the 55 dissertation studies) adult (31 percent, $n = 17$) client system experiencing childbirth (20 percent, $n = 11$). Nurses were the study participants in just three (5 percent) of the 55 dissertations. Data were collected primarily in inpatient facilities (22 percent [$n = 12$] of the studies) or the community (14 percent, $n = 8$).

Additional analysis revealed that several dissertations did not include psychometric data for the instruments used (Table 8-3). Furthermore, just one-half (49 percent, $n = 27$) of the reports included information regarding the appropriateness of the instruments for the population from which the sample was drawn, and only slightly more than two-fifths (44 percent, $n = 24$) included reliability data for the particular study sample.

Abstracts of Master's Theses. The first known Neuman Systems Model–based master's thesis was published in *Master's Abstracts International* in 1985 (Briggs, 1985). These master's theses were conducted by students enrolled in master's programs at 20 different colleges or universities; more than two-fifths (42 percent) were conducted by students at D'Youville College (Table 8-5).

As can be seen in Table 8-4, more than three-quarters (77 percent, $n = 62$) of the 81 master's theses focused on clinical topics, and almost two-thirds (31 percent, $n = 25$) were designed as experiments. Additional analyses revealed that the modal study participant was an individual (in 93 percent [$n = 75$] of the 81 studies) who was a registered nurse (22 percent, $n = 18$). The setting for data collection could not be determined from the content of the thesis abstracts.

The thesis abstracts contained insufficient information to determine the specific Neuman Systems Model phenomena studied or the linkages between Neuman Systems Model concepts and propositions and the study variables. Conclusions regarding the utility of the Neuman Systems Model for the study conducted or the implications of the study findings for the credibility of the Neuman Systems Model were evident in just one-tenth (9 percent, $n = 7$) of the thesis abstracts. The issue of credibility is particularly critical in that one-quarter (25 percent, $n = 4$) of the 16 correlational studies and almost one-half (48 percent, $n = 12$) of the 25 experimental studies yielded results that were not statistically significant. Furthermore, another one-eighth (12 percent, $n = 2$) of the 16 correlational studies and one-eighth (12 percent, $n = 3$) of the 25 experimental studies yielded a combination of statistically significant and nonsignificant results.

The scientific merit of the master's theses could not be determined from the content of the abstracts. The stated purpose of the study was sufficient for understanding in 80 (96 percent) of the 81 thesis abstracts. However, insufficient information was given to determine the adequacy of the explanation of theoretical and clinical significance or the study procedures. Similarly, the appropriateness of the data analysis procedures could not be determined. Sample size ranged from 1 to 549 participants; samples were generally adequate for the study purpose and the research design.

Abstracts Published in Journals. One of the two abstracts published in journals was an instrument development study; the other was a correlational study. Both focused on clinical topics. The content of the instrument development abstract implied that the study focused on Neuman Systems Model prevention interventions; the other study focused on client system coping. The participants in the instrument development study were registered nurses ($N = 144$); the participants in the other study were family caregivers ($N = 122$) of individuals with the medical diagnosis of hepatoma. Given the limitations of abstracts, it was not possible to determine the adequacy of the sample sizes, although the sample for the instrument development study may have been too small for adequate psychometric testing of a new instrument. The instrument development study abstract did, however, include sufficient information to determine that the validity and reliability of the new instrument are adequate. No information about instruments was given in the other abstract. Furthermore, neither abstract included any information about specific linkages between the Neuman Systems Model concepts and propositions and the study variables or any conclusions regarding the credibility of the Neuman Systems Model.

Interpretation.   The finding that just one-half of the journal articles and book chapters and not quite two-thirds of the doctoral dissertations included a linkage between Neuman Systems Model concepts and all study variables and that very few reports included any linkage between Neuman Systems Model relational propositions and propositions about study variables indicates that researchers do not pay sufficient attention to the conceptual aspect of their studies. Researchers must explicate the linkages between the Neuman Systems Model concepts and propositions and their study variables in a clear and concise manner. More specifically, it is *not* sufficient only to mention that the Neuman Systems Model guided the study. Rather, the Neuman Systems Model concepts and propositions selected to guide the study must be identified and explicitly linked to the study variables and hypotheses. Faculty supervising doctoral dissertations and master's theses, journal and book editors, and peer reviewers all are strongly encouraged to require an explicit statement of such linkages as a condition of acceptance of the manuscript. Furthermore, educators are strongly encouraged to include strategies for explicating the linkages in all nursing research courses. See, for example, Fawcett's (1999) template for writing conceptual model–based research proposals and reports, along with Fawcett and Gigliotti's (in press) discussion of how a conceptual model can be used to guide nursing research. The five steps identified by Fawcett and Gigliotti facilitate researchers' understanding of how to clearly and explicitly integrate a conceptual model into research proposals and final reports of the research. Those five steps are listed in Table 8-6.

The Neuman Systems Model emphasis on assessment of perceptions of both the client system and the caregiver (see Appendix C, Table C-1) requires much greater atten-

TABLE 8-6. Using the Neuman Systems Model to Guide Research

Step 1. Develop a comprehensive understanding of the substantive content and research rules of the Neuman Systems Model [see Chapters 1 and 7].

Step 2. Review existing research guided by the Neuman Systems Model.

Step 3. Construct a conceptual–theoretical–empirical structure.

- Select middle-range theory concepts that are in keeping with the content of the Neuman Systems Model.
- Select research methods that clearly reflect the content of the Neuman Systems Model.

Step 4. Clearly communicate the conceptual–theoretical–empirical structure in written proposals and reports of study findings.

- Identify the Neuman Systems Model as the underlying guide for the study.
- Discuss the Neuman Systems Model in sufficient breadth and depth so that the relation of the model to the middle-range theory and the empirical research methods is clear.
- Clearly state the linkages between the relevant Neuman Systems Model concepts and the middle-range theory concepts.
- Clearly state the linkages between the relevant Neuman Systems Model concepts and propositions and the study aims and/or hypotheses.
- Present a diagram of the conceptual–theoretical–empirical structure for the study.

Step 5. Conclude the report of research findings with an evaluation of the empirical adequacy of the middle-range theory that was generated or tested and the credibility of the Neuman Systems Model.

Adapted from Fawcett, J., & Gigliotti, E. (in press). Using conceptual models of nursing to guide nursing research: The case of the Neuman Systems Model. Nursing Science Quarterly, with permission.

tion in Neuman Systems Model–based studies. Researchers could, for example, collect and compare data from the client systems of interest and their nurses or other health care providers. Or researchers could collect data from study participants and could themselves complete the same instruments rating their perceptions of the study participants' situation, and then examine similarities and differences in their respective perceptions, as is done in Neuman Systems Model–based clinical practice.

The analyses also indicate that researchers need to state a hypothesis for each inferential statistical test that is performed. This recommendation recognizes the importance of using the appropriate statistical language, in order to better inform the reader of the researcher's theoretical ideas or conjectures.

Whether the lack of attention to sample size justification revealed by the analyses is a flaw in methodology, a commission of reporting, or an omission due to page limitations in the case of journal articles and book chapters cannot be determined with any certainty. However, the finding that just 8 percent of the journal articles and book chapters included justification of sample size suggests that page limitations may have influenced the inclusion of this information. However, given that sample size justification requires only one or two sentences (see Fawcett, 1999, pp. 165, 168), it is more likely that the exclusion of the information was a commission of reporting. It is recommended that editors and peer reviewers require researchers to include this widely known and important aspect of scientific merit in their reports. More puzzling is the finding that just 44 percent of the doctoral dissertations included sample size justification. Given that a page limitation rarely is imposed on dissertations, the finding suggests that faculty do not require students to include this very important information. It is recommended that faculty impose more rigorous standards of reporting for dissertations. From a more proactive point of view, it is recommended that doctoral students and other researchers accept the responsibility of including sample size justification in their study reports.

The lack of attention to inclusion of psychometric data is particularly troublesome. There is no justifiable reason for the exclusion of validity and reliability data for each instrument in any report of research, especially because such data can be reported in two or three sentences (see Fawcett, 1999, pp. 170–71). It is recommended that all researchers accept the responsibility of including psychometric data in their study reports. If a proactive approach is not successful, then it is recommended that faculty, editors, and peer reviewers require researchers to include these well-known and critical aspects of scientific merit in their reports.

Overall, there was no evidence of sustained programs of nursing research. Rather, the reports reflect primarily "one-shot" studies, many of which were conducted by a single investigator, rather than a team of researchers. Although each study certainly contributes to the advancement of nursing science in general and the Neuman Systems Model in particular, programs of targeted research have the potential to contribute even more. Researchers should, therefore, begin to think about the place of each of their studies within ongoing programs of research. (A prototype program of research is described in Chapter 10.)

Furthermore, teams of researchers with complementary research skills usually are better able than researchers working alone to address the sophisticated research methods required to study the interrelations between all of the phenomena encompassed by the Neuman Systems Model. Researchers are encouraged to build research teams by collaborating with colleagues and seeking continuing consultation with experts for the conceptual, theoretical, and methodological aspects of their research programs.

Researchers also are encouraged to conduct Neuman Systems Model–based "cluster studies," that is, a series of studies conducted simultaneously by two or more researchers who share the same sample and data collection procedures but examine different variables. One researcher could, for example, study the effects of a particular extrapersonal stressor on the physiological client system variable, whereas another researcher could study the effects of the same extrapersonal stressor on the developmental client system variable. Still other researchers could study the effects of that extrapersonal stressor on the psychological, sociocultural, and spiritual client system variables. All of the researchers could use the same sample of, for example, school-aged children, and collaborate on recruitment of study participants and collection of data.

Meta-analysis is a powerful methodology that permits integration of results across a series of related studies (Rosenthal, 1991). Unfortunately, the lack of programmatic Neuman Systems Model–based research precluded meta-analysis of the studies reviewed, which, in turn, precluded conclusions regarding the overall credibility of the Neuman Systems Model and its utility for various areas of nursing research.

Noteworthy is the lack of attention to conclusions regarding the credibility and utility of the Neuman Systems Model in the journal articles and book chapters. Indeed, almost two-thirds (61 percent) of those reports did not include a statement of conclusions regarding the utility or credibility of the model, in contrast to the vast majority (91 percent) of doctoral dissertations, which did include such conclusions. Given the word limitation for abstracts, it is not surprising that such conclusions were evident in just 9 percent of the master's thesis abstracts. However, the finding that some abstracts did include conclusions regarding model credibility and utility indicates that it is possible to make such statements in an abstract. Researchers are, therefore, encouraged to write concise, yet comprehensive abstracts that include all essential information about the conceptual and methodological aspects of studies.

The review findings indicate that academic courses, continuing education workshops, and formal mentoring programs definitely are needed to help researchers to better explicate the linkages between the Neuman Systems Model and their studies and to design programs of targeted Neuman Systems Model–based research, so to ultimately identify and understand factors that contribute to the effectiveness of prevention interventions. In addition, researchers are encouraged to submit manuscripts based on their master's thesis or doctoral dissertation to widely circulated, peer-reviewed journals.

Establishment of networks of researchers and research teams who are interested in filling in gaps and extending knowledge of Neuman Systems Model phenomena can be facilitated by public presentations of the results of Neuman Systems Model studies at conferences, especially the biennial Neuman Systems Model symposia. Network establishment also can be facilitated by the organizational capabilities of the Neuman Systems Model Trustees Group, the society devoted to the continued evolution of the Neuman Systems Model through Neuman Systems Model–based research and practice (see Appendix D), as well as by the creation of an Institute for the Study of the Neuman Systems Model (Smith & Edgil, 1995). In addition, retrieval of publications for reviews of Neuman Systems Model–based research would be greatly facilitated if researchers would forward copies of their research reports to the Neuman Systems Model Archives at Neumann College in Aston, Pennsylvania.

Stage 5: Public Presentation

Public presentation of the integrative review project has been addressed by one presentation and two publications. A paper was presented in April 1999 at the Seventh Biennial International Neuman Systems Model Symposium in Vancouver, Canada. The publications include the present chapter and an article in a peer-reviewed nursing journal (Fawcett & Giangrande, in press).

CONCLUSION

The integrative review presented in this chapter was limited to literature published through 1997. The review should be extended to include all research reports published since that time. Furthermore, funding should be sought for integrative reviews. Funds are especially needed for the purchase of doctoral dissertations and master's theses from University Microfilms, as well as for photocopying of journal articles and book chapters.

ENDNOTES

1. This project was partially funded by Xi Chapter of Sigma Theta Tau International, University of Pennsylvania School of Nursing.
2. A portion of this chapter was previously published in *Nursing Science Quarterly* and is used with permission from Sage Publications, Inc.
3. The assistance of Lois Lowry with initial testing of the code book is gratefully acknowledged.

REFERENCES

Briggs, L. L. (1985). Nursing diagnoses generated from assessment data in a medical or nursing database. *Master's Abstracts International, 23,* 470.

Cooper, H. M. (1989). *Integrating research: A guide for literature reviews* (2nd ed.). Newbury Park, CA: Sage.

Devine, E. C., & Cook, T. D. (1983). A meta-analytic analysis of effects of psychoeducational interventions on length of postsurgical hospital stay. *Nursing Research, 32,* 267–74.

Dunbar, S. B. (1982). The effect of formal patient education on selected psychological and physiological variables of adaptation after acute myocardial infarction. *Dissertation Abstracts International, 43,* 1794B.

Fawcett, J. (1999). *Relationship of theory and research* (3rd ed.). Philadelphia: Davis.

Fawcett, J., & Giangrande, S. K. (2001). Neuman Systems Model–based research: An integrative review project. *Nursing Science Quarterly, 14.*

Fawcett, J., & Gigliotti, E. (in press). Using conceptual models of nursing to guide nursing research: The case of the Neuman Systems Model. *Nursing Science Quarterly.*

Gigliotti, E. (2001). Empirical tests of the Neuman systems model: Relational statement analysis. *Nursing Science Quarterly, 14.*

Heater, B. S., Becker, A. M., & Olson, R. K. (1988). Nursing interventions and patient outcomes: A meta-analysis of studies. *Nursing Research, 37,* 303–307.

Louis, M. (1995). The Neuman model in nursing research: An update. In B. Neuman (Ed.), *The
Neuman Systems Model* (3rd ed., pp. 473–95). Norwalk, CT: Appleton & Lange.

Louis, M., & Koertvelyessy, A. (1989). The Neuman model in research. In B. Neuman (Ed.),
The Neuman Systems Model (2nd ed., pp. 93–114). Norwalk, CT: Appleton & Lange.

Neuman, B. (1982). *The Neuman Systems Model: Application to nursing education and practice.* Norwalk, CT: Appleton & Lange.

Neuman, B. (1989). *The Neuman Systems Model* (2nd ed.). Norwalk, CT: Appleton & Lange.

Neuman, B. (1995). *The Neuman Systems Model* (3rd ed.). Norwalk, CT: Appleton & Lange.

Rosenthal, R. (1979). The "file drawer problem" and tolerance for null results. *Psychological
Bulletin, 86,* 638–41.

Rosenthal, R. (1991). *Meta-analytic procedures for social research* (rev. ed.). Newbury Park,
CA: Sage.

Smith, M. C., & Edgil, A. E. (1995). Future directions for research with the Neuman Systems
Model. In B. Neuman (Ed.), *The Neuman Systems Model* (3rd ed., pp. 509–17). Norwalk,
CT: Appleton & Lange.

Smith, M. L., & Glass, G. V. (1977). Meta-analysis of psychotherapy outcome studies. *American Psychologist, 32,* 752–60.

Wampler, K. S. (1982). Bringing the review of literature into the age of quantification: Meta-
analysis as a strategy for integrating research findings in family studies. *Journal of Marriage
and the Family, 44,* 1009–23.

Ziemer, M. M. (1982). Providing patients with information prior to surgery and the reported
frequency of coping behaviors and development of symptoms following surgery. *Dissertation Abstracts International, 43,* 2165B.

Ziemer, M. M. (1983). Effects of information on postsurgical coping. *Nursing Research, 32,*
282–87.

BIBLIOGRAPHY

List of Research Reports Reviewed (*N* = 200)
Journal Articles (*n* = 59)

Ali, N. S., & Khalil, H. Z. (1989). Effect of psychoeducational intervention on anxiety among
Egyptian bladder cancer patients. *Cancer Nursing, 12,* 236–42.

*Andersen, J. E., & Briggs, L. L. (1988). Nursing diagnosis: A study of quality and supportive
evidence. *Image: Journal of Nursing Scholarship, 20,* 141–44.

Bass, L. S. (1991). What do parents need when their infant is a patient in the NICU? *Neonatal
Network, 10*(4), 25–33.

Beynon, C., & Laschinger, H. K. (1993). Theory-based practice: Attitudes of nursing managers
before and after educational sessions. *Public Health Nursing, 10,* 183–88.

Blank, J. J., Clark, L., Longman, A. J., & Atwood, J. R. (1989). Perceived home care needs of
cancer patients and their caregivers. *Cancer Nursing, 12,* 78–84.

Bowdler, J. E., & Barrell, L. M. (1987). Health needs of homeless persons. *Public Health Nursing, 4,* 135–40.

Bowman, A. M. (1997). Sleep satisfaction, perceived pain and acute confusion in elderly
clients undergoing orthopaedic procedures. *Journal of Advanced Nursing, 26,* 550–64.

Breckenridge, D. M. (1997). Decisions regarding dialysis treatment modality: A holistic perspective. *Holistic Nursing Practice, 12*(1), 54–61.

Breckenridge, D. M. (1997). Patients' perceptions of why, how, and by whom dialysis treatment modality was chosen. *Association of Nephrology Nurses Journal, 24,* 313–21.

Brown, K. C., Sirles, A. T., Hilyer, J. C., & Thomas, M. J. (1992). Cost-effectiveness of a back school intervention for municipal employees. *Spine, 17,* 1224–28.

Bueno, M. N., Redeker, N., & Norman, E. M. (1992). Analysis of motor vehicle crash data in an urban trauma center: Implications for nursing practice and research. *Heart and Lung, 21,* 558–67.

Cantin, B., & Mitchell, M. (1989). Nurses' smoking behavior. *The Canadian Nurse, 85*(1), 20–21.

Carroll, T. L. (1989). Role deprivation in baccalaureate nursing students pre and post curriculum revision. *Journal of Nursing Education, 28,* 134–39.

*Cava, M. A. (1992). An examination of coping strategies used by long-term cancer survivors. *Canadian Oncology Nursing Journal, 2,* 99–102.

Clark, C. C., Cross, J. R., Deane, D. M., & Lowry, L. W. (1991). Spirituality: Integral to quality care. *Holistic Nursing Practice, 5,* 67–76.

Collins, M. A. (1996). The relation of work stress, hardiness, and burnout among full-time hospital staff nurses. *Journal of Nursing Staff Development, 12,* 81–85.

Courchene, V. S., Patalski, E., & Martin, J. (1991). A study of the health of pediatric nurses administering Cyclosporin A. *Pediatric Nursing, 17,* 497–500.

Decker, S. D., & Young, E. (1991). Self-perceived needs of primary caregivers of home-hospice clients. *Journal of Community Health Nursing, 8,* 147–54.

*Fields, W. L., & Loveridge, C. (1988). Critical thinking and fatigue: How do nurses on 8- & 12-hour shifts compare? *Nursing Economic$, 6,* 189–91.

Flannery, J. (1995). Cognitive assessment in the acute care setting: Reliability and validity of the Levels of Cognitive Functioning Assessment Scale (LOCFAS). *Journal of Nursing Measurement, 3,* 43–58.

Fowler, B. A., & Risner, P. B. (1994). A health promotion program evaluation in a minority industry. *Association of Black Nursing Faculty Journal, 5*(3), 72–76.

Freiberger, D., Bryant, J., & Marino, B. (1992). The effects of different central venous line dressing changes on bacterial growth in a pediatric oncology population. *Journal of Pediatric Oncology Nursing, 9,* 3–7.

Gavigan, M., Kline-O'Sullivan, C., & Klumpp-Lybrand, B. (1990). The effect of regular turning on CABG patients. *Critical Care Nursing Quarterly, 12*(4), 69–76.

Gellner, P., Landers, S., O'Rourke, D., & Schlegel, M. (1994). Community health nursing in the 1990s: Risky business? *Holistic Nursing Practice, 8*(2), 15–21.

George, J. (1997). Nurses' perceived autonomy in a shared governance setting. *Journal of Shared Governance, 3*(2), 17–21.

Gifford, D. K. (1996). Monthly incidence of stroke in rural Kansas. *Kansas Nurse, 71*(5), 3–4.

Grant, J. S., & Bean, C. A. (1992). Self-identified needs of informal caregivers of head-injured adults. *Family and Community Health, 15*(2), 49–58.

Gries, M., & Fernsler, J. (1988). Patient perceptions of the mechanical ventilation experience. *Focus on Critical Care, 15,* 52–59.

Hainsworth, D. S. (1996). The effect of death education on attitudes of hospital nurses toward care of the dying. *Oncology Nursing Forum, 23,* 963–67.

Heffline, M. S. (1991). A comparative study of pharmacological versus nursing interventions in the treatment of postanesthesia shivering. *Journal of Post Anesthesia Nursing, 6,* 311–20.

Hinds, C. (1990). Personal and contextual factors predicting patients' reported quality of life: Exploring congruency with Betty Neuman's assumptions. *Journal of Advanced Nursing, 15,* 456–62.

**Hoch, C. C. [nee Schmidt]. (1987). Assessing delivery of nursing care. *Journal of Gerontological Nursing, 13*(1), 10–17.

Johnson, P. (1983). Black hypertension: A transcultural case study using the Betty Neuman model of nursing care. *Issues in Health Care of Women, 4,* 191–210.

Jones, W. R. (1996). Stressors in the primary caregivers of traumatic head injured persons. *AXON, 18,* 9–11.

Kahn, E. C. (1992). A comparison of family needs based on the presence or absence of DNR orders. *Dimensions of Critical Care Nursing, 11,* 286–92.

Koku, R. V. (1992). Severity of low back pain: A comparison between participants who did and did not receive counseling. *American Association of Occupational Health Nurses Journal, 40,* 84–89.

Leja, A. M. (1989). Using guided imagery to combat postsurgical depression. *Journal of Gerontological Nursing, 15*(4), 6–11.

Loescher, L. J., Clark, L., Atwood, J. R., Leigh, S., & Lamb, G. (1990). The impact of the cancer experience on long-term survivors. *Oncology Nursing Forum, 17,* 223–29.

Lowry, L. W., & Anderson, B. (1993). Neuman's framework and ventilator dependency: A pilot study. *Nursing Science Quarterly, 6,* 195–200.

Lowry, L. W., Saeger, J., & Barnett, S. (1997). Client satisfaction with prenatal care and pregnancy outcomes. *Outcomes Management for Nursing Practice, 1*(1), 29–35.

Mackenzie, S. J., & Laschinger, H. K. S. (1995). Correlates of nursing diagnosis quality in public health nursing. *Journal of Advanced Nursing, 21,* 800–808.

*Maligalig, R. M. L. (1994). Parents' perceptions of the stressors of pediatric ambulatory surgery. *Journal of Post Anesthesia Nursing, 9,* 278–82.

*Mannina, J. (1997). Finding an effective hearing testing protocol to identify hearing loss and middle ear disease in school-aged children. *Journal of School Nursing, 13*(5), 23–28.

Montgomery, P., & Craig, D. (1990). Levels of stress and health practices of wives of alcoholics. *Canadian Journal of Nursing Research, 22*(2), 60–70.

**Moody, N. B. (1996). Nurse faculty job satisfaction: A national survey. *Journal of Professional Nursing, 12,* 277–88.

Nortridge, J. A., Mayeux, V., Anderson, S. J., & Bell, M. L. (1992). The use of cognitive style mapping as a predictor for academic success of first semester diploma nursing students. *Journal of Nursing Education, 31,* 352–56.

Nuttall, P., & Flores, F. C. (1997). Hmong healing practices used for common childhood illnesses. *Pediatric Nursing, 23,* 247–51.

Radwanski, M. (1992). Self-medicating practices for managing chronic pain after spinal cord injury. *Rehabilitation Nursing, 17,* 312–18.

Rodrigues-Fisher, L., Bourguignon, C., & Good, B. V. (1993). Dietary fiber nursing intervention: Prevention of constipation in older adults. *Clinical Nursing Research, 2,* 464–77.

Roggensack, J. (1994). The influence of perioperative theory and clinical in a baccalaureate nursing program on the decision to practice perioperative nursing. *Prairie Rose, 63*(2), 6–7.

*Semple, O. D. (1995). The experiences of family members of persons with Huntington's disease. *Perspectives, 19*(4), 4–10.

Sirles, A. T., Brown, K., & Hilyer, J. C. (1991). Effects of back school education and exercise in back injured municipal workers. *American Association of Occupational Health Nursing Journal, 39,* 7–12.

Skipwith, D. H. (1994). Telephone counseling interventions with caregivers of elders. *Journal of Psychosocial Nursing and Mental Health Services, 32*(3), 7–12, 34–35.

Speck, B. J. (1990). The effect of guided imagery upon first semester nursing students performing their first injections. *Journal of Nursing Education, 29,* 346–50.

Vaughn, M., Cheatwood, S., Sirles, A. T., & Brown, K. C. (1989). The effect of progressive muscle relaxation on stress among clerical workers. *American Association of Occupational Health Nurses Journal, 37,* 302–306.

Waddell, K. L., & Demi, A. S. (1993). Effectiveness of an intensive partial hospitalization program for treatment of anxiety disorders. *Archives of Psychiatric Nursing, 7,* 2–10.

**Williamson, J. W. (1992). The effects of ocean sounds on sleep after coronary artery bypass graft surgery. *American Journal of Critical Care, 1,* 91–97.

Wilson, V. S. (1987). Identification of stressors related to patients' psychological responses to the surgical intensive care unit. *Heart and Lung, 16,* 267–73.

**Ziemer, M. M. (1983). Effects of information on postsurgical coping. *Nursing Research, 32,* 282–87.

* From a master's thesis
** From a doctoral dissertation

Book Chapters (*n* = 3)

Louis, M. (1989). An intervention to reduce anxiety levels for nurses working with long-term care clients using Neuman's model. In J. P. Riehl-Sisca (Ed.), *Conceptual models for nursing practice* (3rd ed., pp. 95–103). Norwalk, CT: Appleton & Lange.

Lowry, L. W., & Jopp, M. C. (1989). An evaluation instrument for assessing an associate degree nursing curriculum based on the Neuman Systems Model. In J. P. Riehl-Sisca (Ed.), *Conceptual models for nursing practice* (3rd ed., pp. 73–85). Norwalk, CT: Appleton & Lange.

Purushotham, D., & Walker, G. (1994). The Neuman Systems Model: A conceptual framework for clinical teaching/learning process. In R. M. Carroll-Johnson & M. Paquette (Eds.), *Classification of nursing diagnoses: Proceedings of the tenth conference* (pp. 271–73). Philadelphia: Lippincott.

Doctoral Dissertations (*n* = 55)

Al-Nagshabandi, E. A. H. (1994). An exploration of the physical and psychological responses of surgically-induced menopausal Saudi women using the Neuman Systems Model. *Dissertation Abstracts International, 55,* 1374B.

Barnes-McDowell, B. M. (1997). Home apnea monitoring: Family functioning, concerns, and coping. *Dissertation Abstracts International, 58,* 1205B.

Bemker, M. A. (1997). Adolescent female substance abuse: Risk and resiliency factors. *Dissertation Abstracts International, 57,* 75446B.

Bittinger, J. P. (1996). Case management and satisfaction with nursing care of patients hospitalized with congestive heart failure. *Dissertation Abstracts International, 56,* 3866B.

Burritt, J. E. (1988). The effects of perceived social support on the relationship between job stress and job satisfaction and job performance among registered nurses employed in acute care facilities. *Dissertation Abstracts International, 49,* 2123B.

Cagle, R. (1997). The relationship between health care provider advice and the initiation of breast-feeding. *Dissertation Abstracts International, 57,* 4974B.

Cammuso, B. S. (1994). Caring and accountability in nursing practice in Ireland and the United States: Helping Irish nurses bridge the gap when they choose to practice in the United States. *Dissertation Abstracts International, 55,* 76B.

**Capers, C. F. (1987). Perceptions of problematic behavior as held by lay black adults and registered nurses. *Dissertation Abstracts International, 47,* 4467B.

Chilton, L. L. A. (1997). The influence of behavioral cues on immunization practices of elders. *Dissertation Abstracts International, 57,* 5572B.

Collins, A. S. (1992). Effects of positional changes on selected physiological and psychological measurements in clients with atrial fibrillation. *Dissertation Abstracts International, 53,* 200B.

Downing, B. H. (1995). Evaluation of a computer assisted intervention for musculoskeletal discomfort, strength, and flexibility and job satisfaction of video display operators. *Dissertation Abstracts International, 55,* 3237B.

Dunbar, S. B. (1982). The effect of formal patient education on selected psychological and physiological variables of adaptation after acute myocardial infarction. *Dissertation Abstracts International, 43,* 1794B.

**Flannery, J. C. (1988). Validity and reliability of Levels of Cognitive Functioning Assessment Scale for adults with closed head injuries. *Dissertation Abstracts International, 48,* 3248B.

Fulton, B. J. (1993). Evaluation of the effectiveness of the Neuman Systems Model as a theoretical framework for baccalaureate nursing programs. *Dissertation Abstracts International, 53,* 5641B.

**Gibson, D. E. (1989). A Q-analysis of interpersonal trust in the nurse-client relationship. *Dissertation Abstracts International, 50,* 493B.

Gibson, M. H. (1996). The quality of life of adult hemodialysis patients. *Dissertation Abstracts International, 56,* 5416B.

Glazer, G. L. (1985). The relationship between pregnant women's anxiety levels and stressors and their partners' anxiety levels and stressors. *Dissertation Abstracts International, 46,* 1869B.

Goble, D. S. (1991). A curriculum framework for the prevention of child sexual abuse. *Dissertation Abstracts International, 52,* 2004A.

**Hanson, M. J. S. (1996). Beliefs, attitudes, subjective norms, perceived behavioral control, and cigarette smoking in White, African-American, and Puerto Rican-American teenage women. *Dissertation Abstracts International, 56,* 4240B.

Harbin, P. D. O. (1990). A Q-analysis of the stressors of adult female nursing students enrolled in baccalaureate schools of nursing. *Dissertation Abstracts International, 50,* 3919B.

Hayes, K. V. D. (1995). Diagnostic content validation and operational definitions of risk factors for the nursing diagnosis high risk for disuse syndrome. *Dissertation Abstracts International, 55,* 5284B.

**Heaman, D. J. (1992). Perceived stressors and coping strategies of parents with developmentally disabled children. *Dissertation Abstracts International, 52,* 6316B.

Henze, R. L. (1994). The relationship among selected stress variables and white blood count in severely head injured patients. *Dissertation Abstracts International, 55,* 365B.

Herald, P. A. (1994). Relationship between hydration status and renal function in patients receiving aminoglycoside antibiotics. *Dissertation Abstracts International, 55,* 365B.

Lancaster, D. R. N. (1992). Coping with appraised threat of breast cancer: Primary prevention coping behaviors utilized by women at increased risk. *Dissertation Abstracts International, 53,* 202B.

Lee, P. L. (1996). Caregiver stress as experienced by wives of institutionalized and in-home dementia husbands. *Dissertation Abstracts International, 56,* 4241B.

McDaniel, G. M. S. (1990). The effects of two methods of dangling on heart rate and blood pressure in postoperative abdominal hysterectomy patients. *Dissertation Abstracts International, 50,* 3923B.

Mirenda, R. M. (1996). A conceptual-theoretical strategy for curriculum development in bac-calaureate nursing programs. *Dissertation Abstracts International, 56,* 5421B.

Monahan, G. L. (1997). A profile of pregnant drug-using female arrestees in California: The re-lationships among sociodemographic characteristics, reproductive and drug addiction histo-ries, HIV/STD risk behaviors, and utilization of prenatal care services and substance abuse treatment programs. *Dissertation Abstracts International, 57,* 5576B.

*Moody, N. B. (1991). Selected demographic variables, organizational characteristics, role orientation, and job satisfaction among nurse faculty. *Dissertation Abstracts International, 52,* 1356B.

Norman, S. E. (1991). The relationship between hardiness and sleep disturbances in HIV-infected men. *Dissertation Abstracts International, 51,* 4780B.

Norris, E. W. (1990). Physiologic response to exercise in clients with mitral valve prolapse syndrome. *Dissertation Abstracts International, 50,* 5549B.

Payne, P. L. (1994). A study of the teaching of primary prevention competencies as recom-mended by the report of the PEW Health Professions Commission in bachelor of science in nursing programs and associate in nursing programs. *Dissertation Abstracts International, 54,* 3553B.

Peoples, L. T. (1991). The relationship between selected client, provider, and agency variables and the utilization of home care services. *Dissertation Abstracts International, 51,* 3782B.

Poole, V. L. (1992). Pregnancy wantedness, attitude toward pregnancy, and use of alcohol, to-bacco, and street drugs during pregnancy. *Dissertation Abstracts International, 52,* 5193B.

Pothiban, L. (1993). Risk factor prevalence, risk status, and perceived risk for coronary heart disease among Thai elderly. *Dissertation Abstracts International, 54,* 1337B.

Quinn, A. T. (1992). A hospice death education course: evaluating effectiveness in meeting goals. *Dissertation Abstracts International, 53,* 728A.

Rowe, M. L. (1990). The relationship of commitment and social support to the life satisfaction of caregivers to patients with Alzheimer's disease. *Dissertation Abstracts International, 51,* 1747B.

Rowles, C. J. (1993). The relationship of selected personal and organizational variables and the tenure of directors of nursing in nursing homes. *Dissertation Abstracts International, 53,* 4593B.

Schlosser, S. P. (1985). The effect of anticipatory guidance on mood state in primiparas experi-encing unplanned cesarean delivery. *Dissertation Abstracts International, 46,* 2627B.

*Schmidt, C. S. (1983). A comparison of the effectiveness of two nursing models in decreasing depression and increasing life satisfaction of retired individuals. *Dissertation Abstracts Inter-national, 43,* 2856B.

Sipple, J. E. A. (1989). A model for curriculum change based on retrospective analysis. *Disser-tation Abstracts International, 50,* 1927A.

South, L. D. (1995). The relationship of self-concept and social support in school age children with leukemia. *Dissertation Abstracts International, 56,* 1939B.

Tarmina, M. S. (1992). Self-selected diet of adult women with families. *Dissertation Abstracts International, 53,* 777B.

Tennyson, M. G. (1992). Becoming pregnant: Perceptions of black adolescents. *Dissertation Abstracts International, 52,* 5196B.

Terhaar, M. F. (1989). The influence of physiologic stability, behavioral stability and family sta-bility on the preterm infant's length of stay in the neonatal intensive care unit. *Dissertation Abstracts International, 50,* 1328B.

Thornhill, B. E. (1986). A Q-analysis of stressors in the primipara during the immediate post-partal period. *Dissertation Abstracts International, 47,* 135B.

Underwood, P. W. (1986). Psychosocial variables: Their prediction of birth complications and relation to perception of childbirth. *Dissertation Abstracts International, 47,* 997B.

Vincent, J. L. M. (1988). A Q analysis of the stressors of fathers with an infant in an intensive care unit. *Dissertation Abstracts International, 49,* 3111B.

Watson, L. A. (1991). Comparison of the effects of usual, support, and informational nursing interventions on the extent to which families of critically ill patients perceived their needs were met. *Dissertation Abstracts International, 52,* 2999B.

Webb, C. A. (1988). A cross-sectional study of hope, physical status, cognitions and meaning and purpose of pre- and post-retirement adults. *Dissertation Abstracts International, 49,* 1922A.

**Whatley, J. H. (1989). Effects of health locus of control and social network on risk-taking in adolescents. *Dissertation Abstracts International, 50,* 129B.

*Williamson, J. W. (1990). The influence of self-selected monotonous sounds on the night sleep pattern of postoperative open heart surgery patients. *Dissertation Abstracts International, 51,* 1750B.

Yoder, R. E. (1995). Primary prevention emphasis and self-reported health behaviors of nursing students. *Dissertation Abstracts International, 56,* 747B.

*Ziemer, M. M. (1982). Providing patients with information prior to surgery and the reported frequency of coping behaviors and development of symptoms following surgery. *Dissertation Abstracts International, 43,* 2165B.

Also published as a journal article
**Also published as a journal article but Neuman Systems Model not cited*

Master's Theses (*n* = 81)

Alford, D. L. (1994). Differences in levels of anxiety of spouses of critical care surgical patients when the spouse participates in preoperative care. *Master's Abstracts International, 32,* 222.

Allen, K. S. (1997). The effect of cancer diagnosis information on the anxiety of patients with an initial diagnosis of first cancer. *Master's Abstracts International, 35,* 996.

Anderson, R. R. (1992). Indicators of nutritional status as a predictor of pressure ulcer development in the critically ill adult. *Master's Abstracts International, 30,* 92.

Averill, J. B. (1989). The impact of primary prevention as an intervention strategy. Masters Abstracts International, *27,* 89.

Baloush, N. A. (1991). Social support and maternal reaction in Saudi Arabian women with premature births from a Neuman framework. *Master's Abstracts International, 29,* 432.

Barnes, M. E. (1994). Knowledge, experiences, attitudes, and assessment practices of nurse practitioners with regard to stressors related to childhood sexual abuse. *Master's Abstracts International, 32,* 223.

Baskin-Nedzelski, J. (1992). Job stressors among visiting nurses. Masters Abstracts International, *30,* 79.

Baumle, W. M. (1993). A comparison study of the psychological pain response of persons on long-term intermittent intravenous antibiotic therapy. *Master's Abstracts International, 31,* 1199.

Besseghini, C. (1990). Stressful life events and angina in individuals undergoing exercise stress testing. *Master's Abstracts International, 28,* 569.

Bischoff, S. M. (1988). Job stress in nurses working in correctional settings. *Master's Abstracts International, 26,* 323.

Blount, K. R. (1989). The relationship between the parent's and five to six-year-old child's perception of life events as stressors within the Neuman health care systems framework. *Master's Abstracts International, 27,* 487.

Boyes, L. M. (1994). The effects of permanent night shift versus night shift rotation on job performance in the critical care area. *Master's Abstracts International, 32,* 1366.

*Briggs, L. L. (1985). Nursing diagnoses generated from assessment data in a medical or nursing data base. *Master's Abstracts International, 23,* 470.

Brown, F. A. (1995). The effects of an eight-hour affective education program on fear of AIDS and homophobia in student nurses. *Master's Abstracts International, 33,* 1487.

*Cava, M. A. (1991). A descriptive study of the use of coping strategies to promote wellness by individuals who have survived cancer. *Master's Abstracts International, 29,* 89.

Clevenger, M. D. (1995). Nursing activities and patient control. *Master's Abstracts International, 33,* 1835.

Cole, B. A. (1995). Patient compliance with tuberculosis preventive treatment. *Master's Abstracts International, 33,* 1835.

Columbus, L. A. (1991). Effectiveness of a health promotion program in improving older women's ability to cope. *Master's Abstracts International, 29,* 274.

Cotten, N. C. (1993). An interdisciplinary high risk assessment tool for rehabilitation inpatient falls. *Master's Abstracts International, 31,* 1732.

Cullen, L. M. (1994). Nurses' perceptions of humor as a preventive intervention to promote the health of clients in a health care setting. *Master's Abstracts International, 32,* 592.

Donner, P. L. (1994). Maternal anxiety related to the care of an infant requiring pharmacological management for apnea of prematurity. *Master's Abstracts International, 32,* 937.

Elgar, S. J. (1992). The influence of companion animals on perceived social support and perceived stress among family caregivers. *Master's Abstracts International, 30,* 732.

*Fields, W. L. (1988). The effects of the 12-hour shift on fatigue and critical thinking performance in critical care nurses. *Master's Abstracts International, 26,* 237.

Fillmore, J. A. (1993). The effects of preoperative teaching on anxiety levels of hysterectomy patients. *Master's Abstracts International, 31,* 761.

Finney, G. A. H. (1990). Spiritual needs of patients. *Master's Abstracts International, 28,* 272.

Fukuzawa, M. (1996). Nursing care behaviors which predict patient satisfaction. *Master's Abstracts International, 34,* 1547.

Gaeta, T. V. (1990). A study to determine client satisfaction with home care services. *Master's Abstracts International, 28,* 408.

Geiger, P. A. (1996). Participation in a phase II cardiac rehabilitation program and perceived quality of life. *Master's Abstracts International, 34,* 1548.

Goldstein, L. A. (1988). Needs of spouses of hospitalized cancer patients. *Master's Abstracts International, 26,* 105.

Good, B. A. V. (1993). Efficacy of nursing intervention as secondary prevention of chronic nonorganic constipation in older adult nursing home residents: A replication study. *Master's Abstracts International, 31,* 1736.

Greve, D. L. (1993). An examination of the efficacy of increased fiber and fluids on the establishment of voluntary bowel movements in terminally ill older adults receiving antibiotics. *Master's Abstracts International, 31,* 1203.

Gulliver, K. M. (1997). Hopelessness and spiritual well-being in persons with HIV infection. *Master's Abstracts International, 35,* 1374.

Harper, B. (1993). Nurses' beliefs about social support and the effect of nursing care on cardiac clients' attitudes in reducing cardiac risk status. *Master's Abstracts International, 31,* 273.

Haskill, K. M. (1988). Sources of occupational stress of the community health nurse. *Master's Abstracts International, 26,* 106.

Higgs, K. T. (1995). Preterm labor risk factors identified in an ambulatory perinatal setting with home uterine activity monitoring support. *Master's Abstracts International, 33,* 1490.

Holloway, C. (1995). Stress perceived among nurse managers in community health settings. *Master's Abstracts International, 33,* 1490.

Ivey, B. M. (1994). Social support and the woman with breast cancer: Issues of measurement. *Master's Abstracts International, 32,* 1628.

Johnson, K. M. (1996). Stressors of local Ontario Nurses' Association presidents. *Master's Abstracts International, 34,* 1149.

Kazakoff, K. J. (1991). The evaluation of return to work and retention of employment of cardiac patients following cardiac rehabilitation programs. *Master's Abstracts International, 29,* 450.

Kelleher, J. J. (1991). Health behaviors of HIV positive people. *Master's Abstracts International, 29,* 645.

Klimek, S. C. (1995). Identification and comparison of factors affecting breast self-examination between professional nurses and non-nursing professional women. *Master's Abstracts International, 33,* 516.

Larino, E. A. (1997). Determining the level of care provided by the family nurse practitioner during a deployment. *Master's Abstracts International, 35,* 1376.

Lenhart, E. M. (1994). The effect of preoperative intensive care orientation on postoperative anxiety levels in spouses of coronary artery bypass clients. *Master's Abstracts International, 32,* 1372.

Lesmond, J. S. G. (1993). Clients' perceptions of the effects of social support in their adjustment to breast cancer in a visiting nursing environment in central Ontario, Canada. *Master's Abstracts International, 31,* 276.

*Maligalig, R. M. L. (1994). Parents' perceptions of the stressors of pediatric ambulatory surgery. *Master's Abstracts International, 32,* 597.

Mann, N. J. (1996). Risk behavior of adolescents who have liver disease. *Master's Abstracts International, 34,* 1150.

*Mannina, J. M. (1995). The use of puretone audiometry and tympanometry to identify hearing loss and middle ear disease in school age children. *Master's Abstracts International, 33,* 1823.

Marini, S. L. (1991). A comparison of predictive validity of the Norton scale, the Daly scale, and the Braden scale. *Master's Abstracts International, 29,* 648.

McCue, M. M. (1991). The caregiving experience of the elderly female caregiver of a spouse impaired by stroke. *Master's Abstracts International, 29,* 218.

McMillan, D. E. (1997). Impact of therapeutic support of inherent coping strategies on chronic low back pain: A nursing intervention study. *Master's Abstracts International, 35,* 520.

Micevski, V. (1997). Gender differences in the presentation of physiological symptoms of myocardial infarction. *Master's Abstracts International, 35,* 520.

Miller, C. A. (1988). Effects of support on the level of anxiety for family members and/or significant others of emergency room patients. *Master's Abstracts International, 26,* 177.

Morris, D. C. (1991). Occupational stress among home care first line managers. *Master's Abstracts International, 29,* 443.

Morrison, L. A. (1993). Palliative care volunteers' descriptions of the stressors experienced in their relationship with clients coping with terminal illness at home. *Master's Abstracts International, 31,* 301.

Moynihan, B. A. (1995). A descriptive study of three male adolescent sex offenders. *Master's Abstracts International, 33,* 873.

Murphy, N. G. (1990). Factors associated with breastfeeding success and failure: A systematic integrative review. *Master's Abstracts International, 28,* 275.

Murray, M. M. (1994). Relationships among the frequency of pressure ulcer risk assessment, nursing, interventions, and the occurrence and severity of pressure ulcers. *Master's Abstracts International, 32,* 1630.

Newman, S. K. (1995). Perceived stressors between partnered and unpartnered women. *Master's Abstracts International, 33,* 178.

Nicholson, C. H. (1995). Client's perceptions of preparedness for discharge home following total hip or knee replacement surgery. *Master's Abstracts International, 33,* 873.

Occhi, A. M. (1993). Donation: The family's perspective. *Master's Abstracts International, 31,* 1208.

O'Neal, C. A. S. (1993). Effects of BSE on depression/anxiety in women diagnosed with breast cancer. *Master's Abstracts International, 31,* 1747.

Parker, V. J. (1995). Stress of discharge in men and women following cardiac surgery. *Master's Abstracts International, 33,* 518.

Peper, K. R. (1992). Concerns/problems experienced after discharge from an acute care setting: The patient's perspective. *Master's Abstracts International, 30,* 714.

Petock, A. M. (1991). Decubitus ulcers and physiological stressors. *Master's Abstracts International, 29,* 267.

Porritt See, J. A. S. (1994). The effects of a prenatal education program on the identification and reporting of the stressors of postpartum depression. *Master's Abstracts International, 32,* 1632.

Sabati, N. (1995). Relationship between Neuman's systems model's buffering property of the flexible line of defense and active participation in support groups for women. *Master's Abstracts International, 33,* 179.

St. John-Spadafore, M. J. (1994). The impact of a primary prevention program on women's perceived ability to manage stressors. *Master's Abstracts International, 32,* 943.

Sammarco-Christie, C. A. (1990). The study of stressors of the operating room nurse versus those of the intensive care unit nurse. *Masters Abstracts International, 28,* 276.

Scalzo Tarrant, T. (1993). Improving the frequency and proficiency of breast self examination. *Master's Abstracts International, 31,* 1211.

Scarpino, L. L. (1988). Family caregivers' perception associated with the chemotherapy treatment setting for the oncology client. *Master's Abstracts International, 26,* 424.

*Semple, O. D. (1995). The experiences of family members of patients with Huntington's disease. *Master's Abstracts International, 33,* 1847.

Smith, J. A. (1995). Caregiver wellness following interventions based on interdisciplinary geriatric assessment. *Master's Abstracts International, 33,* 1707.

Story, M. (1993). Stressful life events of women. *Master's Abstracts International, 31,* 1212.

Sullivan, M. M. (1991). Comparisons of job satisfaction scores of school nurses with job satisfaction normative scores of hospital nurses. *Master's Abstracts International, 29,* 652.

Tomson, D. C. (1994). The impact of previous experience in nursing, educational background, and marital status on self-esteem among community health care workers. *Master's Abstracts International, 32,* 1172.

Triggs, D. R. (1992). The influence of a stress management class on job satisfaction and related occupational tensions in registered nurses. *Master's Abstracts International, 30,* 718.

Tudini, J. B. (1992). A survey of the psychological variables of burnout and depression among nurses. *Master's Abstracts International, 30,* 1302.

Vujakovich, M. A. (1996). Family stress and coping behaviors in families of head-injured individuals. *Master's Abstracts International, 34,* 286.

Wilkey, S. F. (1990). The effects of an eight-hour continuing education course on the death anxiety levels of registered nurses. *Master's Abstracts International, 28,* 480.

Wright, J. G. (1997). The impact of preoperative education on health locus of control, self-effi-cacy, and anxiety for patients undergoing total joint replacement surgery. *Master's Abstracts International, 35,* 216.

Zeliznak, C. M. (1991). Sources of occupational stress of the community health nurse. *Master's Abstracts International, 29,* 654.

*Also published as a journal article

Abstracts Published in Journals (*n* = 2)

Carrigg, K. C., & Weber, R. (1997). Development of the Spiritual Care Scale. *Image: Journal of Nursing Scholarship, 29,* 293.

Lin, M., Ku, N., Leu, J., Chen, J., & Lin, L. (1996). An exploration of the stress aspects, coping behaviors, health status and related aspects in family caregivers of hepatoma patients. *Nursing Research (China), 4,* 171–85. [Chinese, English abstract]

nine

The Neuman Systems Model and Research Instruments

Eileen Gigliotti, Jacqueline Fawcett

K nowledge is developed and expanded through the generation, testing, and utilization of theories. Every theory development effort is guided by a particular conceptual model that provides the intellectual and sociohistorical context for thinking about theories, for conducting research to generate and test the theories, and for utilizing the theories in practice. The success of every theory development effort depends in great part on the selection of appropriate research methods, especially the instruments that measure the concepts of the theory. The purpose of this chapter is to present and discuss the instruments that have been used in research guided by the Neuman Systems Model.

THE RESEARCH INSTRUMENTS

Searches of the literature for two integrative reviews of the Neuman Systems Model–based research yielded 212 research reports that are applicable for this chapter. The reports encompassed 60 journal articles, 2 abstracts published in journals, 2 book chapters, 85 master's theses, and 63 doctoral dissertations (Fawcett, 1999; Fawcett & Giangrande, 2001; Gigliotti, 2001). Given the prohibitive cost of obtaining all doctoral dissertations and master's theses, the literature reviewed for this chapter was limited to the 60 journal articles, 1 of the abstracts, and 2 book chapters; the other abstract was not included because sufficient information about the instruments was not available in the abstract, and the complete article was written in Chinese.

The goal of the literature review for this chapter was to identify the instruments used for data collection, the middle-range theory concept measured by each instrument, and the linkage between the instrument and the Neuman Systems Model as stated in each research report. For the purposes of the review, any empirical indicator that was used to measure a middle-range theory concept was regarded as an instrument, including questionnaires, rating scales, visual analog scales, chart reviews, interview schedules, needs assessments, logs, evaluation tools, physiological measures, and intervention protocols.

A total of 121 different instruments were identified (Tables 9-1 to 9-11). The 10 instruments that appear more than once in the tables—the Beck Depression Inventory, the Norbeck Social Support Questionnaire, the State Trait Anxiety Inventory, the Carter Center Institute Health Risk Appraisal, the Health Status Questionnaire, the Cancer Survivors Questionnaire, the Dynamap, the Mini-Mental Status Exam, the Personal Views Survey, and the Patient/Client Perception Interview Guide—were counted only once in the total.

The instruments initially were categorized according to the extent of their linkage with the Neuman Systems Model. Twenty-four different instruments were derived directly from the Neuman Systems Model (Tables 9-1, 9-3, 9-6, 9-8, 9-10). Two of these instruments appear more than once in the tables. The Patient Perception Interview Guide was used to measure patients' perceptions of why, how, and by whom dialysis treatment modality was chosen in one study (see Table 9-8). Data from the same instrument, now labeled the Client Perception Interview Guide, was used to measure factors influencing dialysis treatment modality decision in another study (see Table 9-8). The Cancer Survivors Questionnaire was used in the same study to measure cancer survivors' physiological, psychological, and sociocultural changes and problems/concerns (see Table 9-1), as well as their needs (see Table 9-3).

Seventy-five different instruments were explicitly linked to the Neuman Systems Model (Tables 9-2, 9-4, 9-5, 9-7, 9-9). Four of those instruments were used more than once. The State Trait Anxiety Inventory was used to measure anxiety in three different studies (see Tables 9-4, 9-5, and 9-7) and psychological well-being in one study (see Table 9-7). The Beck Depression Inventory was to measure depression in one study (see Table 9-4), mental health status in another study (see Table 9-7), and psychological well-being in yet another study (see Table 9-7). The Norbeck Social Support Questionnaire was used to measure the client's perception of social support in one study (see Table 9-4) and social support in another (see Table 9-9). The Dynamap was used to measure blood pressure in one study and rate pressure product in another (see Table 9-5).

Two other instruments that were linked to the Neuman Systems Model were used to measure more than one concept within the same study. The Carter Center Institute Health Risk Appraisal was used to measure modifiable health risks (see Table 9-2), as well as health screening data, such as height and weight (see Table 9-4). The Health Status Questionnaire was used to measure chemical hazard exposure (see Table 9-2), lifestyle factors and protective practices (see Table 9-4), and altered health status (see Table 9-5).

The linkage between the Neuman Systems Model and 26 instruments was not explicitly stated in the study report (Tables 9-10 and 9-11). Two of those instruments appear more than once in the tables. The Mini-Mental Status Exam was not linked to a Neuman Systems Model concept when used to measure mental status (see Table 9-11), although this instrument was linked to the Neuman Systems Model concept of tertiary prevention intervention when used to measure mental health status (see Table 9-7). In addition, the Personal Views Survey, which measures hardiness, was not linked to a Neuman Systems Model in one study (see Table 9-11), but was linked to the Neuman Systems Model concept of the psychological client system variable within the flexible line of defense in another study (see Table 9-4). Furthermore, although the two instruments listed in Table 9-10 were directly derived from the Neuman Systems Model, their linkages to specific Neuman Systems Model concepts were not stated in the research reports.

TABLE 9-1. Measurement of Middle-Range Theory Concepts Representing Stressors: Instruments Derived from the Neuman Systems Model

Instrument	Middle-Range Theory Concept	Neuman Systems Model Concept	Population	Study
Smoking Questionnaire	Age, Sex, Education, Work Area, and Setting	Stressors	Nurses	Cantin & Mitchell, 1989
Needs Assessment Interview Schedule	Caregivers' Life Situation	Caregivers' Stressor Perceptions	Primary caregivers of home-hospice clients	Decker & Young, 1991
Neuman Stressors Inductive Interviews	Home Care Needs and Stressors	Clients' and Caregivers' Perceptions of Intrapersonal, Interpersonal, and Extrapersonal Stressors	Cancer patients and caregivers	Blank et al., 1989
Telephone Interview Schedule	Health: Physical, Mental, Social	Care Provider Stressor Perception	Homeless persons	Bowdler & Barrell, 1987
Health Interview Schedule	Economic, General	Client Stressor Perception		
Self-Identified Needs Questionnaire	Self-Identified Needs of Caregivers	Client Stressor Perception	Caregivers of head-injured adults	Grant & Bean, 1992
Hospital and Home Visits	Stressors and Coping Patterns	Physiological, Psychological, Sociocultural, and Developmental Stressors	A 36-year-old woman who had a hypertensive crisis	Johnson, 1983
Semi-Structured Interview Guide	Parents' Perceptions of Stressors	Client's Perception of Intrapersonal, Interpersonal, and Extrapersonal Stressors	Parents of children who had day surgery	Maligalig, 1994
Logs of Problems, Solutions, Actions	Physical and Psychological Problems	Client's Perception of Intrapersonal, Interpersonal, and Extrapersonal Stressors	Caregivers of elders	Skipwith, 1994

TABLE 9-1. Measurement of Middle-Range Theory Concepts Representing Stressors: Instruments Derived from the Neuman Systems Model *(continued)*

Instrument	Middle-Range Theory Concept	Neuman Systems Model Concept	Population	Study
Cancer Survivors Questionnaire (Loescher et al., 1990)	Physiological, Psychological, and Socio-cultural Changes and Problems/ Concerns	Client's Perception of Stressors	Long-term cancer survivors	Loescher et al., 1990
Interview Schedule	Perception of the Intubation Experience	Client Stressor Perception	Mechanically ventilated patients	Gries & Fernsler, 1988
Neuman Model Nursing Assessment Guide	Impact of Aging and Retirement	Client Stressor Perception	Retired individuals	Hoch, 1987
The Perceived Stress Level Tool (Open-Ended Stressor Rank)	Stressors of Wives of Alcoholics	Client's Perception of Interpersonal, Intrapersonal, and Extrapersonal Stressors	Wives of alcoholics	Montgomery & Craig, 1990
Patient Stressor Scale	Surgical Intensive Care Unit Stressors	Client's Perception of Stressors	Surgical intensive care unit patients	Wilson, 1987

The second level of categorization was according to association between the instrument and a Neuman Systems Model concept. The analysis revealed that 26 instruments measured middle-range theory concepts representing perceptions of stressors (Tables 9-1 and 9-2). Nineteen instruments measured middle-range theory concepts representing the lines of defense and/or resistance (Tables 9-3 and 9-4); 24 measured middle-range theory concepts representing client system reactions (Tables 9-3 and 9-5); and 22 measured middle-range theory concepts representing prevention interventions (Tables 9-6 and 9-7). Sixteen instruments measured other middle-range theory concepts that investigators broadly associated with Neuman Systems Model concepts, including client system variables; client system perceptions; person, environment, health, and nursing; wellness/illness; and needs assessment (Tables 9-8 and 9-9).

The third level of categorization was according to the type of instrument—standardized or nonstandardized. Instruments were considered standardized when sufficient evidence of validity and reliability testing was provided in the research report. Italics denote standardized instruments in the tables. The analysis revealed 59 different standardized instruments and 62 nonstandardized instruments.

Finally, commonalities within and across levels of categorization were explored. Twenty-six instruments were used to measure middle-range theory concepts that represented the Neuman Systems Model concept stressors (Tables 9-1 and 9-2). In keeping

TABLE 9-2. Measurement of Middle-Range Theory Concepts Representing Stressors: Instruments Linked to the Neuman Systems Model

Instrument	Middle-Range Theory Concept	Neuman Systems Model Concept	Population	Study
Ventilator Data	Weaning Attempts	Extrapersonal Stressor	Mechanically ventilated patients	Lowry & Anderson, 1993
Pain Analog Scale	Pain	Stressor	Spinal cord-injured patients	Radwanski, 1992
Audit Tool	Health: Physical, Mental, Social, Economic, General	Objective Stressors	Homeless persons	Bowdler & Barrell, 1987
Chart Review (No tool)	Monthly Differences in Environmental Factors	Stressors	Clients admitted to a rural Kansas hospital	Gifford, 1996
Critical Care Family Needs Inventory (Molter, 1979)	Perceived Needs of Family Members	*Client Stressor Perception:* Psychological Developmental Physiological Sociocultural	Family members of critically ill patients	Kahn, 1992
Crash Classification	Role of Trauma Victim	Stressor	Motor vehicle crash victims	Bueno, Redeker, & Norman, 1992
Health Status Questionnaire	Chemical Hazard Exposure	Stressors	Pediatric nurses	Courchene, Patalski, & Martin, 1991
Maternal Smoking Habits Questionnaire	Maternal Smoking History	Stressor	Infants	Flanders-Stepans & Fuller, 1999
Generic Environmental Tobacco Smoke Exposure Questionnaire	Tobacco Smoke Exposure	Stressor		
Carter Center Institute Health Risk Appraisal (Carter Center Institute, 1991)	Modifiable Health Risks	Intrapersonal, Interpersonal, and Extrapersonal Stressors	Black Americans in an industry without a medical department	Fowler & Risner, 1994
The Burden Interview (Zarit, 1990)	Caregiver's Stressors	Client Perception of Stressors	Caregivers of head-injured patients	Jones, 1996
The Stress Diagnostic Survey (Ivancevich, Matteson, & Dorin, 1990)	Job Stress	Stressor	Nurses	Marsh, Beard, & Adams, 1999

TABLE 9-3. Measurement of the Middle-Range Theory Concepts Representing Lines of Defense and Resistance and Client System Response: Instruments Derived from the Neuman Systems Model

Instrument	Middle-Range Theory Concept	Neuman Systems Model Concept	Population	Study
Semi-Structured Interview Schedule	Stressors and Experiences	Lines of Defense and Resistance	Family members of persons with Huntington's disease	Semple, 1995
Cancer Survivors Questionnaire (Loescher et al., 1990)	Needs of Cancer Survivors	Reaction to Stressors	Long-term cancer survivors	Loescher et al., 1990

with Neuman's emphasis on client perception, 14 of the 26 instruments that were used to measure middle-range theory concepts representing stressors were designed to elicit information about the client's perception of specific stressors—7 interview schedules, 2 questionnaires, 2 stressor rating scales, 1 stressor assessment guide, 1 log, and 1 needs inventory. Moreover, 5 of those 14 instruments measure caregivers' perception of stressors.

Of the 26 instruments used to measure middle-range theory concepts representing stressors, 14 (see Table 9-1) were directly derived from and 12 (see Table 9-2) were explicitly linked with the Neuman Systems Model. Furthermore, 22 of the 26 instruments were nonstandardized situation-specific measures; 14 of these were directly derived from the Neuman Systems Model (see Table 9-1) and 8 were explicitly linked with the model (see Table 9-2). As can be seen in Tables 9-1 and 9-2, some middle-range theory concepts that represented stressors were general, such as surgical intensive care unit stressors, home care stressors, and stressors of wives of alcoholics. Other middle-range theory concepts representing stressors were more specific, such as age, sex, education, work area, and setting; caregivers' life situations and needs; physical, mental, social, economic, and general health; physiological, psychological, and sociocultural changes and problems/concepts; intubation experience; impact of aging and retirement; ventilator weaning attempts; role of trauma victim; chemical hazard exposure; maternal smoking history; tobacco smoke exposure; modifiable health risks; and job stress.

Twenty-four instruments were used to measure middle-range theory concepts representing the Neuman Systems Model concept client's response to stressors. Thirteen of those 24 instruments (Tables 9-3 and 9-5) specifically measured middle-range theory concepts representing the initial stress reaction or the central core response—5 measured middle-range theory concepts representing the initial stress reaction as invasion of the normal line of defense; 1 measured a middle-range theory concept representing the initial stress reaction as activation of the lines of resistance; and 7 measured middle-range theory concepts representing a response in the central core. Four of the 6 instruments that measured middle-range theory concepts representing the initial stress reaction as the client's perception of stress level were standardized measures for the middle-range theory concepts of burnout, role stress, pain, and anxiety. All seven (5 standardized, 2 nonstan-

TABLE 9-4. Measurement of the Lines of Defense and Resistance: Instruments Linked to the Neuman Systems Model

Instrument	Middle-Range Theory Concept	Neuman Systems Model Concept	Population	Study
Beck Depression Inventory (Beck et al., 1961)	Depression Level Before and After Hospital Discharge	Flexible Line of Defense	Post-surgical older adults	Leja, 1989
The Maternal Role Involvement Questionnaire (Gigliotti, 1997)	Psychological Involvement– Maternal Role	Flexible Line of Defense– Psychological Variable	Mothers attending college	Gigliotti, 1999
The Student Role Involvement Questionnaire (Gigliotti, 1997)	Psychological Involvement– Student Role	Flexible Line of Defense– Psychological Variable		
Norbeck Social Support Questionnaire (Norbeck, Lindsey, & Carrieri, 1981, 1983)	Client's Perception of Social support	Flexible Line of Defense– Sociocultural Variable		
The JAREL Spiritual Well-Being Scale (Hungelmann et al., 1989)	Spiritual Well-Being	Flexible Line of Defense– Spiritual Variable	Nurses	Marsh, Beard, & Adams, 1999
The Personal Views Survey (Quellette, 1993)	Hardiness	Flexible Line of Defense– Psychological Variable		
Use of Seat Belts	Safety Restraints	Flexible Line of Defense, Normal Line of Defense	Motor vehicle crash victims	Bueno, Redeker, & Norman, 1992
Du Pont Automatic Clinical Analyzer (asa V) and ALC-Pack (ethyl alcohol) (Du Pont Company)	No Alcohol Use	Flexible Line of Defense, Normal Line of Defense		
Health Status Questionnaire	Lifestyle Factors/ Protective Practices	Flexible Line of Defense, Normal Line of Defense	Pediatric nurses	Courchene, Ptalski, & Martin, 1991

TABLE 9-4. Measurement of the Lines of Defense and Resistance: Instruments Linked to the Neuman Systems Model *(continued)*

Instrument	Middle-Range Theory Concept	Neuman Systems Model Concept	Population	Study
FANTASTIC Lifestyle Checklist (Wilson & Ciliska, 1984; Wilson et al., 1983)	Health Practices	Flexible Line of Defense, Normal Line of Defense	Wives of alcoholics	Montgomery & Craig, 1990
Risk/Treatment Factor Data	Hypertension Risk and Treatment Factors	Flexible Line of Defense	Black female caregivers/ noncaregivers	Picot et al., 1999
The Modified Hill Cognitive Style Model Instrument (Hill & Nunney, 1971).	Cognitive Style	Normal Line of Defense	First-semester nursing students	Nortridge et al., 1992
Physical Coping Behavior Scale (Ziemer, 1982, 1983)	Postoperative Coping Behaviors	Lines of Defense	Postoperative patients	Ziemer, 1983
Psychophysiologic Coping Behavior Scale (Ziemer, 1982,1983)				
State-Trait Anxiety Inventory (STAI) (Spielberger, Gorsuch, & Lushene, 1970)			Nurses working with long-term care clients	Louis, 1989
State Anxiety Scale	Anxiety at Present	Flexible Line of Defense		
Trait Anxiety Scale	Anxiety in General	Normal Line of Defense		
Self-Rated Anxiety Status Inventory (Zung, 1971)	Measure of Clinical Disorder	Line(s) of Resistance		
Carter Center Institute Health Risk Appraisal (Carter Center Institute, 1991)	Health Screening Data (Height, Weight, Other)	Flexible Line of Defense, Normal Line of Defense, Lines of Resistance	Black Americans in an industry with no medical department	Fowler & Risner, 1994
Capillary Gas– Liquid Chroma- tographic Assay (Hewlett- Packard model ~~5000~~)	Nicotine/Cotinine	Lines of Resistance	Infants	Flanders-Stepans & Fuller, 1999

TABLE 9-5. Measurement of Middle-Range Theory Concepts Representing Client System Response: Instruments Linked to the Neuman Systems Model

Instrument	Middle-Range Theory Concept	Neuman Systems Model Concept	Population	Study
ABP Monitors (Spacelabs, 1988)	Blood Pressure Responses	Basic Structure	Black female caregivers/ noncaregivers	Picot et al., 1999
The Mental Status Examination (Adams et al., 1978)	Impaired Psychological Response	Psychological Response	Surgical intensive care unit patients	Wilson, 1987
The Perceived Stress Level Tool (Visual Analog)	Stress Level	Client's Perception of Stress	Wives of alcoholics	Montgomery & Craig, 1990
Trauma Score (Champion et al., 1981)	Traumatic Injuries	Stressor Impact	Motor vehicle crash victims	Bueno, Redeker, & Norman, 1992
Health Status Questionnaire	Altered Health Status	Stress Reactions	Pediatric nurses	Courchene, Patalski,& Martin, 1991
Nellcor N-10 Pulse Oxymeter (Nellcor, Inc., 1986)	Pulse Rate/Oxygen Saturation	Central Core Response	Infants	Flanders-Stepans & Fuller, 1999
Dynamap Monitor (Critikon, Inc., 1984)	Blood Pressure	Central Core Response		
Stethoscope	Respirations	Central Core Response		
Mercury-in-glass thermometers	Core Temperature	Central Core Response		
Collected Data (No tool)	Incidence of Pulmonary Complications and Length of Hospital Stay	Impact of Stressors	Patients who had coronary artery bypass graft surgery	Gavigan, Kline-O'Sullivan, & Klumpp-Lybrand, 1990
Chart Review (No tool)	CVA Symptoms	Client Health	Clients admitted to a rural Kansas hospital	Gifford, 1996
Dynamap 1846SX (Critikon, Inc.)	Rate Pressure Product	Central Core Response	Post-anesthesia patients	Heffline, 1991
EMG (Caldwell Quantum 84, Caldwell, Kennewick, WA)	Shivering	Central Core Response		

TABLE 9-5. Measurement of Middle-Range Theory Concepts Representing Client System Response: Instruments Linked to the Neuman Systems Model *(continued)*

Instrument	Middle-Range Theory Concept	Neuman Systems Model Concept	Population	Study
The Appraisal Caregiving Scale (M. Oberst, personal communication, September 1992)	Experienced Stresses	Stress Level/ Reaction to Stressor Exposure	Caregivers of head-injured patients	Jones, 1996
McGill Pain Questionnaire (Melzack, 1975)	Severity of Pain	Penetration of Lines of Defense	City employed back-school participants	Koku, 1992
STAI (Form Y-I; A-State) (Spielberger et al., 1983)	Preoperative and Postoperative Anxiety	Normal Line of Defense Invasion	Egyptian cancer bladder patients	Ali & Khalil, 1989
Observation and Wound Cultures	Infection	Activation of Lines of Resistance	Pediatric oncology patients	Freiberger, Bryant, & Marino, 1992
Perceived Multiple Role Stress Scale (Gigliotti, in press)	Client's Perception of Multiple Role Stress	Normal Line of Defense Invasion	Mothers attending college	Gigliotti, 1999
The Maslach Burnout Inventory (Maslach & Jackson, 1986)	Burnout	Normal Line of Defense Invasion	Nurses	Marsh, Beard, & Adams, 1999
Visual Analog Scales (VAS)	Mood Symptoms	Normal Line of Defense Destabilization	Black female caregivers/ noncaregivers	Picot et al., 1999
Physical Symptoms Report (Ziemer, 1982, 1983)	Patient Reports of Postoperative Symptoms	Stressor Impact	Postoperative patients	Ziemer, 1983
Pain Intensity Scale (Ziemer, 1982, 1983)	Pain Intensity	Stressor Impact		
Distress Scale (Ziemer, 1982, 1983)	Postoperative Distress	Stressor Impact		

TABLE 9-6. Measurement of Middle-Range Theory Concepts Representing Prevention Interventions: Instrument Derived from the Neuman Systems Model

Instrument	Middle-Range Theory Concept	Neuman Systems Model Concept	Population	Study
Telephone Counseling Intervention	Telephone Counseling	Primary, Secondary, and Tertiary Prevention Interventions	Caregivers of elders	Skipwith, 1994

dardized) of the instruments associated with the central core response were physiological measures of such middle-range theory concepts as blood pressure changes, respirations, core temperature, and oxygen saturation levels. Other middle-range theory concepts measured as representatives of client system responses included cancer survivors' needs, impaired psychological response, traumatic injury, altered health status, incidence of pulmonary complications and length of hospital stay, cerebrovascular accident symptoms, shivering, severity of pain, pain intensity, postoperative distress, postoperative symptoms, pre- and postoperative anxiety, infection, and mood symptoms.

Furthermore, 19 instruments measured middle-range theory concepts that represented the Neuman Systems Model concepts lines of defense and/or lines of resistance (Tables 9-3 and 9-4). Eight instruments measured middle-range theory concepts representing the flexible line of defense. Seven of these were standardized instruments measuring the middle-range theory concepts of depression levels, spiritual well-being, anxiety at present, social support, hardiness, and maternal and student role involvement. The one nonstandardized instrument was used to document the middle-range theory concept of risks and treatment factors. Standardized instruments were used to measure the middle-range theory concepts of cognitive style and anxiety in general, as representatives of the normal line of defense. Other standardized instruments were used to measure the middle-range theory concepts of a clinical disorder and nicotine/cotinine levels, as representatives of the lines of resistance. Still other instruments were used to measure the middle-range theory concepts of safety restraints, alcohol use, lifestyle factors/protective practices, and health practices, all of which represented both the flexible and normal lines of defense. Furthermore, other instruments were used to measure the middle-range theory concept of stressors and experiences, and the concept of health screening data, including height and weight, all of which represented both the lines of defense and the lines of resistance.

Moreover, six instruments were used to measure diverse middle-range theory concepts that represented diverse Neuman Systems Model concepts. That is, the same instrument was used to measure different middle-range theory concepts and was used to represent different Neuman Systems Model concepts. In one study, the Cancer Survivors Questionnaire was used to measure cancer survivors' physiological, psychological, and sociocultural changes and problems/concerns, which represented the client's perception of stressors (see Table 9-1), and also was used to measure cancer survivors' needs, which represented client system reaction to stressors (see Table 9-3). In another study, the Carter Center Institute Health Risk Appraisal was used to measure modifiable health risks, which represented intrapersonal, interpersonal, and extrapersonal stressors (see Table 9-2), as well as health screening data, which represented the flexible and normal

TABLE 9-7. Measurement of Middle-Range Theory Concepts Representing Prevention Interventions: Instruments Linked to the Neuman Systems Model

Instrument	Middle-Range Theory Concept	Neuman Systems Model Concept	Population	Study
Beck Depression Inventory (Beck, Rial, & Rickels, 1974)	Mental Health Status	Effectiveness of a Case Management Tertiary Prevention Intervention	Psychiatric patients	Chiverton et al., 1999
Mini-Mental Status Examination (Folstein, Folstein, & McHugh, 1975)	Mental Health Status			
Patient and Caregiver Satisfaction Instruments	Satisfaction with Case Management Program			
Pure Tone Audiometry Tympanometry	Hearing Loss	Primary, Secondary, and Tertiary Intervention	Elementary school children	Mannina, 1997
The Risser Patient Satisfaction Scale (Risser, 1975)	Satisfaction with Prenatal Care	Effectiveness of a Primary Prevention Intervention	Low-income pregnant women	Lowry, Saeger, & Barnett, 1997
Hmong Parenting Interview	Healing Practices	Primary, Secondary, and Tertiary Prevention	Hmong parents	Nuttall & Flores, 1997
The Richards–Campbell Sleep Questionnaire (Richards, 1987)	Sleep Patterns	Effectiveness of a Primary, Secondary, and Tertiary Prevention Intervention	Postoperative patients who had coronary artery bypass graft surgery	Williamson, 1992
Levels of Cognitive Functioning Assessment Scale (Flannery, 1995)	Cognitive Functioning	Tertiary Prevention Intervention	Traumatic brain-injured patients	Flannery, 1995

TABLE 9-7. Measurement of Middle-Range Theory Concepts Representing Prevention Interventions: Instruments Linked to the Neuman Systems Model *(continued)*

Instrument	Middle-Range Theory Concept	Neuman Systems Model Concept	Population	Study
Dynamometer	Back strength	Effectiveness of an Intervention to Strengthen the Lines of Defense	Back-injured city employees	Sirles, Brown, & Hilyer, 1991
Acuflex I Sit-and-Reach Test (Hoeger, Hopkins, & Johnson, 1988)	Back Flexibility			
Pain Self-Report	Pain			
The Nottingham Health Profile (Hunt, McEwen, & McKenna, 1986)	Psychological Well-Being			
Psychological Well Being Schedule (Dupuy, 1984)	Psychological Well-Being			
Spielberger Anxiety Scales (Spielberger et al.,1983)	Psychological Well-Being			
Beck Depression Inventory (Beck, 1967)	Psychological Well-Being			
Cost, Lost Time, and Injury Measures	Injury Control	Effectiveness of an Intervention to Strengthen Resistance	Back-injured municipal employees	Brown et al., 1992
Collected Data (No tool)	Regular Turning	Primary Prevention Intervention	Patients who had coronary artery bypass graft surgery	Gavigan, Kline-O'Sullivan, & Klumpp-Lybrand, 1990
Emerson Model 96H Heat Lamp (Emerson, Cambridge, MA)	Heat Combinations	Nursing Intervention	Postanesthesia Patients	Heffline, 1991

TABLE 9-7. Measurement of Middle-Range Theory Concepts Representing Prevention Interventions: Instruments Linked to the Neuman Systems Model *(continued)*

Instrument	Middle-Range Theory Concept	Neuman Systems Model Concept	Population	Study
The State-Trait Anxiety Inventory (STAI) (Speilberger et al., 1983)	Anxiety	Effectiveness of an Intervention to Protect the Normal Line of Defense	First-semester nursing students	Speck, 1990
Biodot Stress Dots (Biodot International, 1986)	Physiological Stress			
Student performance time and score	Anxiety			
Stress Response Index	Negative Stress Reactions	Effectiveness of an Intervention to Strengthen the Lines of Defense and Resistance	Office workers	Vaughn et al., 1989

lines of defense and the lines of resistance (see Table 9-4). In still another study, the Health Status Questionnaire was used to measure chemical hazard exposure, which represented stressors (see Table 9-2); lifestyle factors/protective practices, which represented the flexible and normal lines of defense (see Table 9-4); and altered health status, which represented stress reactions (see Table 9-5).

In addition, the Beck Depression Inventory was used to measure depression, which represented the flexible line of defense, in one study (see Table 9-4); mental health status, which represented tertiary prevention intervention, in another study (see Table 9-7); and psychological well-being, which represented an intervention designed to strengthen the lines of defense, in yet another study (see Table 9-7). The State-Trait Anxiety Inventory (STAI) was used to measure anxiety, which represented the flexible and normal lines of defense in one study (see Table 9-4), invasion of the normal line of defense in another study (see Table 9-5), and an intervention designed to strengthen the lines of defense in yet another study (see Table 9-7). In still another study, the STAI was used to measure psychological well-being, which represented an intervention designed to protect the normal line of defense (see Table 9-7). The Norbeck Social Support Questionnaire was used to measure social support, which represented interpersonal factors in one study (see Table 9-9) and the sociocultural client system variable of the flexible line of defense in another study (see Table 9-4).

CONCLUSION

The review of instruments indicates that although much excellent work has been done, even more work is needed to forge strong links between the Neuman Systems Model and research instruments. Five recommendations are offered as direction for future work.

TABLE 9-8. Measurement of Middle-Range Theory Concepts Representing Other Neuman Systems Model Concepts: Instruments Derived from the Neuman Systems Model

Instrument	Middle-Range Theory Concept	Neuman Systems Model Concept	Population	Study
Semi-Structured Interview Guide	Parental Needs	Needs Assessment	Parents of infants in a neonatal intensive care unit	Bass, 1991
The Safety Assessment Tool	Demographic Data Risk Factors Safety Issues Incident Prevention/ Intervention	Person Environment Health Nursing	Community health nurses	Gellner et al., 1994
AAS Nursing Curriculum Evaluation Tool (Lowry & Jopp, 1989)	Perception of: Clients Environment Health Nursing	Person Stress/Stressors Wellness/Illness Nursing	Associate degree nursing program students	Lowry & Jopp, 1989
Patient Perception Interview Guide	Patients' Perceptions of Why, How, and by Whom Dialysis Treatment Modality Was Chosen	Client System Perceptions	Men and women with end-stage renal disease	Breckenridge, 1997b
Structured Interview Guide	Trust, Support, Respect	Spiritual Variable	Men and women who had surgery due to cancer or heart disease within past 6 months	Clark et al., 1991
Client Perception Interview Guide	Factors Influencing Dialysis Treatment Modality Decision	Physiological, Psychological, Sociocultural, Developmental, and Spiritual Variables	Men and women with end-stage renal disease	Breckenridge, 1997a
Demographic Profile	Demographic Information	Five Person Variables	Wives of alcoholics	Montgomery & Craig, 1990

TABLE 9-9. Measurement of Middle-Range Theory Concepts Representing Other Neuman Systems Model Concepts: Instruments Linked to the Neuman Systems Model

Instrument	Middle-Range Theory Concept	Neuman Systems Model Concept	Population	Study
Data Collection Form	Demographic Data Perceived Degree of Emotional Support Hospital Follow-up Group	Environmental Forces	Mental health unit patients	Barker, Robinson & Brautigan, 1999
Demographic Data	Age	Intrapersonal Client Variable— Developmental	Mechanically ventilated patients	Lowry & Anderson 1993
	Disease State/ Injury	Intrapersonal Client Variable— Physiological		
Anderson–Lowry Ventilation Scale	Ventilation-Related Anxiety	Intrapersonal Client Variable— Physiological		
The Multi-dimensional Health Locus of Control Scales (Wallston, Wallston, & DeVillis, 1978)	Locus of Control	Intrapersonal Client Variable— Physiological		
One Item Hope Scale (Miller & Powers, 1988)	Hope	Intrapersonal Client Variable— Spiritual		
Norbeck Social Support Questionnaire (NSSQ) (Norbeck, Lindsey, & Carrieri, 1981)	Social Support	Interpersonal Factors		
Self-Control Schedule (Rosenbaum, 1980)	Learned Resourcefulness	Internal Environment–Intrapersonal Factor, and Created Environment	Men and women with lung cancer	Hinds, 1990
Information Styles Questionnaire (Cassileth et al., 1980)	Preferred Style of Obtaining and Responding to Illness-Related Information	Internal Environment–Intrapersonal Factor		
Quality of Life Index (Ferrans & Powers 1985)	Quality of Life	Level of Health		

TABLE 9-10. Other Research Instruments Derived from the Neuman Systems Model: Neuman Systems Model Concepts Not Specified

Instrument	Middle-Range Theory Concept	Neuman Systems Model Concept	Population	Study
Spiritual Care Scale (Carrigg & Weber, 1997)	Spiritual Care Psychosocial Care	Not Stated Not Stated	Nurses	Carrigg & Weber, 1997
Semi-Structured Interview Guide	Major Stress Area	Not Stated	Long-term cancer survivors	Cava, 1992
	Coping Strategies	Not Stated		
	Changes in Lifestyle	Not Stated		
	Views of the Future	Not Stated		
	Expectations of Support from Others	Not Stated		

First, the analysis of instruments should be extended to those used in master's theses and doctoral dissertations. Second, much more attention should be given to the validity of existing instruments with regard to the Neuman Systems Model. More specifically, investigators are urged to select instruments that are valid measures of theory concepts within the context of the Neuman Systems Model. For example, if an instrument is purported to measure the theory concept of health, the researcher must determine whether (a) the instrument actually operationalizes a particular definition of health, such as general physical, mental, and social well-being; and (b) whether the particular definition of health is congruent with the Neuman Systems Model, with its emphasis on health as client system stability, variances from wellness, and reconstitution.

Third, researchers need to examine the logical congruence of existing instruments with Neuman Systems Model concepts and to directly derive instruments from the Neuman Systems Model to measure concepts for which there are no existing logically congruent instruments. The ultimate goal is to accumulate a battery of valid and reliable questionnaires and other research instruments that measure the full spectrum of Neuman Systems Model concepts, including physiological, psychological, sociocultural, developmental, and spiritual client system variables; the central core; the flexible and normal lines of defense and the lines of resistance; the internal, external, and created environments; intrapersonal, interpersonal, and extrapersonal stressors; client system stability, variances from wellness, and reconstitution; and primary, secondary, and tertiary prevention interventions. Furthermore, instruments are needed to measure those concepts for diverse client systems, including individuals, families, communities, and organizations. As they develop Neuman Systems Model–based instruments, researchers should consider the advantages and disadvantages of generic, clinical condition-specific, age- or developmental stage-specific, gender-specific, and culture-specific instruments. In addition, given the Neuman Systems Model emphasis on the perceptions of both client systems and

TABLE 9-11. Other Research Instruments Used in Neuman Systems Model–Based Studies: Neuman Systems Model Concepts Not Specified

Instrument	Middle-Range Theory Concept	Neuman Systems Model Concept	Population	Study
Structured Interview	Surgical Concerns	Not stated	Elderly clients undergoing orthopedic procedures	Bowman, 1997
Mini-Mental Status Exam (Folstein, Folstein, and McHugh, 1975)	Mental Status	Not Stated		
Visual Analog Pain Scale	Pain	Not Stated		
Sleep Satisfaction Scale	Sleep Satisfaction	Not Stated		
Smoking Questionnaire	Smoking Behavior	Not Stated	Nurses	Cantin & Mitchell, 1989
Personal Views Survey (E. W. McCranie & V. Lambert, personal communication)	Hardiness	Not Stated	Nurses	Collins, 1996
The Tedium Burnout Scale (Pines & Aronson, 1981)	Burnout	Not Stated		
The Nursing Stress Scale (Gray-Toft & Anderson, 1981)	Occupational Stress	Not Stated		
Three-Minute Reasoning Test Based on Grammatical Transformation (Baddeley, 1968).	Critical Thinking	Not Stated	Critical care nurses	Fields & Loveridge, 1988
Subjective Symptoms of Fatigue Test (Yoshitake, 1978)	Fatigue Level	Not Stated		

TABLE 9-11. Other Research Instruments Used in Neuman Systems Model–Based Studies: Neuman Systems Model Concepts Not Specified *(continued)*

Instrument	Middle-Range Theory Concept	Neuman Systems Model Concept	Population	Study
The Schutzenhofer Professional Nursing Autonomy Scale (Schutzenhofer & Musser, 1994)	Professional Autonomy	Not Stated	Staff nurses	George, 1997
Three Open-Ended Perception Questions	Professional Practice Perceptions	Not Stated		
Attitudes, Subjective Norms, and Behavioral Intentions of Nurses Toward Care of Dying Persons and Their Families (Waltman, 1990)	Attitudes, Subjective Norms, and Behavioral Intentions Toward Care of Dying Persons and Their Families	Not Stated	Nurses	Hainsworth, 1996
Organizational Characteristics	Organizational Characteristics	Not Stated	Nurse faculty	Moody, 1996
Role Orientation	Role Orientation	Not Stated		
JDI (Smith, Kendall, & Hulin, 1969)	Job Satisfaction	Not Stated		
JIG (Ironson et al., 1989)	Job Satisfaction	Not Stated		
Drug Use for Chronic Pain Management Survey	Drug Use	Not Stated	Spinal cord– injured patients	Radwanski, 1992
Chronic Pain Modifier	Drug Effectiveness	Not Stated		
Perioperative Survey	Amount and Influence of Perioperative Theory	Not Stated	Nurses	Roggensack, 1994

TABLE 9-11. Other Research Instruments Used in Neuman Systems Model–Based Studies: Neuman Systems Model Concepts Not Specified *(continued)*

Instrument	Middle-Range Theory Concept	Neuman Systems Model Concept	Population	Study
The Agoraphobic Cognitions Questionnaire and Body Sensations Questionnaire (Chambless et al., 1984)	Fear of Fear	Not Stated	Patients with anxiety disorders	Waddell & Demi, 1993
The Mobility Inventory for Agoraphobia (Chambless et al., 1985)	Severity of Impaired Functioning	Not Stated		
The Symptom Checklist 90—Revised (Derogatis, 1983)	Psychological Symptom Distress	Not Stated		
Family Functioning Questionnaire (Linder-Pelz et al., 1984)	Level of Family Functioning	Not Stated	Men and women with lung cancer	Hinds, 1990

caregivers, alternate forms of each instrument should be developed to measure the study participant's and the researcher's perceptions or ratings of the phenomenon being measured. The idea of establishing a battery of research instruments follows from Quayhagen and Roth's (1989) pioneering work, which resulted in the identification of a set of existing clinically appropriate questionnaires for Neuman Systems Model–based assessment of physiological, psychological, sociological, developmental, and spiritual client system variables and environmental influences in mature and aging families.

Fourth, the utility of research instruments for use in Neuman Systems Model–based clinical practice needs to be examined. Fifth, the research potential of Neuman Systems Model–based clinical tools (Chapter 4) and Neuman Systems Model–based educational tools (Chapter 14) needs to be determined. The use of research instruments to record clinical information, and the use of clinical tools and educational tools as sources of data for research will greatly facilitate the integration of research, clinical practice, and education.

REFERENCES

Fawcett, J. (1999, April). Neuman Systems Model Research: An Integrative Review. Paper presented at the Seventh Biennial International Neuman Systems Model Symposium, Vancouver, British Columbia, Canada.

Fawcett, J., & Giangrande, S. K. (2001). Neuman Systems Model-based research: An integrative review project. *Nursing Science Quarterly, 14.*

Gigliotti, E. (2001). Empirical tests of the Neuman systems model: Relational statement analysis. *Nursing Science Quarterly, 14.*

Quayhagen, M. P., & Roth, P. A. (1989). From models to measures in assessment of mature families. *Journal of Professional Nursing, 5,* 144–51.

Studies Reviewed

Ali, N. S., & Khalil, H. Z. (1989). Effect of psychoeducational intervention on anxiety among Egyptian bladder cancer patients. *Cancer Nursing, 12,* 236–42.

Barker, E., Robinson, D., & Brautigan, R. (1999). The effect of psychiatric home nurse follow-up on readmission rates of patients with depression. *Journal of the American Psychiatric Nurses Association, 5,* 111–16.

Bass, L. S. (1991). What do parents need when their infant is a patient in the NICU? *Neonatal Network, 10*(4), 25–33.

Blank, J. J., Clark, L., Longman, A. J., & Atwood, J. R. (1989). Perceived home care needs of cancer patients and their caregivers. *Cancer Nursing, 12,* 78–84.

Bowdler, J. E., & Barrell, L. M. (1987). Health needs of homeless persons. *Public Health Nursing, 4,* 135–40.

Bowman, A. M. (1997). Sleep satisfaction, perceived pain and acute confusion in elderly clients undergoing orthopaedic procedures. *Journal of Advanced Nursing, 26,* 550–64.

Breckenridge, D. M. (1997a). Decisions regarding dialysis treatment modality: A holistic perspective. *Holistic Nursing Practice, 12*(1), 54–61.

Breckenridge, D. M. (1997b). Patients' perception of why, how, and by whom dialysis treatment modality was chosen. *Association of Nephrology Nurses Journal, 24,* 313–21.

Brown, K. C., Sirles, A. T., Hilyer, J. C., & Thomas, M. J. (1992). Cost-effectiveness of a back school intervention for municipal employees. *Spine, 17,* 1224–28.

Bueno, M. N., Redeker, N., & Norman, E. M. (1992). Analysis of motor vehicle crash data in an urban trauma center: Implications for nursing practice and research. *Heart and Lung, 21,* 558–67.

Cantin, B., & Mitchell, M. (1989). Nurses' smoking behavior. *The Canadian Nurse, 85*(1), 20–21.

Carrigg, K. C., & Weber, R. (1997). Development of the Spiritual Care Scale. *Image: Journal of Nursing Scholarship, 29,* 293.

Cava, M. A. (1992). An examination of coping strategies used by long-term cancer survivors. *Canadian Oncology Nursing Journal, 2,* 99–102.

Chiverton, P., Tororetti, D., LaForest, M., & Walker, P. H. (1999). Bridging the gap between psychiatric hospitalization and community care: Cost and quality outcomes. *Journal of the American Psychiatric Nurses Association, 5*(2), 46–53.

Clark, C. C., Cross, J. R., Deane, D. M., & Lowry, L. W. (1991). Spirituality: Integral to quality care. *Holistic Nursing Practice, 5,* 67–76.

Collins, M. A. (1996). The relation of work stress, hardiness, and burnout among full-time hospital staff nurses. *Journal of Nursing Staff Development, 12,* 81–85.

Courchene, V. S., Patalski, E., & Martin, J. (1991). A study of the health of pediatric nurses administering Cyclosporine A. *Pediatric Nursing, 17,* 497–500.

Decker, S. D., & Young, E. (1991). Self-perceived needs of primary caregivers of home-hospice clients. *Journal of Community Health Nursing, 8, 147–54.*

Fields, W. L., & Loveridge, C. (1988). Critical thinking and fatigue: How do nurses on 8- & 12-hour shifts compare? *Nursing Economic$, 6,* 189–91.

Flanders-Stepans, M. B., & Fuller, S. G. (1999). Physiological effects of infant exposure to environmental tobacco smoke: A passive observation study. *Journal of Perinatal Education, 8,* 10–21.

Flannery, J. (1995). Cognitive assessment in the acute care setting: Reliability and validity of the Levels of Cognitive Functioning Assessment Scale (LOCFAS). *Journal of Nursing Measurement, 3,* 43–58.

Fowler, B. A., & Risner, P. B. (1994). A health promotion program evaluation in a minority industry. *Association of Black Nursing Faculty Journal, 5*(3), 72–76.

Freiberger, D., Bryant, J., & Marino, B. (1992). The effects of different central venous line dressing changes on bacterial growth in a pediatric oncology population. *Journal of Pediatric Oncology Nursing, 9,* 3–7.

Gavigan, M., Kline-O'Sullivan, C., & Klumpp-Lybrand, B. (1990). The effect of regular turning on CABG patients. *Critical Care Nursing Quarterly, 12*(4), 69–76.

Gellner, P., Landers, S., O'Rourke, D., & Schlegel, M. (1994). Community health nursing in the 1990s: Risky business? *Holistic Nursing Practice, 8*(2), 15–21.

George, J. (1997). Nurses' perceived autonomy in a shared governance setting. *Journal of Shared Governance, 3*(2), 17–21.

Gifford, D. K. (1996). Monthly incidence of stroke in rural Kansas. *Kansas Nurse, 71*(5), 3–4.

Gigliotti, E. (1999). Women's multiple role stress: Testing Neuman's flexible line of defense. *Nursing Science Quarterly, 12,* 36–44.

Grant, J. S., & Bean, C. A. (1992). Self-identified needs of informal caregivers of head-injured adults. *Family and Community Health, 15*(2), 49–58.

Gries, M., & Fernsler, J. (1988). Patient perceptions of the mechanical ventilation experience. *Focus on Critical Care, 15,* 52–59.

Hainsworth, D. S. (1996). The effect of death education on attitudes of hospital nurses toward care of the dying. *Oncology Nursing Forum, 23,* 963–67.

Heffline, M. S. (1991). A comparative study of pharmacological versus nursing interventions in the treatment of postanesthesia shivering. *Journal of Post Anesthesia Nursing, 6,* 311–20.

Hinds, C. (1990). Personal and contextual factors predicting patients' reported quality of life: Exploring congruency with Betty Neuman's assumptions. *Journal of Advanced Nursing, 15,* 456–62.

Hoch, C. C. (1987). Assessing delivery of nursing care. *Journal of Gerontological Nursing, 13,* 1–17.

Johnson, P. (1983). Black hypertension: A transcultural case study using the Betty Neuman model of nursing care. *Issues in Health Care of Women, 4,* 191–210.

Jones, W. R. (1996). Stressors in the primary caregivers of traumatic head injured persons. *AXON, 18,* 9–11.

Kahn, E. C. (1992). A comparison of family needs based on the presence or absence of DNR orders. *Dimensions of Critical Care Nursing, 11,* 286–92.

Koku, R. V. (1992). Severity of low back pain: A comparison between participants who did and did not receive counseling. *American Association of Occupational Health Nurses Journal, 40,* 84–89.

Leja, A. M. (1989). Using guided imagery to combat postsurgical depression. *Journal of Gerontological Nursing, 15*(4), 6–11.

Loescher, L. J., Clark, L., Atwood, J. R., Leigh, S., & Lamb, G. (1990). The impact of the cancer experience on long-term survivors. *Oncology Nursing Forum, 17,* 223–29.

Louis, M. (1989). An intervention to reduce anxiety levels for nurses working with long-term care clients using Neuman's model. In J. P. Riehl-Sisca (Ed.), *Conceptual models for nursing practice* (3rd ed., pp. 95–103). Norwalk, CT: Appleton & Lange.

Lowry, L. W., & Anderson, B. (1993). Neuman's framework and ventilator dependency: *A pilot study. Nursing Science Quarterly, 6,* 195–200.

Lowry, L. W., & Jopp, M. C. (1989). An evaluation instrument for assessing an associate degree nursing curriculum based on the Neuman systems model. In J. P. Riehl-Sisca (Ed.), *Conceptual models for nursing practice* (3rd ed., pp. 73–85). Norwalk, CT: Appleton & Lange.

Lowry, L. W., Saeger, J., & Barnett, S. (1997). Client satisfaction with prenatal care and pregnancy outcomes. *Outcomes Management for Nursing Practice, 1*(1), 29–35.

Maligalig, R. M. L. (1994). Parents' perceptions of the stressors of pediatric ambulatory surgery. *Journal of Post Anesthesia Nursing, 9,* 278–82.

Mannina, J. (1997). Finding an effective hearing testing protocol to identify hearing loss and middle ear disease in school-aged children. *Journal of School Nursing, 13*(5), 23–28.

Marsh, V., Beard, M. T., & Adams, B. N. (1999). Job stress and burnout: The mediational effect of spiritual well-being and hardiness among nurses. *Journal of Theory Construction and Testing, 3,* 13–19.

Montgomery, P., & Craig, D. (1990). Levels of stress and health practices of wives of alcoholics. *Canadian Journal of Nursing Research, 22,* 60–70.

Moody, N. B. (1996). Nurse faculty job satisfaction: A national survey. *Journal of Professional Nursing, 12,* 277–88.

Nortridge, J. A., Mayeux, V., Anderson, S. J., & Bell, M. L. (1992). The use of cognitive style mapping as a predictor for academic success of first semester diploma nursing students. *Journal of Nursing Education, 31,* 352–56.

Nuttall, P., & Flores, F. C. (1997). Hmong healing practices used for common childhood illnesses. *Pediatric Nursing, 23,* 247–51.

Picot, S. J. F., Zauszniewski, J. A., Debanne, S. M., & Holston, E. C. (1999). Mood and blood pressure responses in black female caregivers and noncaregivers. *Nursing Research, 48,* 150–61.

Radwanski, M. (1992). Self-medicating practices for managing chronic pain after spinal cord injury. *Rehabilitation Nursing, 17,* 312–18.

Roggensack, J. (1994). The influence of perioperative theory and clinical in a baccalaureate nursing program on the decision to practice perioperative nursing. *Prairie Rose, 63*(2), 6–7.

Semple, O. D. (1995). The experiences of family members of persons with Huntington's disease. *Perspectives, 19*(4), 4–10.

Sirles, A. T., Brown, K., & Hilyer, J. C. (1991). Effects of back school education and exercise in back injured municipal workers. *American Association of Occupational Health Nursing Journal, 39,* 7–12.

Skipwith, D. H. (1994). Telephone counseling interventions with caregivers of elders. *Journal of Psychosocial Nursing and Mental Health Services, 32*(3), 7–12, 34–35.

Speck, B. J. (1990). The effect of guided imagery upon first semester nursing students performing their first injections. *Journal of Nursing Education, 29,* 346–50.

Vaughn, M., Cheatwood, S., Sirles, A. T., & Brown, K. C. (1989). The effect of progressive muscle relaxation on stress among clerical workers. *American Association of Occupational Health Nurses Journal, 37,* 302–306.

Waddell, K. L., & Demi, A. S. (1993). Effectiveness of an intensive partial hospitalization program for treatment of anxiety disorders. *Archives of Psychiatric Nursing, 7,* 2–10.

Williamson, J. W. (1992). The effects of ocean sounds on sleep after coronary artery bypass graft surgery. *American Journal of Critical Care, 1,* 91–97.

Wilson, V. S. (1987). Identification of stressors related to patients' psychological responses to the surgical intensive care unit. *Heart and Lung, 16,* 267–73.

Ziemer, M. M. (1983). Effects of information on postsurgical coping. *Nursing Research, 32,* 282–87.

Standardized Instruments

Adams, M., Hanson, R., Norkool, D., et al. (1978). Working with the confused or delirious patient: Psychological responses in critical care units. *American Journal of Nursing, 78,* 1504–12.

Baddeley, A. D. (1968). A 3-minute reasoning test based on grammatical transformation. *Psychonomic Science, 10,* 341–42.

Beck, A. (1967). *Depression: Causes and treatment.* Philadelphia: University of Pennsylvania Press.

Beck, A. T., Rial, W. Y., & Rickels, K. (1974). Short form of the Depression Inventory: Cross validation. *Psychosocial Reports, 34,* 1184–86.

Beck, A. T., Ward, C. H., Menderson, M., Mock, J., & Erbaugh, J. (1961). An inventory for measuring depression. *Archives of General Psychiatry, 4,* 561–71.

Biodot International, Inc. (1986). *Biodot Fact Sheet.* Indianapolis, IN: Biodot International, Inc.

Carrigg, K. C., & Weber, R. (1997). Development of the spiritual care scale. *Image: Journal of Nursing Scholarship, 29,* 293.

Carter Center Institute (1991). *Health risk appraisal.* Atlanta, GA: Emory University.

Cassileth, B. R., Zupkis, R. V., Sutton-Smith, K., & March, V. (1980). Information and participation preferences among cancer patients. *Annals of Internal Medicine, 92,* 832–36.

Chambless, D. L., Caputo, G. C., Bright, P., & Gallagher, R. (1984). Assessment of fear of fear in agoraphobics: The body sensations questionnaire and the agoraphobic cognitions questionnaire. *Journal of Consulting and Clinical Psychology, 52,* 1090–97.

Chambless, D. L., Caputo, G. C., Jasin, S. E., Gracely, E. J., & Williams, C. (1985). The mobility inventory for agoraphobia. *Behavior Research and Therapy, 23*(1), 35–44.

Champion, H. R., Sacco, W. J., Carnazzo, A. J., Copes, W., & Fouty, W. J. (1981). Trauma Score. *Critical Care Medicine, 9,* 672–76.

Critikon, Inc. (1984). *Dinamap adult/pediatric and neonatal vital signs monitor model 1846 operation manual.* Tampa, FL: Critikon, Inc.

Derogatis, L. R. (1983). *Description and bibliography for the SCL90-R and other instruments of the psychopathology rating scale series.* Towson, MD: Clinical Psychometric Research.

Du Pont Automatic Clinical Analyzer (asa V) and ALC-Pack (ethyl alcohol). Wilmington, DE: Du Pont Corporation.

Dupuy, H. (1984). The psychological well-being index. In Wenger, N., Mattson, M., Furburg, C., & Elinson, J. (Eds.) *Assessment of quality of life in clinical trials of cardiovascular therapies.* New York: LeJacq Publishing, Inc.

Ferrans, C. E., & Powers, M. J. (1985). Quality of life index: Development and psychometric properties. *Advances in Nursing Science, 8*(1), 15–24.

Flanders-Stepans, M. B., & Fuller, S. G. (1999). Physiological effects of infant exposure to environmental tobacco smoke: A passive observation study. *The Journal of Perinatal Education, 8,* 10–21.

Flannery, J. (1995). Cognitive assessment in the acute care setting: Reliability and validity of the Levels of Cognitive Functioning Assessment Scale (LOCFAS). *Journal of Nursing Measurement, 3,* 43–58.

Folstein, M. F., Folstein, S. E., & McHugh, P. R. (1975). "Mini-Mental State": A practical method for grading the cognitive state of patients for the clinician. *Journal of Psychiatric Research, 12,* 189–98.

Gigliotti, E. (1997). The relations among maternal and student role involvement, perceived social support and perceived multiple role stress in mothers attending college: A study based on Betty Neuman's systems model. *Dissertation Abstracts International, 58*(01), B. (University Microfilms No. 9718709).

Gigliotti, E. (in press). Development of the perceived multiple role stress scale (PMRS). *Journal of Nursing Measurement.*

Gray-Toft, P., & Anderson, J. G. (1981). Stress among hospital nursing staff: Its causes and effects. *Social Science and Medicine, 15,* 639–47.

Hill, J. E., & Nunney, D. N. (1971). *Personalizing educational programs utilizing cognitive style mapping.* Bloomfield Hills, MI: Oakland Community College Press.

Hoeger, W., Hopkins, D., & Johnson, L. (1988). *Assessment of muscle flexibility.* Addison, IL: Novel Products.

Hungelmann, J., Kenkel-Rossi, E., Klassen, L., Stollenwerk, R. (1989). Development of the JAREL Spiritual Well-Being Scale. In R. M. Carroll-Johnson (Ed.), *Classification of Nursing Diagnoses Proceedings of the Eighth Conference North American Nursing Diagnosis Association* (pp. 393–98). Philadelphia: Lippincott.

Hunt, H., McEwen, J, & McKenna, S. (1986). *Measuring health status.* London: Croom Helm.

Ironson, G. H., Smith, P. C., Brannick, M. R., Gibson, W. M., & Paul, K. B. (1989). Construction of a job in general scale: A comparison of global, composite and specific measures. *Journal of Applied Psychology, 74,* 193–200.

Ivancevich, J. M., Matteson, M. T., & Dorin, F. (1990). *Research on the stress diagnostic survey.* Houston, TX: F.D. Associates.

Loescher, L. J., Clark, L., Atwood, J. R., Leigh, S., & Lamb, G. (1990). The impact of the cancer experience on long-term survivors. *Oncology Nursing Forum, 17,* 223–29.

Linder-Pelz, S., Levy, S., Tamir, A., & Epstein, L. M. (1984). A measure of family-functioning for health care practice and research in Israel. *Journal of Comparative Family Studies, 15,* 211–30.

Lowry, L. W., & Jopp, M. C. (1989). An evaluation instrument for assessing an associate degree nursing curriculum based on the Neuman systems model. In J.P. Riehl-Sisca (Ed.), *Conceptual models for nursing practice* (3rd ed., pp. 73–85). Norwalk, CT: Appleton & Lange.

Maslach, C., & Jackson, S. E. (1986). *The Maslach Burnout Inventory Manual* (2nd ed). Palo Alto, CA: Consulting Psychologists Press.

Melzack, R. (1975). The McGill Pain Questionnaire: Major properties and scoring methods. *Pain, 1,* 275–99.

Miller, J. F., & Powers, M. L. (1988). Development of an instrument to measure hope. *Nursing Research, 37,* 6–9.

Molter, N. (1979). Needs of relatives of critically ill patients: A descriptive study. *Heart and Lung, 8,* 332–39.

Nellcor, Inc. (1986). *User's Manual: Nellcor N-10 Portable Pulse Oximeter.* Hayward, CA: Nellcor, Inc.

Norbeck, J. S., Lindsey, A. M., & Carrieri, V. L. (1981). The development of an instrument to measure social support. *Nursing Research, 30,* 264–69.

Norbeck, J. S., Lindsey, A. M. & Carrieri, V. L. (1983). Further development of the Norbeck Social Support Questionnaire: Normative data and validity testing. *Nursing Research, 32,* 4–9.

Quellette, S. C. (1993). Inquiries into hardiness. In L. Goldberger & S. Breznitz (Eds.), *Handbook of stress: Theoretical and clinical aspects* (2nd ed., pp.16–37). New York: Free Press.

Pines, A., & Aronson, E. (1981). *Career burnout: Causes and cures.* New York: Free Press.

Richards, K. (1987). Techniques for measurement of sleep in critical care. *Focus on Critical Care, 14,* 34–40.

Risser, N. L. (1975). Development of an instrument to measure patient satisfaction with nursing care in primary settings. *Nursing Research, 24,* 45–52.

Rosenbaum, M. (1980). A schedule for assessing self-control behaviors: Preliminary findings. *Behavior Therapy, 11,* 109–21.

Schutzenhofer, K., & Musser, D. (1994). Nurse characteristics and professional autonomy. *Image: Journal of Nursing Scholarship, 26,* 201–204.

Smith, P. C., Kendall, L. M., & Hulin, C. L. (1969). *The measurement of satisfaction in work and retirement.* Chicago: Rand McNally.

Spacelabs, Inc. (1988). *Operations/technical manual 90207 ambulatory blood pressure monitor.* Redman, WA: Spacelabs.

Spielberger, C. D., Gorsuch, R. L., & Lushene, R. E. (1970). *STAI manual for the State-Trait Anxiety Inventory.* Palo Alto, CA: Consulting Psychologists Press.

Spielberger, C., Gorsuch, R., Lushene, R., Vagg, P., & Jacobs, G. (1983). *Manual for the State-Trait Anxiety Inventory.* Palo Alto, CA: Consulting Psychologists Press.

Wallston, K. A., Wallston, B. S., & DeVillis, R. D. (1978). Development of the multidimensional health locus of control (MHLC) scales. *Health Education Monographs, 6*(2), 160–70.

Waltman, N. L. (1990). Attitudes, subjective norms, and behavioral intentions of nurses toward dying patients and their families. *Oncology Nursing Forum, 17*(Suppl. 3), 55–62.

Wilson, D. M., & Ciliska, D. (1984). Lifestyle assessment: Development and use of the FANTASTIC Checklist. *Canadian Family Physician, 30,* 1527–32.

Wilson, D., Evans, C. E., Marshall, J., et al. (1983). The FANTASTIC Lifestyle Questionnaire: Development and preliminary evaluation. In F. Landry (Ed.), *Health risk estimation, risk reduction and health promotion* (pp. 665–70). Ottawa: Canadian Public Health Association.

Yoshitake, H. (1978). Three characteristic patterns of subjective fatigue symptoms. *Ergonomics, 21,* 231–33.

Zarit, S. H. (1990, June). *Concepts and measures in family caregiving research.* Paper presented at the Conference of Conceptual and Methodological Issues in Family Caregiving Research, Toronto, Ontario, Canada.

Ziemer, M. M. (1982). Providing patients with information prior to surgery and the reported frequency of coping behaviors and development of symptoms following surgery. *Dissertation Abstracts International, 43,* 2165B.

Ziemer, M. M. (1983). Effects of information on postsurgical coping. *Nursing Research, 32,* 282–87.

Zung, W. K. (1971). A rating instrument for anxiety disorders. *Psychosomatics, 12,* 371–79.

ten

Using the Neuman Systems Model to Guide Nursing Research in the United States

Diane M. Breckenridge

This chapter presents a description of how the Neuman Systems Model has been used to plan and implement a program of research in the United States. I am a clinical nurse specialist in nephrology nursing who has worked with the Neuman Systems Model since the mid-1970s, and identified a phenomenon of particular research interest when I began doctoral studies 10 years ago, after 15 years of clinical nursing practice. That phenomenon of interest—how, why, and by whom treatment modalities are chosen—has been the basis of my ongoing program of nursing research, which has been guided by the Neuman Systems Model.

FROM NURSING PRACTICE TO NURSING RESEARCH

Fawcett (2000) contends that the nursing science dimension of the professional discipline of nursing is accomplished by nursing research. The product of nursing research is development and dissemination of conceptual–theoretical–empirical (C-T-E) systems of nursing knowledge. Fawcett further contends that there is a reciprocal relationship between nursing research and nursing practice, as well as a reciprocal relationship between C-T-E system development and dissemination and C-T-E system utilization and clinical evaluation. The reciprocal relationship is evident in that clinical practice problems catalyze research and the results of research provide solutions for these clinical problems. The catalyst for my program of research was the clinical question of how, why, and by whom treatment modalities are chosen. The results of the research (Breckenridge, 1995a, 1995b, 1997a, 1997b, 1999) are middle-range theories that are beginning to provide information from the patient's perspective that will foster development of prevention interventions that will promote optimal client system stability.

I am one of the first nurses in the United States to become a master's degree–prepared nephrology clinical nurse specialist. I submitted my view of nephrology nursing practice to Jacqueline Fawcett and Betty Neuman in the late 1970s, who encouraged me to develop a nursing discipline–specific Neuman Systems Model–based health care focus and framework for nephrology nursing practice. This Neuman-based health care focus and framework for nursing practice (Breckenridge 1982, 1989, 1995b) can be used as a generic framework for various patient populations and for others to emulate in their own practice. Similarly, the Neuman Systems Model–based nursing assessment format for renal clients, which I developed with my colleagues (Breckenridge, Cupit, & Raimondo, 1982) can be used as a prototype for development of Neuman Systems Model–based assessment formats for other clinical populations.

My program of research, which began during doctoral study, followed from my clinical work with renal clients. My research program expanded to include clients with prostate cancer during a postdoctoral fellowship. The phenomenon of interest for both patient populations has been patient-focused decision making for treatment options in the discipline-specific practice areas of nephrology and oncology nursing. My overall goal has been to conduct discipline-specific research (Mitchell, 1994) using discipline-specific methodologies (Thorne, Kirkham, & MacDonald-Emes, 1997), and to engage in discipline-specific practice (Smith, 1995) that will enhance the professional discipline of nursing in the United States.

The program of research began with a descriptive theory–generating qualitative study (Breckenridge, 1995), using the interpretive method of naturalistic inquiry (Glaser & Strauss, 1967; Sandelowski, 1995a, 1995b; Strauss & Corbin, 1990). Degner and Beaton's (1987) life–death decisions in health care framework and the Neuman Systems Model (Neuman, 1982, 1989, 1995) guided the research. Inasmuch as the Neuman Systems Model directs researchers to study patients' perceptions, the study was concerned primarily with patients' perceptions of how, why, and by whom their dialysis treatment modality was chosen. The conceptual model concepts of interest were patients' perceptions from the Neuman Systems Model and control over the type of treatment from the Degner and Beaton framework. Data were collected using the Patient Perception Interview Guide. Analysis of the data led to the discovery of the middle-range descriptive classification theory, "Patient's Choice of a Treatment Modality versus Selection of Patient's Treatment Modality" (Figure 10-1) (Breckenridge, 1997b). Fawcett's (1999) analysis of the theory revealed that it was made up of two multidimensional concepts (Figure 10-2).

My secondary analysis of the study data focused on the extent to which the study participants' responses reflected the five Neuman Systems Model client system variables (Breckenridge, 1997a). That analysis revealed that all five client system variables were evident in the participant's responses and led to an expansion of the theory (Figure 10-3).

I then extended my research focus from renal nursing to the more comprehensive area of genitourinary–renal nursing. During postdoctoral work, I replicated the original renal dialysis treatment modality study (Breckenridge, 1997b) with prostate cancer patients who resided in New Jersey or Pennsylvania. The Patient Perception Interview Guide for Prostate Cancer Decision Making (Table 10-1) was used to elicit study participants' perceptions of how, why, and by whom the prostate cancer treatment modality they received was chosen. This interview guide is similar to the guide used in the original

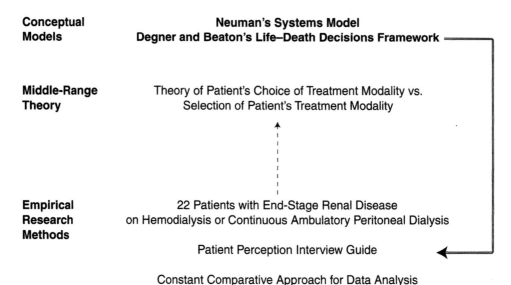

FIGURE 10-1. Conceptual–theoretical–empirical structure for study of renal patients' decision making.

renal dialysis treatment modality study. Analysis of the data revealed a middle-range de-scriptive classification theory of self-decision influencing factors. The core category of the theory of prostate cancer treatment modality decision making was self-decision. Fur-ther analysis of the data revealed four themes that represent factors that influence self-decision: provider influence, immediate family influence, friends/relatives influence, and

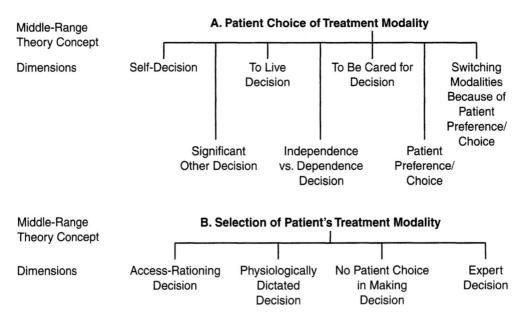

FIGURE 10-2. Concepts of the theory of patient's choice of treatment (**A**) versus selection of treatment modality (**B**) and their dimensions.

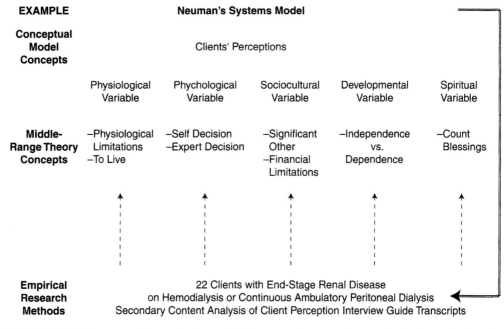

FIGURE 10-3. Conceptual–theoretical–empirical structure for secondary analysis of renal patients' decision making.

TABLE 10-1. The Patient Perception Interview Guide

1. Please tell me how the prostate treatment that you have received or are receiving was selected? Possible probes:
   a. What options were presented to you or did you consider? What did you view as the pros and cons of each option?
   b. What factors did you think about or weigh when making your decision?
   c. Please walk me through the way the decision was made.
      –To what extent did your own opinions influence the selection of treatment?
      –To what extent did your physician's recommendations influence the selection of treatment?
      –To what extent did your nurse influence the selection of treatment?
      –To what extent did a social worker influence the selection of treatment?
      –To what extent did your family influence the selection of treatment?
      –To what extent did someone else (who?) influence the selection of treatment?
      –To what extent did your insurance coverage influence the selection of treatment?
   d. What kind of information was made available to you? What were the sources? Did you actively seek information about the treatment options? If so, what kinds of things did you do? With whom did you talk in order to learn more about the treatment options?
2. What do you like about the treatment you received and/or are receiving?
3. What are the drawbacks to the treatment you received and/or are receiving?
4. Is the treatment you received and/or are receiving still your preferred choice? If no, please explain what other option you would prefer and why you now prefer that option?

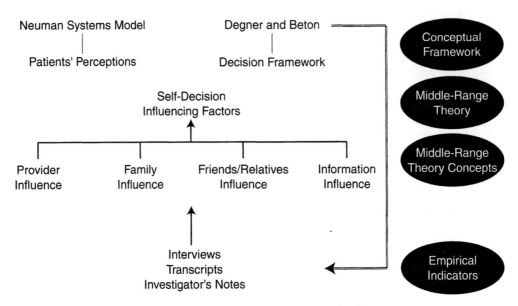

FIGURE 10-4. Conceptual–theoretical–empirical structure for study of prostate cancer patients' decision making.

information influence (Figure 10-4) (Breckenridge, 1999). Next, I replicated the prostate cancer treatment modality study with prostate cancer patients who resided in Missouri. Analysis of the data from this study revealed the same core category of self-decision and the same four themes—provider influence, immediate family influence, friends/relatives influence, and information influence. Another theme also was identified in the responses of the Missouri study participants. This theme represented a spiritual influence on self-decision. The spiritual influence was clearly evident in participants' statements that they made their decisions about prostate cancer treatment modality with "the strong presence of God."

I continued postdoctoral work as an oncology research fellow and completed a secondary content analysis of the data from the two prostate cancer studies. The study participants' responses again reflected the five Neuman Systems Model client system variables (Figure 10-5). Additional research has involved a secondary analysis of the data from the renal and the prostate cancer studies. Once again, the responses reflected all five Neuman Systems Model client system variables (Figure 10-6).

CONCLUSION

The use of the Neuman Systems Model has led to a clear and consistent focus on clients' perceptions of how, why, and by whom treatment modality decisions were made. Moreover, the five Neuman Systems Model client system variables have provided a consistent coding schema for data from two distinct client populations—renal dialysis patients and prostate cancer patients. The nursing discipline–specific middle-range theories that have been generated from the studies represent knowledge that can be used for nursing discipline-specific nephrology practice with renal dialysis patients and for nursing discipline–specific oncology practice with prostate cancer patients. In particular, the

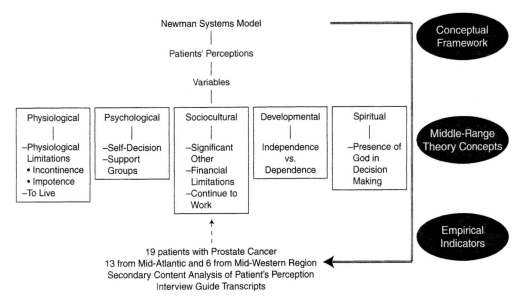

FIGURE 10-5. Conceptual–theoretical–empirical structure for secondary analysis of prostate cancer patients' decision making.

knowledge gained from the studies enhances nurses' understanding of treatment modality decision making and will lead to the development of prevention interventions that foster expression of patients' perceptions of what is involved in decisions about treatment modalities.

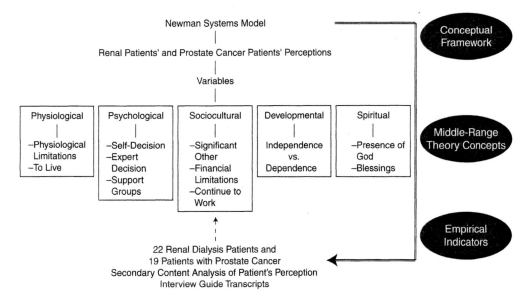

FIGURE 10-6. Conceptual–theoretical–empirical structure for secondary analysis comparing renal patients' and prostate cancer patients' perspective on treatment option decision making.

REFERENCES

Breckenridge, D. M. (1982). Adaptation of Neuman health-care systems model for the renal client. In B. Neuman (Ed.), *The Neuman Systems Model: Application to nursing education and practice* (pp. 267–77). Norwalk, CT: Appleton-Century-Crofts.

Breckenridge, D. M. (1989). Primary prevention as an intervention modality for the renal client. In B. Neuman (Ed.), *The Neuman Systems Model:* (2nd ed., pp. 397–406). Norwalk, CT: Appleton & Lange.

Breckenridge, D. M. (1995a). Nephrology practice and directions for nursing research. In: B. Neuman (Ed.), *The Neuman Systems Model* (3rd ed., pp. 499–507). Norwalk, CT: Appleton & Lange.

Breckenridge, D. M. (1995b). Patient's Choice . . . Is It? A Qualitative Study of Patients' Perceptions of Why, How, and by Whom Dialysis Treatment Modality Was Chosen. Unpublished doctoral dissertation, University of Maryland.

Breckenridge, D. M. (1997a). Decisions regarding dialysis treatment modality: A holistic perspective. *Holistic Nursing Practice, 12*(1), 54–61.

Breckenridge, D. M. (1997b). Patients' perceptions of why, how, and by whom dialysis treatment modality was chosen. *American Nephrology Nurses Association Journal, 24,* 313–19.

Breckenridge, D. M. (1999). Patient Participation in Treatment Decisions for Prostate Cancer. Paper presented at the American Cancer Society 5th National Conference on Cancer Nursing Research, Newport Beach, CA.

Breckenridge, D. M., Cupit, M. C., & Raimondo, J. (1982, January/February). Systematic nursing assessment tool for the CAPD client. *Nephrology Nurse, 24,* 26–27, 30–31.

Degner, L. F., & Beaton, J. I. (1987). *Life–death decisions in health care.* New York: Hemisphere.

Fawcett, J. (1999). *The relationship of theory and research* (3rd ed.). Philadelphia: Davis.

Fawcett, J. (2000). *Analysis and evaluation of contemporary nursing knowledge: Nursing models and theories.* Philadelphia: Davis.

Glaser, B., & Strauss, A. L. (1967). *The discovery of grounded theory: Strategies for qualitative research.* New York: Aldine.

Mitchell, G. (1994). Discipline-specific inquiry: The hermeneutics of theory-guided nursing research. *Nursing Outlook, 42,* 224–28.

Neuman, B. (1982). *The Neuman Systems Model: Application to nursing education and practice.* Norwalk, CT: Appleton-Century-Crofts.

Neuman, B. (1989). *The Neuman Systems Model* (2nd ed.). Norwalk, CT: Appleton & Lange.

Neuman, B. (1995). *The Neuman Systems Model* (3rd ed.). Norwalk, CT: Appleton & Lange.

Sandelowski, M. (1995a). Sample size in qualitative research. *Research in Nursing and Health, 18,* 179–83.

Sandelowski, M. (1995b). Qualitative analysis: What it is and how to begin. *Research in Nursing and Health, 18,* 371–75.

Smith, M. C. (1995). The core of advanced practice nursing. *Nursing Science Quarterly, 8,* 2–3.

Strauss, A., & Corbin, J. (1990). *Basics of qualitative research: Grounded theory procedures and techniques.* Newbury Park, CA: Sage.

Thorne, S., Kirkham, S. R., & MacDonald-Emes, J. (1997). Interpretive description: A noncategorical qualitative alternative for developing nursing knowledge. *Research in Nursing and Health, 20,* 169–77.

eleven

Using the Neuman Systems Model to Guide Nursing Research in Thailand

Linchong Pothiban

The Neuman Systems Model is one of just a few nursing conceptual models that are well known in Thailand. The model was first introduced to Thai nursing circa 1974 in a nursing theory course taught at Mahidol University in Bangkok. That course initially was offered only to master's program students, but now both undergraduate and master's program students take nursing theory courses.

Although students learn about the Neuman Systems Model and other nursing conceptual models, and although the curricula of some schools of nursing in Thailand are based on nursing conceptual models, they rarely are used to guide nursing practice. Furthermore, although students now are learning how to apply nursing conceptual models under the guidance of clinical instructors, many professional nurses lack the theoretical knowledge and clinical skills required to use a conceptual model as a guide for their practice. Similarly, nursing conceptual models rarely are used to guide nursing research in Thailand.

This chapter describes the use of the Neuman Systems Model in nursing research in Thailand.[1] A review of Neuman Systems Model–based nursing research is presented, followed by the report of a Neuman Systems Model–based study conducted by the author.

NEUMAN SYSTEMS MODEL–BASED NURSING RESEARCH IN THAILAND

A review of literature was undertaken to determine the use of nursing conceptual models as guides for Thai nursing research. The review was limited to the 1,720 research papers that were available in the library at the Faculty of Nursing, Chiang Mai University, Chiang Mai, Thailand. Just 274 (15.9 percent) of the 1,720 studies were based on nursing conceptual models, and only 7 (2.6 percent) of the 274 studies were based on the Neuman Systems Model. Two of the 7 were doctoral dissertations (Pothiban, 1993; Sukvattananan, 1997) and 5 were master's theses (Lawang, 1999; Maraphen, 1999; Petchraung, 1999; Rattanalum et al., 1999; Siridumrong, 1999).

Pothiban (1995) conducted a descriptive study to identify the prevalence of risk factors, risk status, and perceived risk for coronary heart disease (CHD) among Thai elderly people. The study was designed to obtain data that could be used for planning primary prevention interventions for clients with CHD. Sukvattananan (1992) examined the relation of extrapersonal stressors, including parental lifestyle, child training, and socioeconomic status, to the health status of preschoolers in the Bangkok metropolitan area.

Siridumrong (1999) used the Neuman Systems Model to categorize the health problems of mothers during the postpartum period. Lawang (1999) identified the physiological, psychological, sociocultural, developmental, and spiritual problems and health care needs of homebound diabetic parents residing in the Bangkok metropolitan area. Petchraung (1999) examined factors related to the physiological, psychological, sociocultural, developmental, and spiritual needs for home care of patients with essential hypertension.

Maraphen (1999) studied the severity of health care problems of heroin addicts seeking care at narcotic clinics in the Bangkok metropolis administration. Rattanalum and colleagues (1999) studied the effects of Neuman Systems Model–based home visits on mothers with 1- to 3-year-old children suffering from acute upper respiratory tract infection.

Although the number of Neuman Systems Model–based studies conducted by Thai nurses may be underestimated due to the limited literature available for this review, it is obvious that there is a paucity of Neuman Systems Model–based Thai nursing research. Clearly, more Neuman Systems Model–based research is needed to more fully understand the health of the Thai people.

REPORT OF A NEUMAN SYSTEMS MODEL–BASED STUDY IN THAILAND

Toward that end, the author conducted an exploratory descriptive study designed to (a) examine the congruence of health as described by Thai elderly clients with health as defined by the Neuman Systems Model, and (b) identify stressors and stressor reactions, as well as the status of the flexible line of defense and the lines of resistance of Thai elderly clients.

Study Methods

The sample was limited to Thai individuals 60 years of age and over, who had intact memory and resided in Chiang Mai municipality. Participants were recruited from the Health Promotion Center for the Elderly, Faculty of Nursing, Chiang Mai University, and at a Health Care Center in Chiang Mai municipality.

The study participants included 24 females and 3 males, ranging in age from 61 to 77 years. Two participants were single, 9 were married, and 16 were widowed. All participants were Buddhist. Their education ranged from grade 4 to college graduate. All participants gave verbal voluntary agreement.

Data were collected by means of focus group interviews and in-depth interviews. Data collectors were three doctoral students and three nursing instructors who knew the study participants. Content analysis was used to analyze the data.

The Meaning of Health

The study participants viewed health as a state of physiological, psychological, and spiritual stability demonstrated by being free from disease, illness, or symptoms; being able to function; and being happy and peaceful. For some participants, the physical state of being healthy was being free from disease, illness, or any symptoms and being strong and active. One participant stated: "I am healthy; I don't have any disease."

Conversely, one participant explained: "I am not completely healthy [because] I have many diseases—cataracts, arthritis, and cervical spondylosis—and I don't feel as good as before." Similarly, another participant commented, "My health is not really good. I don't feel well. The pain in my shoulder and arms is more frequent now."

In contrast, some participants stated that they were healthy while having some disease. One participant, who had cancer, stated: "I am healthy. I can go everywhere I want. I can eat more now." Another participant, who had hypertension, commented, "I am healthy because I can still work. I take medication for my blood pressure every day and it is normal now." These and most other participants regarded health as being able to perform self-care, that is, being able to eat, walk, sleep, work, or do what they wanted to do independently. Similarly, some participants viewed being able to go to the temple and perform religious activities as an indicator for being healthy.

Participants' views of health as a psychological state were reflected in their descriptions of being healthy as a state of feeling good, happiness, having nothing to worry about, being able to think clearly. The participants' descriptions of having good relationships with others, being loved and respected by their own children, and having children or grandchildren around also reflected a view of health as a psychological state.

All participants mentioned that they felt unhealthy when their physical condition changed from normal or was worse than normal; their unhealthy state reflected the instability of the whole body system. All participants also mentioned that their health state was the result of merit and kamma (karma) performed in their last life. People who earn merit are always in good health, whereas those who have negative kamma are in bad health.

Stressors Experienced by Elderly Thai People

In this study, a stressor was defined as a thing that could cause trouble to the individual or could make the individual unhappy. The major stressors reported by the study participants included family problems, physical problems, behavioral problems, economic problems, emotional problems, and social problems. The physical, behavioral, economic, and emotional problems can be categorized as intrapersonal stressors; the family problems, as interpersonal stressors; and the social problems, as extrapersonal stressors.

Family problems that were stressors included children or grandchildren matters, such as children's being stubborn, impolite, ignoring their suggestions; children's behaviors that were not consistent with the elderly person's expectations; children's trouble; or conflicts among children. Other family problem stressors were sickness and death of family members. Examples of participants' comments reflecting family problem stressors are:

> I don't know when my grandson will stop drinking. It makes me feel very unhappy.

> I give many suggestions to them [the children], but they never listen. They may not want me to get involved. That hurts.

> My children don't get along well with each other like other people's children. I think a lot about this.

Noteworthy were the participants' comments that problems pertaining to their grandchildren did not affect them as much as other problems. They explained that they loved and cared for their grandchildren more than their children.

Physical problems that were stressors included diseases or illnesses, disabilities, and physical changes due to aging, such as loss of eyesight or hearing. Behavioral problems that were stressors encompassed lack of exercise; bad eating habits, such as consuming food with high fat and high sodium content and foods that were too spicy; drinking alcohol; smoking; not taking care of self; and working too hard.

Economic problems that were stressors included being poor, having low income, and having no food to eat. Emotional problems that were stressors included being greedy, feeling anger, and loneliness. Social problems that were stressors encompassed being abandoned, living alone, having no one to turn to, and being abused.

Reactions to Stressors

Study participants' reactions to stressors were determined by asking them "What happens when you are under stress or having trouble?" The participants reported psychological and physiological reactions. The psychological reactions were feeling upset, angry, irritable, sad, regretful, lonely, depressed, and not feeling like talking or seeing anybody. The physiological reactions included headaches, tightness in the chest, shortness of breath, chest pains, palpitations, dizziness, feeling uncomfortable, not feeling like eating, and being exhausted.

Lines of Resistance

For the purpose of the study, the lines resistance referred to what could help a person to reduce stress and revert back to normal. The study participants' responses indicated that the nature of the stressor determined what could be done. When confronted with such physical problem stressors as injury, disease, and symptoms, the study participants indicated that physical strength would help to get rid of the abnormality that happened within the body. The participants identified factors that facilitated physical strength, such as lifestyle and learned behaviors. They indicated that they had learned how to behave to relieve symptoms from previous experiences.

When confronted with emotional problem stressors, the lines of resistance encompassed several different factors. One factor was the ability to reappraise the situation and to let go of feeling too much concern. In particular, all participants believed that stress happened because a person appraises a situation as stressful. Therefore, it was very important to reappraise the situation, see it as being changeable over time, and see that all problems have solutions. One participant commented:

> I was so unhappy because my son's business was not good. He invested a lot of money in it and now he has lost all his money. He has family to take care of. I thought a lot about this. I could not help him by giving him money because I didn't have enough money. What I did was support him. Then I realized that whatever will be, will be. He might fail this time and be successful next time. This is life. Thinking like this makes me feel better.

Another participant stated: "I used to worry a lot about my son. He got drunk every day. I told him to stop drinking but he never listened. I told myself that I had already done what I should but he chose to continue. Well! It is his choice. He will learn from what happens sooner or later. I feel okay now."

Another factor was a strong religious belief and acceptance of the "law of kamma." All participants mentioned that what happened in their life was because of kamma or what they did in the past that bears fruit in the present. Therefore, they had to understand the situation and deal with that problem consciously and calmly. The participants also saw that merits made during their life could help against stressful feelings.

Still another factor was the ability to be distracted from a stressful situation by getting involved in other activities, such as talking with others, exercise, watching television, working, gardening, planting, and raising pets. Some participants mentioned that all of those activities required concentration, which helped them to forget their stress.

Flexible and Normal Lines of Defense

The study participants were asked what protected them from stress. That question reflects the flexible line of defense and normal lines of defense. Factors within the normal lines of defense mentioned by the participants were physical strength and mental strength. Typical comments that reflected physical strength were:

> If I am as strong as before, I will not get ill easily like this.

> Whenever I felt exhausted, I am so irritable.

With regard to mental strength, the participants identified factors that protected them from feeling stress, including hardiness, being optimistic, not being too sensitive, not being too obsessive, letting go of stressful things easily, being reasonable, being moderate, not being too serious, and having family support.

Factor within the more dynamic flexible line of defense mentioned by the participants were eating appropriate foods, including lots of vegetables, low-fat foods, and not much meat; being physically active and continuing to work; having enough rest and sleep; and being calm and peaceful.

Discussion of Study Findings

The study participants viewed health as a state of physiological, psychological, and spiritual well-being. Furthermore, health was viewed as the degree of stability of the wholistic self at some point in time, resulting from positive kamma. The study participants' view of health is consistent with the Neuman Systems Model.

The inclusion of the study participants' spiritual beliefs as part of their view of health is rooted in Buddhist doctrine. In Buddhism, people understand the reality of life under the law of kamma. Every one is subject to his or her own kamma, heir to the effects of his or her own will and actions. This understanding leads to the suppression of egocentric contemplation and results in the attainment of a state of equanimity (Somdet Phra Nyanasamvara, 1997) and helps the person to remain calm in the face of difficulties in life (Tongprateep, 2000). The understanding that suffering is caused by desires, concerns, or bonds to factors causing stress also comes from Buddhism. Buddhists believe that letting go of the bonds will relieve the suffering. Therefore, managing one's own heart is a key to a peaceful mind, which the study participants identified as a line of resistance to stress.

The study results indicated that family problems were the major stressors for this sample of elderly Thai clients. The participants' responses revealed the characteristics of family in Thai culture—an extended family with prominent close relationships among family members. Therefore, the main concern of the elderly is the family, especially the children or grandchildren. Most study participants mentioned that they always got more involved with their grandchildren than with their children; their grandchildren always got their attention. The bond with grandchildren seemed to be very tight and could cause a lot of suffering.

The study findings also indicated that the flexible and normal lines of defense were consistent with the Neuman Systems Model. Psychological strength was viewed as the major buffer for the normal state. The beliefs that that a healthy mind results in a healthy body and that spirit controls mind and mind controls body are in keeping with Buddhism. These beliefs also are consistent with the Neuman Systems Model, especially with regard to the interaction of the spiritual and physiological client system variables.

Implications for Future Utilization of the Neuman Systems Model in Thai Nursing Research

The results of the study revealed the major role of spiritual factors in all parts of the client system and confirmed Neuman's statement that the spiritual variable permeates all other client system variables. Knowledge of spirituality is, however, still limited and needs to be investigated cross-culturally.

Furthermore, inasmuch as the study results cannot be generalized to other groups of Thai people, similar studies should be conducted using various other groups. In addition, all concepts of the Neuman Systems Model should be explored further, as should the present study finding that a healthy state can be perceived even when the client has some disease. Prevention interventions that will help ill clients feel capable and peaceful should be developed.

The study reported here is just one example of Neuman Systems Model–based Thai nursing research. It is recommended that other studies be designed to test the following hypotheses, which are derived from the Neuman Systems Model, in various Thai populations:

- Factors considered as flexible lines of defense can predict the health state of the client.
- Risk factor modification can predict the health state of the client.
- Empowerment programs can strengthen the flexible and normal lines of defense.
- Strengthening the lines of resistance can maintain the health state of the client.
- Factors considered as lines of resistance can reduce stress or can be related negatively to stress.
- Primary prevention can prevent health deviation and retain a healthy state.
- Secondary prevention can reduce stress and increase a client's comfort.
- Tertiary prevention can decrease duration of hospitalization and the incidence of complications among ill clients.

CONCLUSION

Nursing is regarded as a professional discipline (Donaldson & Crowley, 1978), and nurses work together with other health care professionals to provide direct service to individuals and groups of individuals (Johnson, 1959). Neuman (1995) maintains that the ultimate goals of nursing are to retain, attain, and maintain the optimal health of individuals and groups. Nurses have to apply unique knowledge to achieve these goals in practice. Nursing knowledge is developed primarily by means of nursing research. But research without theory does not contribute to the advancement of nursing knowledge. Rather, research and theory must be integrated to advance nursing knowledge. The relationship between theory and research may be thought of as a double helix (Fawcett, 1978). The core of the double helix is the pairing of theory development with the research process. Theory directs research, and research findings shape the development of theory. To advance the body of nursing knowledge, therefore, all phases of the research process have to be guided by a nursing conceptual model or a theory.

The Neuman Systems Model is one conceptual model that can be used to guide nursing research (see Chapter 7). As more nurses in Thailand and other countries appreciate the need to develop a unique body of nursing knowledge, use of the Neuman Systems Model as a guide for nursing research needs to be encouraged. This chapter and other chapters in this book have contributed to understanding the utility of the Neuman Systems Model for research (see Chapters 8, 9, and 10) and practice (see Chapters 2 through 6). Nursing leaders in Thailand and elsewhere must contribute their support and the resources necessary to advance conceptual model–based research in general and Neuman Systems Model–based research in particular.

ENDNOTE

1. The assistance of Dr. Kanokporn Sucamvang, Ms. Waraporn Lertponwilaikul, Ms. Varin Binhosen, Ms. Vallapa Khunsongkiat, and Ms. Supap Areeua with data collection is acknowledged and greatly appreciated.

REFERENCES

Donaldson, S. K., & Crowley, D. M. (1978). The discipline of nursing. *Nursing Outlook, 26,* 113–20.

Fawcett, J. (1978). The relationship between theory and research: A double helix. *Advances Nursing Science, 1*(1), 46–62.

Johnson, D. E. (1959). The nature of a science in nursing. *American Journal of Nursing, 59,* 291–94.

Lawang, W. (1999). Problems and health care needs of diabetic patients staying at home in the Bangkok metropolitan area. Unpublished master's thesis, Mahidol University, Bangkok, Thailand.

Maraphen, R. (1999). Health care problems: Heroin addicts seeking care. Unpublished master's thesis. Mahidol University, Bangkok, Thailand.

Neuman, B. (1995). *The Neuman Systems Model* (3rd ed.). Norwalk, CT: Appleton & Lange.

Petchraung, N. (1999). Factors related to the needs for home care of patients with essential hypertension. Unpublished master's thesis, Mahidol University, Bangkok, Thailand.

Pothiban, L. (1993). Risk factor prevalence, risk status and perceived risk for coronary heart disease. *Nursing Newsletter, 22*(1), 1–11.

Rattanalum, W., Sukvattananan, V., Siengsanor, C., & Ruchirarat, D. (1999). The effect of Neuman System Model on mothers with 1–3 year old children suffering from acute upper respiratory tract infection in Muang District, Nakornnayok province, *Journal of Public Health Nursing, 13,* 70–79.

Siridumrong, N. (1999). Factors related to health problems of mothers during the postpartum period at home. Unpublished master's thesis. Mahidol University, Bangkok, Thailand.

Somdet Phra Nyanasamvara, H. H. (1997). What did the Buddha teach? In K. Soonsawad, T. Tepsithar, & V. Amornvorapipatana (Eds.), *Visakha Buja B.E. 2540* (pp. 7–15). Bangkok: Sahadhamika.

Sukvattananan, V. (1997). The relationship between parental life style, child training in personal hygiene, and health status of the preschoolers in Bangkok metropolitan area. Unpublished doctoral dissertation, Mahidol University, Bangkok, Thailand.

Tongprateep, T. (2000). The essential elements of spirituality among rural Thai elders. *Journal of Advanced Nursing, 31,* 197–203.

THE NEUMAN
SYSTEMS MODEL AND
NURSING EDUCATION

twelve

Guidelines for Neuman Systems Model–Based Education for the Health Professions

Diana M. L. Newman, Betty Neuman, Jacqueline Fawcett

The Neuman Systems Model was developed as a way to organize clinical course content (Neuman & Young, 1972). The potential of the model for use as a guide for the entire curriculum soon was recognized. Later, the potential of the model as a guide for education in other health care disciplines was recognized (Toot & Schmoll, 1995). When used as a guide for education, the focus of the four nursing metaparadigm concepts is modified. *Person* becomes the learners in the educational program, and *environment* becomes the surroundings of the learners, the teacher–learner interactions, and the settings in which education for the health professions takes place. *Health* becomes the curriculum that promotes teachers' ability to communicate content effectively and efficiently, and learners' ability to comprehend and apply content, as well as the advancement of the health care discipline of interest. *Nursing* becomes the teaching, learning, and advising strategies used by teachers.

This chapter identifies guidelines for Neuman Systems Model–based education for the health professions. The chapter also presents prototype curricula for associate degree, baccalaureate degree, and master's degree nursing education programs based on the Neuman Systems Model.

THE NEUMAN SYSTEMS MODEL EDUCATION GUIDELINES

Rudimentary guidelines for Neuman Systems Model–based nursing education were extracted from the content of the model several years ago (Fawcett, 1989) and were refined over time (Fawcett, 1995, 2000). The refinements in the guidelines were the direct result of the growing literature about the use of the Neuman Systems Model in nursing education programs (see especially Johnson, 1989; Lowry, 1988, 1998; Mirenda, 1986; Neuman, 1985, 1995; Ross, Bourbonnais, & Carroll, 1987; Strickland-Seng, Mirenda, & Lowry, 1996). The most recent refinements, which are the result of dialogue among the three authors of this chapter, are presented in Table 12-1. Although the guidelines initially were targeted to nursing education, our interest in the multidisciplinary use of the Neuman Systems Model called for the extrapolation of the guidelines to education for all health professions. Consequently, the guidelines listed in Table 12-1 have been written for educators and students in all health care disciplines.

The first guideline stipulates that the focus of a Neuman Systems Model–based educational program is on the client system's reaction to environmental stressors. This means that the curriculum must emphasize clients' perceptions of intrapersonal, interpersonal, and extrapersonal stressors, and that the curriculum must take into account the possibility of both noxious and beneficial stressors. The first guideline also stipulates that the purpose of education for the health professions is to facilitate the design and use of primary, secondary, and tertiary prevention-as-intervention modalities by learners and teachers, and to assist client systems to retain, attain, and maintain optimal wellness. This means that, in concert with the first aspect of this guideline, the ultimate goal of the curriculum is to help learners to implement prevention interventions that will strengthen clients' lines of defense and resistance against environmental stressors.

The second guideline stipulates that the content of a Neuman Systems Model–based curriculum encompasses all of the concepts of the model. This means that the content of program courses encompasses individual, family, and community client systems; physiological, psychological, sociocultural, developmental, and spiritual variables; the central

TABLE 12-1. Guidelines for Neuman Systems Model–Based Education

1. Focus of the Curriculum	The focus of a Neuman Systems Model–based educational program is on the client system's reaction to environmental stressors. The purpose of education for the health professions is to facilitate the design and use of primary, secondary, and tertiary prevention-as-intervention modalities by learners and teachers to assist client systems to retain, attain, and maintain optimal wellness.
2. Nature and Sequence of Content	The content of a Neuman Systems Model–based curriculum encompasses all of the concepts of the model. The sequence of content may be guided by the complexity of interactions among the concepts or by the prevention-as-intervention modalities.
3. Settings for Education for the Health Care Professions	Education can occur in vocational and technical programs, hospital-based nursing diploma programs, associate degree programs, baccalaureate programs, and graduate programs.
4. Characteristics of Learners	Learners who meet the requirements for any type of nursing education program must have the ability to engage in high-level critical thinking. Learners also must be willing to engage in both cooperative and independent learning.
5. Teaching–Learning Strategies	Teaching–learning strategies include a variety of modalities that foster critical thinking, as well as cooperative and independent learning.

core; the flexible and normal lines of defense and the lines of resistance; the internal, external, and created environments; intrapersonal, interpersonal, and extrapersonal stressors; client system stability, variances from wellness, and reconstitution; and primary, secondary, and tertiary prevention interventions.

The second guideline also stipulates that the sequence of content may be guided by the complexity of interactions among the Neuman Systems Model concepts or by the prevention-as-intervention modalities. This means that the content of the Neuman Systems Model should direct the sequence of content. For example, the concepts of the Neuman Systems Model can be introduced in first-level courses and then explored in depth in subsequent courses. The emphasis on concepts varies according to the focus of each course and the client system of interest. Integration of concepts occurs from the beginning to the end of the program and increases in complexity toward the final course. The final course in the program emphasizes the complex integration of all Neuman Systems Model concepts in a wholistic manner.

The third guideline stipulates that education can occur in vocational and technical programs, hospital-based nursing diploma programs, associate degree programs, baccalaureate programs, and graduate programs. This guideline alerts educators to consider how best to ensure consistency between the Neuman Systems Model–based curriculum and the terminal objectives of the program.

The fourth guideline stipulates that learners who meet the requirements for any type of Neuman Systems Model–based educational program for the health professions must have the ability to engage in high-level critical thinking. Learners also must be willing to engage in both cooperative and independent learning. This means that learners must be able to offer constructive criticism and engage in logical reasoning. They also must be willing to share information, ask questions, consider different perspectives, and construct knowledge from discourse.

The fifth guideline stipulates that teaching–learning strategies include a variety of modalities that foster critical thinking, as well as cooperative and independent learning. Specific strategies include the use of a visual representation of the content of the Neuman Systems Model (Johnson, 1989) and *The Nurse Theorists: Portraits of Excellence—Betty Neuman* videotape or CD (Neuman, 1988). Classroom teaching–learning strategies include lectures and discussion about the individual, the family, and the community-as-client systems; small group activities, such as games, crossword puzzles, and simulation games (Busch & Lynch, 1998); keeping a journal of thoughts and questions about the model; and case studies of simulated client situations to test learners' assessment and decision-making skills. Clinical experiences are in various hospital-, home-, and community-based settings and focus on use of the Neuman Systems Model Process Format with diverse individual, family, and community client systems.

IMPLEMENTING THE NEUMAN SYSTEMS MODEL IN NURSING EDUCATION PROGRAMS

The Context of Nursing Education

Nursing education in the twenty-first century presents challenges and opportunities for nurse educators unlike those of the twentieth century. These challenges and opportunities arise from uncharted territory and a paradigm shift. In the past, federal and state governments were viewed as the primary resources for societal needs, such as health care, education, and transportation. For example, federal legislation created the Medicare and Medicaid programs, which are funded with federal tax dollars (Lindeman, 2000). In the late twentieth century, it became apparent that there were insufficient federal funds to meet the many social, economic, health care, and education demands of citizens in the United States. Congress's failure to pass legislation that would introduce national health care reform in 1994 reinforced the notion that the market, rather than the federal government, is the preferred manager of escalating health care costs in the United States. Managed care plans, for-profit hospitals, and health plans currently are growing faster than the not-for-profit sector. Thus, the market has control over health care revenue and utilization factors. As a consequence, nurse educators must design programs to prepare students to practice in the competitive, market-driven world of health care (Lindeman, 2000).

Furthermore, nurse educators must structure learning experiences in an environment of rapidly changing technology (Lindeman, 2000). Indeed, technology has universally revolutionized both professional and nonprofessional education for learners of all ages. Distance learning and online education are common teaching–learning strategies, and interactive technology allows nurses to manage patients from afar. Such technology provides opportunities that may increase access to health care for many people and prevent hospitalizations.

Changing demographics in the United States, such as an increase in nonwhite populations and immigrants, the lowering of the birth rate, and the increase in the number of older persons, particularly those over 85 years of age, also have an impact on nursing education. Indeed, nurse educators have to take into account the diverse learning styles of multicultural students and the health-related values and beliefs of a multicultural patient population (Lindeman, 2000).

Moreover, the knowledge explosion has had an impact on nursing education. The ever-expanding body of knowledge must be understood and evaluated for applicability to nursing education. Moreover, nurse educators have to remain flexible and open in their approach to knowledge development, dissemination, and application.

The Accrediting Organizations

Nurse educators assign great value to accreditation of nursing education programs, which currently is carried out by the Commission on Collegiate Nursing Education (CCNE)—the accrediting arm of the American Association of Colleges of Nursing (AACN)—and the National League for Nursing Accrediting Commission (NLNAC). The CCNE accredits baccalaureate and master's degree programs; the NLNAC accredits associate, baccalaureate, and master's degree programs.

The essential knowledge, values, and professional behaviors expected of baccalaureate nursing program graduates have been delineated by the ACCN (1998) (Table 12-2). The AACN recommendations for content for master's programs in advanced practice nursing are listed in Table 12-3. The recommended content for master's programs is based on the premise that the "primary focus of the master's education program should be the clinical role" (AACN, 1998, p. 3). Clinical roles in advanced practice nursing encompass nurse practitioner, nurse anesthetist, nurse–midwife, and clinical nurse specialist (AACN, 1998). Moreover, advanced practice nursing includes application of the content areas of the case management process and educational theories and methods (AACN, 1998). The CCNE has used the essentials listed in Table 12-2 and the content recommendations

TABLE 12-2. American Association of Colleges of Nursing: Essentials of Professional Nursing Education—Baccalaureate Nursing Programs, 1998

Liberal Education

Professional Values: Altruism, Autonomy, Human Dignity, Integrity, Social Justice

Core Competencies: Critical Thinking, Communication, Assessment, Technical Skills

Core Knowledge: Health Promotion, Risk Reduction, and Disease Prevention; Illness and Disease Management; Information and Health Care Technologies; Ethics; Human Diversity; Global Health Care; Health Care Systems and Policy

Role Development: Provider of Care, Designer, Manager, Coordinator of Care; Member of a Profession

---

listed in Table 12-3 to define professional nursing standards and to identify guidelines for the accreditation of baccalaureate and master's degree nursing programs.

The NLNAC uses performance indicators to document the educational effectiveness of associate, baccalaureate, and master's degree nursing programs. The performance indicators are delineated in four required outcomes and various optional outcomes. The four required outcomes are critical thinking, communication, therapeutic intervention, and patterns of employment. The optional outcomes are professional development, personal development, attainment of credentials, organization or work environment, scholarship, service, and nursing unit defined. The faculty of any educational program requesting accreditation by the NLNAC must address the four required outcomes and two of the optional outcomes (NLNAC, 1997).

Critical Thinking

Critical thinking has been identified by both the AACN and the NLNAC as essential for educational effectiveness in nursing education. The importance of critical thinking to

TABLE 12-3. American Association of Colleges of Nursing: Essential Content of Master's Education for Advanced Practice Nursing, 1996

Graduate Curriculum Core Content

Research

Policy, Organization, and Financing of Health Care: Health Care Policy, Organization of the Health Care Delivery System, Health Care Financing

Ethics

Professional Role Development

Theoretical Foundations of Nursing Practice

Human Diversity and Social Issues

Health Promotion and Disease Prevention

Advanced Practice Nursing Core

Advanced Health/Physical Assessment
Advanced Physiology and Pathophysiology
Advanced Pharmacology

nursing education is attested to by the frequency with which the topic appears in the literature.

Colucciello (1997) suggested that nurses can "ultimately enhance the quality of their practice by examining their thinking" (p. 237). The use of lecture and discussion as a teaching–learning strategy may inhibit critical thinking by limiting the reciprocal exchange of knowledge between teacher and student, especially if minimal discussion occurs. Furthermore, if processes of reasoning are discouraged, consideration of various points of view will be limited. Indeed, any strategy that encourages passive learning will lessen inquiry and present few challenges to students' thinking. In contrast, critical thinking is promoted by teaching–learning strategies that foster truth seeking, open-mindedness, analytic skills, systematic thinking, self-confidence, inquisitiveness, and maturity (Colucciello, 1997). Critical thinking also is promoted by questions that call for clarity and depth of thinking rather than mere recitation of facts.

The Neuman Systems Model and Nursing Education

The Neuman Systems Model is an appropriate framework for nursing curricula in the twenty-first century. More specifically, the Neuman Systems Model provides an organized, specific, cohesive, and systems-based framework to guide the design and implementation of nursing education programs within the context of a market-driven economy and health care environment, increased use of technology, a multicultural society, the knowledge explosion, requirements of accrediting bodies for undergraduate and graduate education, and the emphasis on critical thinking. The following section presents ideal curricula for Neuman Systems Model–based baccalaureate degree, associate degree, and master's degree nursing education programs. Every class for every course in these curricula includes consideration of the five Neuman Systems Model client system variables (physiological, psychological, sociocultural, developmental, and spiritual). In addition, all nursing process content is consistent with the Neuman Systems Model Nursing Process Format, such that students are taught how to elicit client perceptions and to document their own perceptions, and consideration is given to intrapersonal, interpersonal, and extrapersonal stressors, the five client system variables, and strengths and weaknesses of the lines of defense and resistance. The students also learn how to collect clinical information for nursing diagnosis, set nursing goals, and implement and evaluate nursing outcomes.

The Ideal Neuman Systems Model–Based Baccalaureate Nursing Education Program

Baccalaureate degree nursing programs prepare graduates for the roles of provider of care, designer of care, manager of care, coordinator of care, and member of the nursing profession (AACN, 1998). Inherent in these practice roles are a liberal education, as well as the professional values, core competencies, and core knowledge listed in Table 12-2.

The ideal Neuman Systems Model–based baccalaureate nursing program comprises 126 credits—42 nursing credits, 33 allied requirement credits, 17 general elective credits, and 34 core requirements. The allied requirements include courses in microbiology, human anatomy and physiology, inorganic and organic chemistry, introductory statistics, general psychology, nutrition, and principles of sociology. The microbiology, anatomy and physiology, and chemistry courses all include a one-credit laboratory session.

The core requirements include a campus-wide freshman experience, along with courses in effective writing with computers, public speaking, English literature, art or music, one or more foreign languages, history, diversity, ethics, philosophy, and religion (Neumann College Department of Nursing, 2000) The general elective courses can be from any discipline.

The nursing courses begin in the spring of the sophomore year (Table 12-4). The first course, Foundations of Professional Nursing, is a three-credit course, with three hours of classroom instruction each week. The content of this course includes nursing history, the ways of knowing in nursing, and an introduction to the Neuman Systems Model and the Neuman Systems Model Process Format. The course also includes basic content related to individual, family, and community client systems. Assignments include interviews with one individual and one family using the Neuman Systems Model Process Format.

Ten credits in nursing courses are taken during the first semester of the junior year. The nursing course, Primary Preventions 1, is taken at this time. This 3.5-credit course includes 2 credit hours of classroom instruction and 1.5 credit hours of clinical experience with elderly clients and their families each week; classroom instruction is 2 clock hours and the clinical experience is 5 clock hours per week. Inasmuch as the focus of the course is on primary prevention interventions, the clients must be well. Alternatively, clients may be recovering from illness, because the tertiary prevention interventions they require lead back to primary prevention interventions when considering the client's condition in relation to environmental stressors. Clinical experiences with both well and recovering clients is consistent with the Neuman Systems Model focus on primary prevention as health promotion, health maintenance, and illness prevention; and tertiary prevention as wellness maintenance or return to wellness following treatment. Clinical sites for Primary Preventions 1 include skilled nursing facilities, senior centers, and community nursing centers where senior citizens are found.

Primary Preventions 2, which also is taken in the first semester of the junior year, is a 3.5-credit course that emphasizes the developing family as the client system. The credit and clock hour allocations for classroom and clinical experiences are the same as for Primary Preventions 1. The specific clinical foci are antepartal, intrapartal, and postpartal care of low-risk pregnant women and their families. Clinical sites for this course include the labor, delivery, and postpartum units of hospitals; birthing centers; antepartal and postpartal clinics; and clients' homes. Assignments for Primary Preventions 1 and 2 include the application of the Neuman Systems Model Process Format to three different clients for each course and a teaching–learning project for each course. Content about cultural diversity is threaded throughout these courses. Paper and pencil tests measure the students' comprehension of didactic course content.

Another first semester junior year course is Health Assessment and Modalities 1. This three-credit course is made up of 2 credits of classroom instruction and 1.5 laboratory credit hours; classroom instruction is 2 clock hours and the laboratory experience is 3 clock hours each week. The course content encompasses health assessment; hygiene; comfort measures; safety; body mechanics; documentation; and medication calculation, preparation, and administration.

Ten credits in nursing courses also are taken during the second semester of the junior year. The focus of this semester is universal stressors, such as change, intolerance, excess/deprivation, and loss. The courses Secondary Preventions 1 and Secondary Preventions 2 have the same credit allocations for classroom instruction and clinical experiences

TABLE 12-4. Topical Outline of the Ideal Neuman Systems Model–Based Baccalaureate Nursing Program

Year, Semester, and Course	Topic
Sophomore Year, Spring Semester	
Foundations of Professional Nursing	History of Nursing
	Philosophy of Nursing
	Ways of Knowing
	Introduction to the Neuman Systems Model
	The Nursing Process
	The Research Process
	Individual, Family, and Community Client Systems
Junior Year, Fall Semester	
Primary Preventions 1 (Later Maturity)	Developmental Concepts Across the Life Span
	Sociocultural Concepts of Later Maturity
	Spiritual Assessment Across the Life Span
	Psychological Assessment of the Older Adult
	Nursing Care of the Client in Later Maturity
	Alzheimer's Disease; Dementia, Depression, Delirium
	Health Concerns of Young and Middle-Aged Adults
	Assessment of Client Sexuality
	Primary and Early Secondary Prevention for the Adult Client at Risk for Developing Soft Tissue Trauma (prevention and treatment of bedsores)
	Teaching–Learning Process
	Primary and Early Secondary Preventions for the Adult Client Experiencing Pain
	The Client in the Community—Health Planning, Wellness
	Occupational Health
	Continuity of Care Through Discharge Planning
Primary Preventions 2 (The Developing Family)	Primary and Early Secondary Preventions for the Childbearing Family: Antepartum, Labor and Delivery, Normal Newborn, Postpartum, Parent–Infant Attachment/Bonding
	Primary Prevention: Infancy, Toddler, Preschooler, School Age, Adolescent
	Prevention of Childhood Communicable Disease
	Childbearing Family
	Sexuality and Reproductive Decision Making
Health Assessment and Modalities 1	Safety
	Medical Asepsis/Universal Precautions
	Body Mechanics, Alignment
	Range of Motion
	Positioning

TABLE 12-4. Topical Outline of the Ideal Neuman Systems Model–Based Baccalaureate Nursing Program *(continued)*

Year, Semester, and Course	Topic
Junior Year, Fall Semester *(continued)*	
Health Assessment and Modalities 1 *(continued)*	Hygiene, Comfort
	Bed Making
	Medications
	Nutrition, Elimination
	Documentation
	Vital Signs
	Health Assessment: Interviewing and the Health History—General Survey; Skin, Hair, and Nails; Assessment of Abdomen, Anus, Rectosigmoid Region; Respiratory System; Cardiovascular System; Breasts and Regional Lymphatics; Peripheral Vascular System; Eyes and Ears; Face, Head, and Neck; Female Genitalia; Male Genitalia; Musculoskeletal System; Neurological System
Junior Year, Spring Semester	
Secondary Preventions 1 (Stressors: Adults and Children)	Fluid and Electrolytes (Adult and Child)
	Alterations in Gastrointestinal Functions (Adult and Child)
	Alterations in Genetic Patterns
	Alterations in Metabolism (Adult, Pregnancy, Child)
	Alteration in Respiration (Child)
	Alteration in Circulation (Child)
	Infection and Immunity (Child)
	Infection and Communicable Diseases (Adult and Child)
	Alteration in Nervous System (Child)
	Loss/Developmental (Grief Response in Children)
	Impaired Physical Mobility (Adult and Child)
Secondary Preventions 2 (Stressors: Mental Health)	Therapeutic Relationships
	Change Modalities
	Impact of Illness on the Family
	Anxiety Disorders
	Alterations Related to Stress
	Alterations in Relatedness (Schizophrenia)
	Crisis Intervention
	Loss/Alteration in Mood
	Clients with Serious Mental Illness
	Clients with Emotional Problems
	Clients, Families, and Violence
	Eating Disorders
	Substance Abuse
	Dissociative Disorders
	Personality Disorders
Introduction to Nursing Research	Overview of Nursing Research
	Research Problems, Questions, Purposes, and Hypotheses

TABLE 12-4. Topical Outline of the Ideal Neuman Systems Model–Based Baccalaureate Nursing Program *(continued)*

Year, Semester, and Course	Topic
Junior Year, Spring Semester *(continued)*	
Introduction to Nursing Research *(continued)*	Conceptual Models
	Review of the Literature
	Quantitative and Qualitative Designs
	Populations, Samples, Measurement, and Data Collection
	Data Analysis—Understanding Statistics
	Ethics in Nursing Research
	Research Utilization
Senior Year, Fall Semester	
Tertiary Preventions 1 (Complex Stressors; Adults as Clients)	Coronary Artery Disease
	Congestive Heart Failure
	Vascular Disorders
	Hematologic Disorders
	Hypertension
	Cerebral Vascular Disease
	Clients with Respiratory Disorders
	Clients with Artificial Airways
	Client on a Ventilator
	Client with Cancer
	Client with Burns
Tertiary Preventions 2 (Complex Stressors: Community as Client)	Health Education
	Caseload Management
	Community Health: High-Risk Aggregate
	Environmental Health and Safety; Consumerism
	Concepts of Home Health Nursing
	Hospice
	World Health Organization
	Global Health Issues
Economic, Legal, and Political Issues in Nursing and Health Care	Medicare, Medicaid, Managed Care
	Insurance Companies
	Financing of Nursing and Health Care
	Nurse Practice Acts
	Health Care Policy
	Local, Regional, National, and International Political Influences on Nursing and Health Care
Senior Year, Spring Semester	

Note: Wholistic Nursing 1 and Wholistic Nursing 2 share the same classroom content. However, the practicum for Wholistic Nursing 1 is in institutions, and in the community for Wholistic Nursing 2

Wholistic Nursing 1 (Integration of Preventions: Adult as Client)	Concepts of Rehabilitation/Reconstitution
	Rehabilitation Across the Life Span
	Chronic Illness
	Brain Injury

TABLE 12-4. Topical Outline of the Ideal Neuman Systems Model–Based Baccalaureate Nursing Program *(continued)*

Year, Semester, and Course	Topic
Senior Year, Spring Semester *(continued)*	
Wholistic Nursing 2	Spinal Cord Injury
(Community as Client)	Urologic Problems; Acute and Chronic Renal Failure
	Client with HIV/AIDS
	Leadership
	Conflict Resolution
	Student-Led Seminars
Independent Study	Students Select Topic:
	Research Assistant for Faculty Research Project
	Community Nursing Center
	High-Risk Population
	Health Care Policy
	Other

as Primary Preventions 1 and 2. Clinical experiences for Secondary Preventions 1 are with adults and children and their families; the client populations include adults and children with diabetes, orthopedic problems, and gastrointestinal problems. Clinical sites include adult and pediatric acute care units of hospitals. Other sites for clinical experiences may be homes or outpatient units in which adult and pediatric acute care patients are found. Clinical experiences for Secondary Preventions 2 are with adults with acute and chronic mental health and psychiatric problems and their families. Clinical sites include inpatient and outpatient psychiatric units and clients' homes. Students participate in the implementation of a variety of prevention interventions, including individual and group therapy and crisis intervention. Assignments for Secondary Preventions 1 and 2 include three nursing care plans and weekly process recordings for each course. In addition, the students submit one written report of a Neuman Systems Model–based assessment of a family with an ill member during the semester. The family may be a real or fictional one found in an assigned book, movie, or video, or a real family seen as part of the student's clinical experiences. Classroom content is evaluated by paper-and-pencil tests.

The other nursing course taken in the second semester of the junior year is Introduction to Nursing Research. This didactic three-credit course, with three hours of classroom instruction each week, focuses on the basic research process and research critique. Students critique reports of research that is based on the Neuman Systems Model or another conceptual model of nursing. Students in good academic standing may participate in faculty research projects as data collectors, with permission of the faculty. Assignments include written research critiques and paper-and-pencil tests.

Ten credits in nursing courses are again taken in the first semester of the senior year. Tertiary Preventions 1 and Tertiary Preventions 2 have the same credit allocation as the clinical nursing courses taken in the junior year. The focus of Tertiary Preventions 1 is on clients with cardiac, renal, and neurological problems and their families, who are experiencing complex stressors. The course emphasizes maximizing and maintaining optimal levels of wellness for clients who have experienced a crisis and for whom some degree of reconstitution/rehabilitation has occurred, as well as assisting clients who are dying and their families. Course content includes study of selected stressors causing acute and chronic illness over the life span (Neumann College Department of Nursing, 2000). Assignments include three nursing care plans and paper-and-pencil tests of didactic content. Tertiary Preventions 2 focuses on clients and their families in the community. Emphasis is placed on the significance of community-based nursing to assist clients to attain, maintain, and retain health. Clinical experiences occur in visiting nurse services, schools, community nursing centers, and home care agencies. Assignments once again include three nursing care plans and paper-and-pencil tests.

The other first-semester senior year nursing course is Economic, Legal, and Political Aspects of Health Care. This three-credit course includes content about Medicare, Medicaid, and managed care; legal aspects of nursing and health care, including health policy; and current political issues affecting nursing and health care. Assignments include visits to local and state legislators to discuss current economic, legal, and political issues; classroom debates about current issues; and a written report about an economic, legal, or political issue that affects nursing and health care, along with paper-and-pencil tests.

Ten credits in nursing courses are once again taken in the second semester of the senior year. Wholistic Nursing 1 and Wholistic Nursing 2 carry the same credit allocation as other clinical nursing courses. Wholistic Nursing 1 focuses on leadership management experiences with groups of learners and clients. The experiences typically occur in inpatient settings with students alternating in the roles of leader and team member; students may select the particular setting for this experience from medical–surgical units, postpartal units, and inpatient psychiatric units. Assignments include written reports about the roles of health care providers in a nursing unit. Wholistic Nursing 2 focuses on leadership in the assessment of community-based high-risk populations, such as clients with high-risk pregnancies, clients with acquired immune deficiency syndrome (AIDS), the frail elderly, clients newly emigrated to the United States, migrant workers, or those particular populations at risk in the community served by the nursing education program. Assignments include written reports about a particular population, using the Neuman Systems Model as a framework for assessment. Classroom experiences for both courses are student-led seminars. Paper-and-pencil tests evaluate didactic content.

The final nursing course in the curriculum is a two-credit independent study. Typical experiences for this course include but are not limited to working with faculty on a research project, working in a community nursing center, and following a bill that will have an impact on nursing and health care in the legislature. Students negotiate specific assignments with the faculty member who oversees the independent study work. Faculty and on-site preceptors are available to facilitate the student's learning.

The required nursing courses are augmented by elective courses in pharmacology, pathophysiology, and spirituality. Throughout their educational experiences, the students must engage in reflection, critical thinking, inquiry, and syntactical learning. Research is an essential part of all educational experiences, and a required aspect of classroom and clinical learning.

The Ideal Neuman Systems Model–Based Associate Degree Nursing Program

Associate degree nursing programs prepare graduates for the roles of provider of care, manager of care, and member of the nursing profession. Inherent in these practice roles are

TABLE 12-5. Topical Outline of the Ideal Neuman Systems Model–Based Associate Degree Nursing Program

Foundations of Professional Behaviors (3 credits)	The Philosophy of Nursing Ways of Knowing The Neuman Systems Model The Nursing Process Introduction to Nursing Research
Nursing Preventions Laboratory (2 credits)	Safety Body Mechanics, Range of Motion Hygiene Comfort Medication Administration Medical and Surgical Asepsis Parenteral Modalities Vital Signs Documentation
Pharmacology (2 credits)	General Principles of Pharmacology Drug Standards and Medication Computation Terminology Classifications Common Medications
Primary Preventions (4 credits)	Wellness Across the Life Span from Birth to Death Nursing Process with Well Clients—Child Through the Elderly Impact of the Family on Health Client Teaching–Learning
Primary Preventions Laboratory (2 credits)	Implementation of Nursing Process with Children and Adults Clinics Nursing Homes Uncomplicated Pregnancy, Labor and Delivery, Well Child Care
Secondary Preventions (4 credits)	Nursing Process with Clients— Flexible Line of Defense Penetrated Adults and Children with Cardiovascular, Respiratory, Endocrine, Elimination, Integumentary, Reproductive, Mental Health, or Psychiatric Stressors
Secondary Preventions Laboratory (2 credits)	Implementation of Nursing Process in Hospitals, Clinics, Psychiatric Units, and Other Inpatient and Outpatient Settings
Tertiary Preventions (4 credits)	Nursing Process with Adult and Child Clients with Complex Stressors Neurological and Psychological Stressors Long-Term Chronic Illness Death and Dying Principles of Rehabilitation and Reeducation

TABLE 12-5. Topical Outline of the Ideal Neuman Systems Model–Based Associate Degree Nursing Program *(continued)*

Tertiary Preventions Laboratory (2 credits)	Application of Nursing Process with Adults and Children in Rehabilitation Center, Clinics, and Other Inpatient and Outpatient Settings
Wholistic Nursing Laboratory (5 credits)	Integration of Primary, Secondary, and Tertiary Preventions with Clients Across the Life Span

The learner develops leadership and organizational skills through supervision of peers and other nursing personnel in various inpatient settings. This is a precepted clinical experience with a weekly seminar.

Nursing and Health Care Policy (3 credits)	Impact of Ethics, Legal Issues, Financial Concerns, Health Policy, Social and Political Concerns on Nursing
Independent Study	

Learner-designed project with a written and clinical component. Faculty-guided project in which student selects a clinical area and practices according to performance criteria. Evaluation by faculty, clinical preceptor, and written work.

the core components of professional behaviors, communication, assessment, clinical decision making, caring interventions, teaching and learning, collaboration, and managing care (National League for Nursing, 2000). The ideal associate degree nursing program comprises 70 credits—37 nursing credits, 12 biological science credits, 9 social science credits, 6 English credits, 3 general elective credits, and 3 humanities/fine arts credits (Cecil Community College, 1999). A topical outline of the nursing courses for the ideal associate degree nursing program is presented in Table 12-5 (Cecil Community College, 1999).

The Ideal Neuman Systems Model–Based Master's Degree Nursing Program

The primary focus of master's degree education in contemporary nursing is preparation of a clinician, the so-called advanced practice nurse (APN) (AACN, 1996). Commonly used titles for APNs are nurse practitioner, nurse anesthetist, nurse–midwife, and clinical nurse specialist (AACN, 1996). The clinician also must also have knowledge of case management, educational theories, and research. Master's degree education in contemporary nursing also addresses preparation of community health nurses and nurse administrators. Programs that prepare community health nurses focus on populations and aggregates, rather than individuals and families. Programs that prepare nurse administrators focus on organizations.

An example of the curriculum for an ideal master's degree nursing education program is outlined in Table 12-6. The Neuman Systems Model can be used as a curriculum guide for master's degree nursing education with virtually any client system; the example is for elderly individuals as the client system. The curriculum is designed to prepare gerontological nurse practitioners (GNPs) and clinical nurse specialists (CNSs) in long-term care. Master's degree advance practice nursing programs for other age groups, such as pediatric or adult health, would require relevant modifications in the curriculum given in the example.

The GNP program comprises 46 credits, and the CNS program comprises 40 credits. Both GNP and CNS students take several of the same courses—Models and Theories

TABLE 12-6. Topical Outline of an Example of an Ideal Neuman Systems Model–Based Master's Degree Nursing Program: Gerontological Nurse Practitioner (GNP) and Clinical Nurse Specialist (CNS) in Long-Term Care

Course	Topic
The following courses are required of all students:	
Models and Theories of Advanced Nursing Practice	Structure of Nursing Knowledge
	Conceptual–Theoretical–Empirical Structure
	Knowledge Development and Concept Analysis
	Neuman's Systems Model
	Roy's Adaptation Model
	Johnson's Behavioral Systems Model
	King's General Systems Framework
	Levine's Conservation Model
	Rogers's Science of Unitary Human Beings
	Orem's Self-Care Framework
	Nursing Theories: Watson, Leininger, Newman, Orlando, Parse, Peplau
Roles of the Nurse in Advanced Nursing Practice	Societal Changes That Affect Nursing Roles
	Role Theory, Role Conflict, Role Strain, Role Confusion
	Marketing the APN Role
	Collaborative Practice
	Educator Role
	Research Role
	Practice Role
	APN Roles: Nurse Practitioner, Clinical Nurse Specialist, Nurse–Midwife, Nurse Anesthetist
	Entrepreneur
	Parish Nurse
	Case Manager
Research Process 1	History of Nursing Research
	Research Utilization Models
	Quantitative Research
	Qualitative Research
	Ethics in Research
	Research Problems and Purposes
	Review of the Literature
	Conceptual Models of Nursing
	Conceptual–Theoretical–Empirical Structures for Research
	Questions and Hypotheses
	Sampling and Designs
	Concepts of Measurement
	Validity and Reliability
	Data Collection and Data Processing
	Introduction to SPSS

TABLE 12-6. Topical Outline of an Example of an Ideal Neuman Systems Model–Based Master's Degree Nursing Program: Gerontological Nurse Practitioner (GNP) and Clinical Nurse Specialist (CNS) in Long-Term Care *(continued)*

Course	Topic
Research Process 1 *(continued)*	Statistical Theory
	Type I and Type II errors
	Descriptive and Exploratory Analysis
	Inferential Statistics
	Qualitative Data Collection and Analysis
	Critical Appraisal of Nursing Research Proposals
	Interpretation of Outcomes
	Dissemination of Research Findings
	Draft Research Proposal
Research Process 2	Grant Resources
	Grant Application Process
	Development of a Grant Proposal
	Analysis of Designs in Published Research
	ANOVA, MANOVA, ANCOVA
	Repeated Measures
	Sample Size, Effect Size, Power
	Regression Analysis: Linear, Multiple, Logistic
	Path Analysis
	Structural Equation Modeling
	Canonical Correlation
	Causal Models
	Discriminant Analysis
	Chi-Square, Kruskal–Wallis, Mann–Whitney U, t-test
	Complete Research Proposal with Pilot Testing
Health Policy, Legal and Ethical Issues in Advanced Practice Nursing	Historical Perspectives
	Political, Legal, and Ethical Dimensions of Health Care Issues
	Attendance at Legislative Session
	Student Seminars
Advanced Pharmacology	Legal Aspects of Drug Prescription, Administration, Dispensing, and Sales
	Role of Food and Drug Administration in Pharmaceuticals in the United States
	Mechanisms of Prescribing and Providing Medications
	Demographics of Drug Use in the Elderly
	Causes of and Interventions for Polypharmacy

The following content is included for all medications in all categories:

Mechanism of action—absorption, distribution, metabolism, and excretion
Indications for use in common episodic and chronic health problems of the elderly
Potential interactions with aging physiology

TABLE 12-6. Topical Outline of an Example of an Ideal Neuman Systems Model–Based Master's Degree Nursing Program: Gerontological Nurse Practitioner (GNP) and Clinical Nurse Specialist (CNS) in Long-Term Care *(continued)*

Course	Topic
	The following content is included for all medications in all categories: (continued)
	Potential interactions with other drugs, foods, disease and health state, ethnic and cultural background
	Differentiation of adverse effects—side, idiosyncratic, allergic
	Different formulations and their effects
	Appropriate and critical client education
	Necessary modifications of dose for physiological changes
	Monitoring techniques/requirements
	Considerations for prescription, including cost–benefit analysis
	Potential client adaptations to regime and indications of same
	Antihypertensives
	Antiarrhythmics
	Antianginals
	Analgesics
	Anti-inflammatory and arthritis-related drugs
	Hormonal and metabolic preparations
	Antidiabetics
	Gastrointestinal drugs
	Respiratory drugs
	Antidepressants, anxiolytics, and hypnotics
	Antineoplastics
	Antimicrobials
	Neurological system drugs
	Common over-the-counter preparations
Advanced Pathophysiology	Biological Theories of Aging
	Mechanisms of Disease
	Genetic Basis of Longevity and Disease
	Aging, Immune Function, and Immunological Disorders
	Cell Growth, Proliferation, and Aging

The following content is included for each organ system:

Analysis of relationship between normal physiology and specific disease alterations
Description of etiology, natural history, aging, and manifestation of disease
Correlation of pathophysiology with client signs and symptoms
Correlation of pathophysiology with diagnostic data

> Neurological Function and Dysfunction in Aging Adults
> Aging Cardiovascular System in Health and Disease
> Musculoskeletal System Function and Dysfunction
> Aging Gastrointestinal System
> Common Syndromes Secondary to Sociocultural Factors
> Hematological System
> Respiratory System and the Older Adult

TABLE 12-6. Topical Outline of an Example of an Ideal Neuman Systems Model–Based Master's Degree Nursing Program: Gerontological Nurse Practitioner (GNP) and Clinical Nurse Specialist (CNS) in Long-Term Care *(continued)*

Course	Topic
	Renal Function and Urinary Tract in Aging
	Integumentary System
	Reproductive System
	Endocrine Functioning and Aging
Advanced Health and Physical Assessment	

Content includes:

Application of the five Neuman System Model client system variables (physiological, psychological, sociocultural, developmental, spiritual) in health assessment
Analysis of findings to determine change in health status
Identification and documentation of salient findings
Description of comprehensive history and physical
Organization of assessment components to facilitate information gathering and client comfort
Finesse in the use of techniques and equipment
Selection of appropriate diagnostic tests to evaluate the older adult's health status
Correlation of test results with client history and physical findings

> Interview and Health History
> Psychosocial Assessments
> Environmental Assessment
> Integumentary System and Hematology
> Head and Neck, Eyes, Ears, Nose, and Throat
> Laboratory Evaluation of Hormone and Toxicology Levels
> Breasts, Thorax, and Lungs
> Laboratory Tests for Infectious Processes
> Cardiovascular System
> Abdomen
> Reproductive System—Male and Female
> Musculoskeletal System
> Neurological System
> Head-to-Toe Physical Exam
> Comprehensive Gerontological Physical Assessment

The following courses are required of GNP students:

Primary and Secondary Preventions   Health Promotion and Protection
   with Older Adults   Principles of Secondary Prevention

The following content is included for each topic:

The five Neuman System Model client system variables
Risk analysis and reduction
Anticipatory guidance and client/family education
Cultural considerations
Critical thinking and diagnostic reasoning
Identification of health care needs
Appropriate interviewing and physical assessments
Selection of appropriate assessment methodologies and tests
Documentation and presentation to colleagues

TABLE 12-6. Topical Outline of an Example of an Ideal Neuman Systems Model–Based Master's Degree Nursing Program: Gerontological Nurse Practitioner (GNP) and Clinical Nurse Specialist (CNS) in Long-Term Care *(continued)*

Course	Topic
The following content is included for each topic: (continued)	
Referrals and use of community resources	
Family and social support network considerations	
Clinical therapeutics appropriate for health concerns	
Client education and joint decision making	
Management of care across health care settings	
	Supporting and Promoting Functional Mobility
	Screening, Specific Protection, and Diabetes Mellitus
	Cardiovascular Problems
	Mental Health and Substance Abuse
	Rest, Sleep, and Genitourinary Problems
	Skin and Thermal Regulation
	Respiratory Problems
	Gastrointestinal Disorders
	Home Remedies, Homeopathy, Alternative Modalities
Tertiary Prevention for Older Adults	
The following content is included for each topic:	
The five Neuman System Model client system variables	
Cultural considerations	
Critical thinking and diagnostic reasoning	
Identification of health care needs	
Appropriate interviewing and physical assessments	
Selection of appropriate assessment methodologies and tests	
Documentation and presentation to colleagues	
Referrals and use of community resources	
Family and social support network considerations	
Clinical therapeutics appropriate for health concerns	
Client education and joint decision making	
Management of care across health care settings	
	Heart Failure
	Obstructive and Restrictive Airway Disorders
	Neurological Disorders
	Sensory Losses and Disorders
	Anemias and Leukemias
	Palliative Care
	Musculoskeletal Disorders
	Incontinence
	Dementias
Capstone Practicum	Negotiating the Clinical Placement
	Developing Personal Objectives
	Preparing a Curriculum Vita and Professional Résumé
	Credentialing

TABLE 12-6. Topical Outline of an Example of an Ideal Neuman Systems Model–Based Master's Degree Nursing Program: Gerontological Nurse Practitioner (GNP) and Clinical Nurse Specialist (CNS) in Long-Term Care *(continued)*

Course	Topic
The following courses are required of all CNS students:	
Clients with Health Care Challenges Across the Life Span	
The five Neuman Systems Model client system variables serve as the conceptual basis for this course.	
	Knowledge from Nursing and Adjunctive Disciplines Related to Chronic Illness, Transitory and Long-Term Care
	Illness Trajectories for Individuals and Families
	Caregiver Burden
	CNS Role as Clinician, Educator, and Researcher with Clients with Transitory and Long-Term Care
Special Health Care Challenges in Transitional and Long-Term Care	High Risk, Multicultural Populations in Underserved Areas
	Critical Pathway Development Using Corbin and Strauss Trajectory Framework and Neuman Systems Model
	Concepts Related to Transitional and Long-Term Care—Loss, Hope, Uncertainty, Suffering, Stigma, Adherence, Stress, Independence/Dependence, Powerlessness, Alternative Therapies, Financing, Special Technologies, Care and Placement Options, Sexuality
Clinical Practicum (Taken concurrently with Special Health Challenges in Transitional and Long-Term Care) Individually planned practice experiences consistent with learner and program objectives, whenever possible. Consideration is given to practice sites where underserved, vulnerable, at-risk, populations are located.	
	Apply Previously Acquired and Skills in Diverse Settings
	Expand Level of Expertise in a Selected Area of Advanced Nursing Practice
Electives in the CNS Curriculum Concepts of Advanced Practice Geropsychiatric Nursing	Neuman Systems Model Five Client System Variables
	Theories from Adjunctive Disciplines
	Impact of Geropsychiatric Disorders on History Taking, Physical Assessment, Functional Assessment of the Elderly Client and Family
	Depression, Suicide, and Bereavement
	Delirium and Dementia
	Management/Treatment of Geropsychiatric Client with Delirium, Depression, and Dementia by the APN

TABLE 12-6. Topical Outline of an Example of an Ideal Neuman Systems Model–Based Master's Degree Nursing Program: Gerontological Nurse Practitioner (GNP) and Clinical Nurse Specialist (CNS) in Long-Term Care *(continued)*

Course	Topic
Electives in the CNS Curriculum	
Concepts of Advanced Practice	
Geropsychiatric Nursing	Analysis of the Needs of Families of Elderly Persons with Geropsychiatric Disorders
	Substance Abuse
	Care of Mentally Ill Persons in the Home
	Analysis of the Vulnerability of the Geropsychiatric Client
	Pharmacotherapeutic, Pharmacokinetic, and Pharmacodynamic Properties of Drugs Used in the Treatment of Elderly Clients with Geropsychiatric Disorders
	Multidisciplinary and Community-Based Approaches to the Care of the Geropsychiatric Client
	Special Topics in Family Functioning and Support for Families with Geropsychiatric Clients by the APN
	Special Topics in the Management and Treatment of the Geropsychiatric Client by the APN
Case Management in Advanced Nursing Practice	Definition of Case Management, Historical Perspectives, Trends
	Case Management Models
	Case Manager Role
	Case Management Process and Planning
	Case Management Tools, Clinical Pathways
	Continuous Quality Management, Standards of Practice
	Measurement, Outcomes, Evaluation
	Case Management Research
	Legal and Ethical Issues in Case Management
	Health Insurance/Economics
	Health Policy, Legislation, Regulations
	Home Care, Community Resources

of Advanced Practice Nursing; Roles of the Nurse in Advanced Nursing Practice; Research Process 1; Research Process 2; Health Policy, Legal, and Ethical Issues in Advanced Nursing Practice; Advanced Pharmacology; Advanced Pathophysiology; and Advanced Health and Physical Assessment. Advanced Health and Physical Assessment, which includes a laboratory, is a four-credit course; each of the others is a three-credit course.

The CNS students take several courses that are specific to their role and functions—Clients with Health Care Challenges Across the Life Span, Special Health Care Challenges with Clients in Transitional and Long-Term Care, and Clinical Practicum. Each is a three-credit course. Elective courses available to CNS students include Case Management in Advanced Nursing Practice and Concepts of Advanced Practice Geropsychiatric Nursing, each of which is a three-credit course. The specific courses taken by GNP students are Primary and Secondary Preventions with Older Adults (seven credits), Tertiary Preventions with Older Adults (five credits), and Capstone Practicum (nine credits).

CONCLUSION

Application of the guidelines for Neuman Systems Model–based education for the health professions that were presented in this chapter is evident in Chapters 15 and 16. An integrated review of the published reports of use of the Neuman Systems Model in nursing education is the subject matter of Chapter 13. In addition, the educational tools that have been derived from the Neuman Systems Model are discussed in Chapter 14.

REFERENCES

American Association of Colleges of Nursing (1998). *The essentials of baccalaureate education for professional nursing practice.* Washington, DC: Author.

American Association of Colleges of Nursing (1996). *The essentials of master's education for advanced practice nursing.* Washington, DC: Author.

Busch, P., & Lynch, M. H. (1998). Creative teaching strategies in a Neuman-based baccalaureate curriculum. In L. Lowry (Ed.), *The Neuman Systems Model and nursing education: Teaching strategies and outcomes* (pp. 59–69). Indianapolis: Sigma Theta Tau International Center Nursing Press.

Cecil Community College (1999). *General catalog 1999–2000.* North East, MD: Author.

Colucciello, M. K. (1997). Critical thinking skills and dispositions of baccalaureate nursing students—a conceptual model for evaluation. *Journal of Professional Nursing, 13,* 236–45.

Fawcett, J. (1989). *Analysis and evaluation of conceptual models of nursing* (2nd ed.). Philadelphia: Davis.

Fawcett, J. (1995). *Analysis and evaluation of conceptual models of nursing* (3rd ed.). Philadelphia: Davis.

Fawcett, J. (2000). *Analysis and evaluation of contemporary nursing knowledge: Nursing models and theories.* Philadelphia: Davis.

Johnson, S. E. (1989). A picture is worth a thousand words: Helping students visualize a conceptual model. *Nurse Educator, 14*(3), 21–24.

Lindeman, C. A. (2000). The future of nursing education. *Journal of Nursing Education, 39*(3) 5–12.

Lowry, L. (1988). Operationalizing the Neuman Systems Model: A course in concepts and process. *Nurse Educator, 13*(3), 19–22.

Lowry, L. (Ed.). (1998). *The Neuman Systems Model and nursing education: Teaching strategies and outcomes.* Indianapolis: Sigma Theta Tau International Center Nursing Press.

Mirenda, R. M. (1986). The Neuman Systems Model: Description and application. In P. Winstead-Fry (Ed.), *Case studies in nursing theory* (pp. 127–66). New York: National League for Nursing.

National League for Nursing Accreditation Commission. (1997). *Interpretive guidelines for standards and criteria: Baccalaureate and higher degree programs in nursing* (rev. ed.). New York: Author.

National League for Nursing. (2000). *Educational competencies for graduates of associate degree nursing programs.* Sudbury, MA: Jones and Bartlett.

Neuman, B. (1985, August). Betty Neuman. Paper presented at conference on Nursing Theory in Action, Edmonton, Alberta, Canada (audiotape).

Neuman, B. (1988). *The nurse theorists: Portraits of excellence—Betty Neuman.* Athens, OH: Fuld Institute for Technology in Nursing Education (videotape and compact disc).

Neuman, B. (1995). *The Neuman Systems Model* (3rd ed.). Norwalk, CT: Appleton & Lange.

Neuman, B., & Young, R. J. (1972). A model for teaching total person approach to patient problems. *Nursing Research, 21,* 264–69.

Neumann College Department of Nursing. (2000). *Self-study report submitted to the National League for Nursing Accrediting Commission.* Aston, PA: Neumann College.

Ross, M. M., Bourbonnais, F. F., & Carroll, G. (1987). Curricular design and the Betty Neuman Systems Model: A new approach to learning. *International Nursing Review, 34,* 75–79.

Strickland-Seng, V., Mirenda, R., & Lowry, L. W. (1996). The Neuman Systems Model in nursing education. In P. Hinton Walker & B. Neuman (Eds.), *Blueprint for use of nursing models* (pp. 91–140). New York: NLN Press.

Toot, J. L., & Schmoll, B. J. (1995). The Neuman Systems Model and physical education curricula. In B. Neuman (Ed.), *The Neuman Systems Model* (3rd ed., pp. 213–46). Norwalk, CT: Appleton & Lange.

thirteen

The Neuman Systems Model and Education: An Integrative Review

Lois W. Lowry

Integrative reviews provide an overview and critique of the existing literature; they are most helpful when there is a great deal of literature on a particular subject. The Neuman Systems Model has been widely used in education for over 20 years, as evidenced by the extensive list of references at the end of this chapter. One purpose of this chapter is to review the literature about the use of the Neuman Systems Model as a guide for education. The second purpose is to report the results of a follow-up of all known Neuman Systems Model–based educational programs to determine the current status of the model in those programs.

The review was guided by Fawcett's (1989) four rules for using a conceptual model for curriculum development:

1. The first rule identifies the distinctive focus of the curriculum and the purposes to be filled by nursing education.
2. The second rule identifies the general nature and sequence of the content to be presented.
3. The third rule identifies the settings in which nursing education occurs and the characteristics of the students.
4. The fourth rule identifies the teaching–learning strategies to be employed. (p. 31)

BACKGROUND

Neuman (1995) noted that she recognized the need for an organizing framework for the content of graduate programs in nursing. Accordingly, she developed the Neuman Systems Model "to provide a unity, or focal point, for student learning" (p. 674). Neuman's commitment to the dissemination of the Neuman Systems Model led to her national and international consultation to schools of nursing and frequent lectures at theory conferences.

When the National League for Nursing (NLN) mandated the use of conceptual models for nursing curriculum in the mid-1970s, the acceptance and use of the Neuman Systems Model accelerated in the United States. Schools of nursing in Canada and San Juan, Puerto Rico, then began to adopt the model, followed over the next 10 years by schools in the Scandinavian countries, England, Australia, Holland, Kuwait, Taiwan, and Thailand. Since the NLN eliminated the requirement of a specific conceptual framework for curriculum development in the early 1990s, faculties have tended to adopt eclectic frameworks. Some schools of nursing that were originally Neuman Systems Model–based now report that some of the model concepts have been retained, although they no longer use the model exclusively. It is evident, however, that the Neuman Systems Model has been and continues to be useful for educators.

METHOD

An integrated review is a nonexperimental study design in which information obtained from the literature is systemically categorized and summarized. Conclusions are drawn to inform the reader about the present state of knowledge about a subject and to highlight future directions (Cooper, 1989). This review followed guidelines that mandate a rigorous methodology (Ganong, 1987).

Sample

The sample consisted of all articles and book chapters published from 1980 to 2000 that focused on the Neuman Systems Model and education, as well as three accreditation self-study reports from Neuman Systems Model–based educational programs. The 94 publications that were retrieved were categorized into three topical areas: (1) commentaries about the efficacy of using the model for education ($n = 15$), (2) practical applications of the Neuman Systems Model as a curricular or course framework for nursing education ($n = 54$), and (3) teaching–learning strategies or evaluation processes for students and faculty ($n = 25$). All 94 articles, chapters, and self-studies were reviewed and are included in the chapter references; however, all publications were not included in the tables. For example, if two or more publications addressed the same program and were published within the same time frame, the most informative publication was cited in the tables. A few short commentaries, such as those by Neuman (1998) and Mirenda and Wright (1987), were not included in the tables.

The literature review was augmented by a survey of 45 program that were contacted to ascertain current use of the Neuman Systems Model. Only those schools that were accredited by the NLN (U.S. schools) and could be contacted by telephone or electronic mail were approached.

Instruments

A data collection tool for each category of literature was designed for the project. Each tool included specific items derived from Fawcett's (1989) rules for use of conceptual models in education. The first category, commentaries about the efficacy of using the

Neuman Systems Model in education, is based on the first rule—focus and purpose of the curriculum. The data collection tool items included: author and date of commentary, type of educational program, theme of commentary, and expected outcome.

The second category, application of the Neuman Systems Model as a curricular and/or course framework, is based on Fawcett's (1989) second and third rules—nature and sequence of the content, the settings for educational programs, and characteristics of the students. The eight items included in the data collection tool for this category are: author and date of reference, college or university and location, date Neuman Systems Model was adopted, Neuman Systems Model used as curriculum framework, Neuman Systems Model used for a specific course or specialty, inclusion of Neuman Systems Model concepts (e.g., open systems, client system variables, stress, reaction to stress, lines of defense, the three levels of prevention), curriculum/course plan provided, and specific tools included. The last five items were coded as yes or no. If item 5, course or specialty, or item 8, tools, was coded as yes, specific names were given. This tool was used to review literature that addressed baccalaureate, graduate, multilevel, associate, and international programs.

The third category, teaching–learning strategies and evaluation processes for students, is based on Fawcett's (1989) fourth rule, which addresses inclusion of elements in curriculum design. The data collection tool included the following five items: author and date of reference, college or university, course using the strategy or curriculum, name of the strategy, and tools provided. This category of publications also includes strategies for faculty teaching and learning; the few relevant discussions are discussed in the narrative. Detailed information about educational tools is given in Chapter 14.

A telephone or electronic mail survey was conducted to determine current use of the Neuman Systems Model by programs known to have used the Neuman Systems Model in the past. The 45 schools selected for the survey were known through published reports or conference presentations to have used the Neuman Systems Model. The survey requested the information listed in Table 13-1.

DATA ANALYSIS AND RESULTS

Descriptive statistics, aggregation of findings, and identification of trends are the appropriate data analysis techniques for this integrative review. Data from each category (commentaries, educational programs, and teaching–learning strategies) are compiled in the respective tables.

Commentaries

Table 13-2 presents the results of the review of the 15 commentaries about the efficacy of using the Neuman Systems Model for education, arranged from the earliest publica-

TABLE 13-1. Survey Instrument

When did you originally adopt the model?

Do you use the Neuman Systems Model today?
    If yes, is it used as a curriculum framework or for a specific course?
    If not, what is your framework?
    Date of change

TABLE 13-2. Commentaries About the Efficacy of Neuman Systems Model (NSM)–Based Education

Author(s)/Year	Type of Educational Program	Theme	Expected Outcome
Arndt, 1982	Nursing Service Administration	Systems concepts appropriate for administration	NSM useful in administration
Bower, 1982	Baccalaureate Curriculum	NSM as knowledge component of conceptual framework	Neuman-based curriculum
Harty, 1982	Continuing Education (CE)	NSM as structure for CE	Interdisciplinary coordination
Baker, 1982a	Continuing Education Psych/Mental Health	NSM framework for psych nurses	Enhanced practice
Baker, 1982b	Staff Development	NSM framework for psychosocial needs of chronic obstructive pulmonary disease patient	Better care by staff
Capers, 1986	Continuing Education	Differentiation of models and theories	Enhanced understanding
Reed-Sorrow, Harmon, & Kitundu, 1989	Baccalaureate	Computer-programmed learning of NSM	Computer literacy
Roberts, 1994	Staff in-service	In-service education using NSM	Effective process
Lowry & Newsome, 1995	Associate degree (AD)	Comparison of six AD programs	Predict future progress
Mirenda, Seng, & Lowry, 1995	AD, BS, MS	Overview of NSM use	Continued utility
Strickland-Seng, Mirenda, & Lowry, 1996	AD and BS	Blueprint for Model–based curricula	Consistent format
Lowry, 1998a	AD, BS, MS	NSM and educative–interpretive paradigm	Enhanced understanding
Lowry, 1998b	AD, BS, MS	Predictions for future model use	Continued utility
Newsome & Lowry, 1998	AD, BS, MS	Overview of evaluation models	Enhanced understanding
Lowry et al., 2000	Interdisciplinary graduate	NSM as framework for interdisciplinary education	Enhanced collaboration

tion to the most recent. These publications provide general information about the model and recommend its use for baccalaureate, associate degree, and graduate programs, interdisciplinary courses, and continuing education for staff. The five articles published in 1982 give specific guidelines for developing curricula from the perspective of the Neuman Systems Model. These publications represent the then current thinking about how a conceptual model provides the direction for generating content and behavioral objectives for nursing education programs. Strickland-Seng, Mirenda, and Lowry (1996) updated that thinking with a conceptual-model–based blueprint for educational programs. Lowry (1998a, d) explained how the Neuman Systems Model can be used in an educative–interpretative paradigm in which students and faculty are partners in the educational process. Lowry and colleagues (2000) described a Neuman Systems Model–based interdisciplinary graduate program.

Educational Programs

The results of the review of publications addressing educational programs are given in Tables 13-3, 13-4, and 13-5. Fifty-two different programs were described in these publications—37 (61 percent) from the United States, and 15 (39 percent) from other countries. The Neuman Systems Model was first used in baccalaureate programs, with four schools adopting the model in the late 1970s, and eight in the 1980s (Table 13-3). Two consortia, each of which encompassed three schools, adopted the model when the consortia were formed (Mrkonich, Miller, & Hessian, 1989; Nelson, Hansen, & McCullagh, 1989). Seven of the baccalaureate programs have a religious affiliation; the faculty in these programs noted that the inclusion of the spiritual variable influenced their decision to select the Neuman Systems Model. All of the baccalaureate programs used the Neuman Systems Model as a curriculum framework.

Graduate and multilevel programs are listed in Table 13-4; multilevel refers to schools that use the Neuman Systems Model at more than one level of education. A total of nine graduate programs have used the model for a specific specialty. Texas Woman's University, on three campuses, and Northwestern State University were the first to use the Neuman Systems Model for advanced practice specialties, beginning in 1976. Supported by a national grant, the Neuman Systems Model was used to frame a program in gerontic nursing in 1968 that organized the curriculum from the education of nurse aides to master's prepared nurses (Gunter, 1982). As the Neuman Systems Model gained wider acceptance throughout the 1980s, three universities used the model in several levels of nursing education—California State University, Fresno; University of Nevada, Las Vegas; and the University of Texas at Tyler.

Four associate degree programs first started using the Neuman Systems Model in the early 1980s (Lowry & Green, 1989), and three others adopted the model for the curriculum framework in the 1990s (Table 13-5). The programs at Lander University (Sipple & Freese, 1989) and the University of Nevada, Las Vegas (R. Witt, personal communication, May 5, 2000) originally were associate degree programs; they transitioned to Neuman Systems Model–based baccalaureate programs in the 1980s. Los Angeles County Medical Center transitioned from a diploma to an associate degree program (Hilton & Grafton, 1995). Currently, the Neuman Systems Model is used in nine associate degree programs; the most recent adoption was by Gulf Coast Community College in Florida (P. Aylward, personal communication, August 21, 2000).

TABLE 13-3. Application of the Neuman Systems Model (NSM) in Baccalaureate Programs

Author/Date	College/University/State	Date Model Adopted	Curriculum Framework	Course Only	NSM Concepts	Curriculum/Course Plan	Tools
Lebold & Davis, 1982	Saint Xavier College, Chicago, IL	1974	Yes	No	Yes	Yes	No
Knox, Kilchenstein, & Yakulis, 1982	University of Pittsburgh, PA	1977	Yes	No	Yes	Yes	No
Conners, 1982	University of Missouri, Kansas City, MO	1979	Yes	No	Yes	No	No
Mirenda, 1986a, b, c	Neumann College, Aston, PA	1980	Yes	No	Yes	Yes	No
Nichols, Dale, & Turley, 1989	University of Wyoming, Laramie, WY	1980	Yes	No	Yes	Yes	Yes: Path analysis
Mrkonich, Miller, & Hessian, 1989	Minnesota InterCollegiate Nursing Consortium (MINC) St. Paul, MN—College of St. Catherine; Gustavus Adolphus College; St. Olaf College	1985	Yes	No	Yes	Yes	No
Bruton & Matzo, 1989	St. Anselm College, Manchester, NH	1985	Yes	No	Yes	Yes	No
Nelson, Hansen, & McCullagh, 1989	Tri-College University (TCU)—North Dakota State University; Concordia College, Mequon, WI	1986	Yes	No	Yes	Yes	No
Sipple & Freese, 1989	Lander University, Greenwood, SC	1987	Yes	No	Yes	No	No
Strickland-Seng, 1995	University of Tennessee, Martin, TN	1988	No	Yes	Yes	Yes	Yes: Clinical evaluation
Glazebrook, 1995	Minnesota Intercollegiate Nursing Consortium (MINC), St. Paul, MN	1986 (revised)	Yes	No	Yes	Yes	No

TABLE 13-4. Application of the Neuman Systems Model (NSM) in Graduate and Multilevel Programs

Author/Date	University/State	Date Model Adopted	Specialty or Level	NSM Concepts	Curriculum/ Course Plan	Tools
			Graduate Programs			
Neuman & Wyatt, 1980	Ohio University, Athens, OH	1980	Nursing Service Administration	Yes	Yes	No
Johnson et al., 1982	Texas Woman's University, Dallas, TX	1977	Psych/Mental Health Medical/ Surgical Maternal/Child Community Health	Yes	Yes	Yes: Nursing process
Conners, Harmon, & Langford, 1982	Texas Woman's University, Houston, TX	1976	Medical/Surgical	Yes	No	Yes: Assessment, Teaching, Primary Prevention
Tollett, 1982	Texas Woman's University, Houston, TX	1976	Geriatrics/Gerontology	Yes	Yes	No
Moxley & Allen, 1982	Northwestern State University, Natchitoches, LA	1980	Advanced Practice	Yes	Yes	No
Conners, 1982	University of Missouri, Kansas City, MO	1980	Advanced Practice	Yes	No	Yes: Case study
Toot & Schmoll, 1995	Grand Valley State University, MI	1992	Physical Therapy	Yes	Yes	No
			Multilevel			
Gunter, 1982	Texas Woman's University, Houston, TX	1968	Gerontic: Aide, LPN, BS, MS	Yes	Yes	No
Louis, Witt, & LaMancusa, 1989	University of Nevada, Las Vegas, NV	1979	AD, BS, MS	Yes	No	No
Stittich, Avent, & Patterson, 1989	California State University, Fresno, CA	1989	BS, MS: Education, Admin., CNS, NP	Yes	Yes	No
Stittich, Flores, & Nuttall, 1995	California State University, Fresno, CA	1989	BS, MS	Culture	No	No
Klotz, 1995	University of Texas, Tyler, TX	1982	BS, MS	Yes	Yes	Yes: Case study

TABLE 13-5. Application of the Neuman Systems Model (NSM) in Associate Degree Programs

Author/Date	College/State	Date Model Adopted	Curriculum Framework	Course Only	NSM Concepts	Curriculum/ Course Plan
Lowry, 1988	Cecil Community College, North East, MD	1981	Yes	Yes: Introduction	Yes	Yes
Lowry & Green, 1989	University of Nevada, Las Vegas, NV	1980	Yes	No	Yes	Yes
	Indiana University–Purdue University, Ft. Wayne, IN	1982	Yes	No	Yes	Yes
	Cecil Community College, North East, MD	1981	Yes	No	Yes	Yes
	Santa Fe Community College, Gainesville, FL	1985	Yes	No	Yes	Yes
	Yakima Valley Community College, Yakima, WA	1985	No	Yes: Gerontology	Yes	Yes
Hilton & Grafton, 1995	Los Angeles County Medical Center, Los Angeles, CA	1989	Yes	No	Yes	Yes
Bloch & Bloch, 1995	Los Angeles County Medical Center, Los Angeles, CA	1989	No	Yes: Introduction and Culture	Yes	Yes
Accreditation Self-Study, 1990	Athens Technical College, Athens, GA	1990	Yes	No	Yes	Yes
Accreditation Self-Study, 1993	Central Florida Community College, Ocala, FL	1993	Yes	No	Yes	Yes
Accreditation Self-Study, 1999	Southern Adventist University, Collegedale, TN	1998	Yes	No	Yes	Yes

223

Programs based on the Neuman Systems Model that are located outside the United States are listed in Table 13-6. Faculty at 10 baccalaureate programs in Canada have written about their use of the model. The Neuman Systems Model is used by the Department of Psychiatric Nursing at Douglas College in Vancouver, British Columbia, for advanced practice nursing education (M. Tarko, personal communication, May 15, 2000) (see Chapter 6). Some of the Canadian programs are affiliated with community agencies that also use the Neuman Systems Model (Craig, 1995). Three Colleges of Caring Sciences in Sweden use the model for primary health care—Eskilstuna, Jonkoping, and Orobro (Engberg, 1995). The programs at Aarhus University in Denmark (Johanson, 1989) and the University of South Australia (McCulloch, 1995) also have adopted the model.

Teaching–Learning Strategies

A summary of teaching–learning strategies used by educators in Neuman Systems Model–based programs is given in Table 13-7. The first nine publications, from the late 1980s, present descriptions of such strategies as content for client assessment (Beyea & Matzo, 1989; Johnson, 1989), case studies (Story & DuGas, 1988), and small group activities (Karmels, 1993; Lowry, 1988), which were used to assist students to "think Neuman" and to organize data accordingly. The next 16 publications, from a monograph on teaching–learning strategies written 10 years later, present descriptions of a variety of activities whose primary goal was to foster critical thinking and to encourage active learning in the classroom (Lowry, 1998c). Three publications include clinical evaluation tools (Beckman, Boxley-Harges, Bruick-Sorge & Eichenauer, 1998b; Evans, 1998; Strickland-Seng, 1998). Three others include explanations of end-of-program evaluation tools and examples of items from the tools (Beckman et al., 1998b; Freese & Scales, 1998; Lowry, 1998a). Three other reports describe ways to introduce faculty to the model and ways to maintain faculty interest (Conners, 1989; Lowry & Jopp, 1989; Lowry et al., 1998).

Survey Results

Responses to the survey were received from 34 programs located in the United States and two programs in other countries. The survey revealed that the Neuman Systems Model is used at Douglas College, in Vancouver, British Columbia, Canada, for Advanced Practice Psychiatric Nursing (see Chapter 6), and at the Dutch Reformed College for Higher Education in the Netherlands for the baccalaureate program (see Chapter 16). The responses from programs in the United States are summarized in Table 13-8. Twenty-three programs continue to use the Neuman Systems Model, and 11 have changed to an eclectic approach. Five programs using the model have multilevel programs—three are baccalaureate and graduate, and two are practical nursing and associate degree programs. Twelve schools have baccalaureate programs, six have associate degree programs, and one offers a diploma.

Texas Woman's University faculty adopted the model for their graduate nursing specialties at several campuses in the 1970s and provided detailed descriptions of the curriculum. Today, the model is used only in the baccalaureate program (P. Stutz, personal communication, April 28, 2000). In addition, Barnes College at the University of Missouri no longer uses the model for its graduate program (C. Koch, personal communication, May 13, 2000).

TABLE 13-6. Application of the Neuman Systems Model (NSM) in International Programs

Author/Date	University/State	Date Model Adopted	Curriculum Framework	Level	NSM Concepts	Curriculum/ Course Plan	Tools
Ross, Bourbonnais, & Carroll, 1987	University of Ottawa, Canada	1984	No	Baccalaureate, fourth year	Yes	Yes	No
Johansen, 1989	Aarhus University, Denmark	1983	Yes	Advanced Nursing	Yes	No	Yes: Documentation form
Laschinger, Maloney, & Tranmer, 1989	Queen's University, Canada	1984	Yes	Baccalaureate	Yes	Yes	Yes: Care plan
Dyck et al., 1989	University of Saskatchewan, Canada	1985	Yes	Baccalaureate	Yes	Yes	No
McCulloch, 1995	University of South Australia	1987	Yes	Baccalaureate	Yes	Yes	No
Damant, 1995	England	1990s	Yes	Multiprofessional	Yes	No	No
Craig, 1995	University of Prince Edward Island	1992	No	Baccalaureate	Yes	No	No
	University of Calgary	1990	No	Baccalaureate	Yes	No	No
	Brandon University	1990	No	Baccalaureate	Yes	No	No
	University of Moncton	1990	No	Baccalaureate	Yes	No	No
	University of Windsor	1992	No	Post RN	Yes	No	No
	University of Toronto (all Canada)	1992	No	Baccalaureate	Yes	No	No
Beddome, 1995	Okanagan University, British Columbia, Canada	1992	Yes	Baccalaureate	Community as Client	No	Yes: Community assessment
Peternelj-Taylor & Johnson, 1996	University of Saskatchewan, Canada	1990	Yes	Baccalaureate; Psych–Mental Health	Yes	No	No
Engberg, Bjälming, & Bertilson, 1995	Sweden	1990s	Yes	Supervisors, District Nurses	Community	No	Yes: Documentation form
Engberg, 1995	Eskiltuna, Jonkoping, Orobro, Sweden	1990s	No	Baccalaureate	Yes	No	No

225

TABLE 13-7. Teaching–Learning Strategies and Evaluation

Author/Date	College/University/ State or Country	Course/Curriculum	Strategy	Tools
Lowry, 1988	Cecil Community College, North East, MD	Introduction to NSM	Journaling small groups	No
Story & DuGas, 1988	University of Ottawa, Canada	Continuing Education	One-day workshop	Case studies
Beyea & Matzo, 1989	St. Anselm's College, Manchester, NH	Older Adult	Elder assessment	Functional health pattern assessment
Johnson, 1989	Cecil Community College, North East, MD	Clinical Practica	Assessment of five variables	Pie-shaped diagram
Lowry & Jopp, 1989	Cecil Community College, North East, MD	Curriculum	Evaluations of graduates	Lowry-Jopp Neuman Model Evaluation Instrument
Major, 1989	Great Britain	Medical/Surgical	Classification of diagnoses	Taxonomy
Edwards & Kittler, 1991	Simmons College, Boston, MA	Rehabilitation Nursing	Clinical in rehab hospital	No
Karmels, 1993	Texas Technical University, Lubbock, TX	Nursing Theory	Game	No
Stittich, Flores, & Nuttall, 1995	California State University, Fresno, CA	Curriculum	Integrate culture	Case studies
Freiburger, 1998a, b	Indiana University–Purdue, Fort Wayne, IN	Curriculum	Cooperative learning Stories Recode/chunk Reframing	No No No No
Beckman et al., 1998a	Indiana University–Purdue University, Ft. Wayne, IN	Level One courses Level Two courses	Role play Analysis/synthesis Stressor penetration Case studies Oral presentations	Yes Nursing diagnosis, tool NSM diagram Yes Yes
Beckman et al., 1998b	Indiana University–Purdue University, Ft. Wayne, IN	Clinicals Curriculum	Data collection and organization Student performance evaluation Program evaluation outcomes	Yes Nursing assessment guide Clinical performance tool Lowry-Jopp Neuman Model Evaluation Instrument

TABLE 13-7. Teaching–Learning Strategies and Evaluation *(continued)*

Author/Date	College/University/ State or Country	Course/Curriculum	Strategy	Tools
Busch & Lynch, 1998	St. Anselm's College, Manchester, NH	Curriculum	Games Puzzles Questioning Analogies Simulations Case study Journaling	Yes Yes Yes Yes Yes Yes Yes
Chang & Freese, 1998	Lander University, Greenwood, SC	Culture course	Video Analysis	No Yes
Evans, 1998	Yakima Valley College, Yakima Valley, WA	Curriculum	Fourth-generation process	Clinical transition
Freese & Scales, 1998	Lander University, Greenwood, SC	Curriculum	Program evaluation	Program evaluation instruments
Freiburger, 1998b	Indiana University–Purdue University, Ft. Wayne, IN	Nursing Issues course	Question/answer Cooperative learning Videotape–critical thinking	Yes Yes No
Hassell, 1998	Lander University, Greenwood, SC	Family and Community courses	Case studies Community assessment	Assessment tool
Lowry, 1998	Cecil Community College, North East, MD	Curriculum	Program evaluation	Lowry-Jopp Neuman Model Evaluation Instrument
McHolm & Geib, 1998	Malone College, OH	Health Assessment	Date collection and analysis	Assessment tool
Nuttall, Stittich, & Flores, 1998	California State University, Fresno, CA	Curriculum	Clinical judgement	No
Strickland-Seng, 1998	University of Tennessee, Martin, TN	Curriculum	Clinical evaluation	Instruments
Sutherland & Forrest, 1998	Santa Fe Community College, Gainesville, FL	Courses	Self-awareness Active listening Term paper	Yes Yes Yes
Weitzel & Wood, 1998	SUNY, Brockport, NY	Community Health Nursing	Self-paced learning	Modules
Lowry & Martin, 2000	United States	Community Health	Team MED	Community as client

TABLE 13-8. Current Use of NSM by Schools

College/University	Level of Education	Date of Model Adoption	Current Use	Date of Change	Current Framework
Athens Area Technical Institute, Athens, GA	AD	1990	Yes	NA	NA
Barnes College of Nursing, University of Missouri, St. Louis, MO	BS	1989	No	1992	Eclectic
California State University, Fresno, CA	BS/MS	1989	Yes	NA	NA
Cecil Community College, North East, MD	AD	1981	Yes	NA	NA
Central Florida Community College, Oceola, FL	AD	1994	Yes	NA	NA
Daemen College, Amherst, NY	RN-BS	1993	No	1997	Eclectic
Delta State University, Cleveland, MS	BS/MS	1990	No	1997	Eclectic
Gulf Coast Community College, Panama City, FL	PN/AD	2000	Yes	NA	NA
Fitchburg State College, Fitchburg, MA	BS	1992	Yes	NA	NA
Holy Names College, Oakland, CA	BS	1994	Yes	NA	NA
Indiana University–Purdue University, Ft. Wayne, IN	AD	1984	Yes	NA	NA
Lander University, Greenwood, SC	BS	1985	Yes	NA	NA
Loma Linda University, Loma Linda, CA	BS/MS	1992	Yes	NA	NA
Los Angeles County Medical Center, Los Angeles, CA	AD	1989	Yes	NA	NA
Louisiana College, Pineville, LA	BS	1984	Yes	NA	NA
Mansfield College, Mansfield, PA	BS	1987	Yes	NA	NA
McNeese University, Lake Charles, LA	AD/BS/MS	1980	No	1995	Eclectic
Methodist Hospital School of Nursing, Memphis, TN	DIP	1989	No	1992	Eclectic
Milligan College, Milligan College, TN	BS	1994	Yes	NA	NA
Minnesota Intercollegiate Consortium, St. Olaf, MN	BS	1986	Yes	NA	NA
Neumann College, Aston, PA	BS	1980	Yes	NA	NA
Santa Fe Community College, Gainesville, FL	PN/AD	1985	Yes	NA	NA
Seattle Pacific College, WA	BS	1982	Yes	NA	NA

TABLE 13-8. Current Use of NSM by Schools *(continued)*

College/University	Level of Education	Date of Model Adoption	Current Use	Date of Change	Current Framework
Simmons College, Boston, MA	BS/MS	1982	No	1998	Eclectic
Southern Adventist University, Collegedale, TN	AD	1999	Yes	NA	NA
St. Anselm's College, Manchester, NH	BS	1985	Yes	NA	NA
St. Xavier College, Chicago, IL	BS	1974	No	1996	Eclectic
Texas Woman's University, Houston, TX	BS only	1979	Yes	NA	NA
Union College, Lincoln, NE	BS	1989	No	1996	Eclectic
University of Nevada, Las Vagas, NV	BS/MS only	1979	Yes	NA	NA
University of Oklahoma, Oklahoma City, OK	BS	1978	No	1980	Eclectic
University of Pittsburgh, PA	BS	1977	No	1994	Eclectic
University of Tennessee, Martin, TN	BS	1989	Yes	NA	NA
University of Texas, Tyler, TX	BS/MS	1982	No	1998	Eclectic

DISCUSSION

The purpose of this integrated review was to explore how the Neuman Systems Model has been used to guide education from 1980 to 2000. The literature reflects a broad spectrum of themes, from commentaries about the model to applications in different levels of nursing education, as well as specific teaching–learning strategies used by educators. The publications of the 1980s presented a more prescriptive approach to the use of the Neuman Systems Model in the design of curriculum, probably influenced by the NLN mandate to use conceptual models as curriculum frameworks. The systems approach of the Neuman Systems Model was then and continues to be very appealing to faculties and applicable to the educational process. The breadth of the model and easily understood vocabulary positively influence acceptance of the model by members of other disciplines (Lowry et al., 2000; Toot & Schmoll, 1995). Through the years, more baccalaureate programs adopted the model than any other level of education, although the model increased in popularity with associate degree programs in the 1990s. The model is especially favored by church-related institutions because of the inclusion of the spiritual variable. Faculty from Neumann College, a Franciscan school, reported that they were the first to suggest that the spiritual variable be added to the model (R. Mirenda, personal communication, April 26, 2000). Two Adventist colleges (Union and Southern) now use the Neuman Systems Model, and the model may be considered for adoption by all of the nursing programs in Adventist-related schools (P. Hunt, personal communication, May 22, 1999). Four associate degree programs adopted the model in the early 1980s, and another five adopted it in the 1990s. This is an appropriate level of nursing education to emphasize one nursing model, so that students are well versed in theory-based nursing when they begin to practice. Furthermore, associate degree program students who continue with higher education have a firm theoretical foundation on which to build as they progress.

Nurse educators who reported using the Neuman Systems Model for a curriculum framework have explained how they introduce, describe, and define the concepts of the model to the students in introductory courses. Some of the publications include a detailed explanation of how the model guides specific courses in the curriculum (Bloch & Bloch, 1995; Lowry, 1988; Ross, Bourbonnais, & Carroll, 1987; Strickland-Seng, 1995).

Programs outside the United States tended to adopt the model from the mid-1980s until the 1990s, concomitant with Betty Neuman's consultations and her appearances at international conferences (Neuman, 1995, p. 680). The increasing number of international presentations at the biennial Neuman Systems Model symposia indicates that international interest in and use of the model is continuing.

Programs that use the Neuman Systems Model have reported using such creative strategies as journaling, group activities, and games to teach nursing within the context of the model. A few ($n = 8$) discussions of teaching–learning strategies were published in the late 1980s and early 1990s. A recent monograph (Lowry, 1998c) includes 14 chapters that address teaching–learning strategies. These publications provide excellent examples for specific courses, such as community health (Hassell, 1998; Weitzel & Wood, 1998), culture (Chang & Freese, 1998), and issues (Freiburger, 1998a, b). Inasmuch as evaluation is an important component of the accreditation process, it is important for programs to evaluate the curriculum framework and its effect on student learning. Three schools have reported program evaluation processes (Beckman et al., 1998a,b; Freese & Scales, 1998; Lowry, 1998b).

The survey provided information about the current use of the Neuman Systems Model by 17 programs that had been described previously in the literature and 17 other programs that had not been described in publications. Two-thirds ($n = 23$) of the 34 programs continue to use the model in its entirety as a curriculum framework. The programs that have changed from using the model exclusively ($n = 11$) to an eclectic framework retain some Neuman Systems Model concepts. For example, a systems approach is retained by Delta State College (M. Probst, personal communication, May 11, 2000); stressors, by Union College (M. McArthur, personal communication, May 5, 2000); and the three levels of prevention by McNeese University (A. Fields, personal communication, June 3, 2000). In addition, the Neuman Systems Model is used as a framework for community health courses at Delta State College, (M. Probst, personal communication, May 11, 2000), Fitchburg State College, (B. Cammuso, personal communication, March 20, 2000), and Union College. Reasons given for shifting to an eclectic approach included the following: No one model is perfect for all nursing situations, the curriculum is richer with an eclectic approach, there is no one consistent way to explain the model in the literature, and a new dean came to the school. The trend toward eclectic curricula has been noted in many schools of nursing since the NLN withdrew its mandate for using conceptual models as curricula frameworks. Graduate programs, almost exclusively, are eclectic, frequently relegating discussions of nursing models and theories to a general core course. When a Neuman Systems Model–based graduate program retains the model as the curriculum framework, it is within an institution that also has a baccalaureate program, such as Loma Linda University; California State University, Fresno; and the University of Nevada, Las Vegas.

CONCLUSION

This integrated review of the literature provides evidence that the Neuman Systems Model has been and continues to be a very useful guide for education. Although the trend is toward eclecticism in nursing education today, the Neuman Systems Model has served many programs well throughout the years. The faculty of those programs that have moved away from exclusive use of the model claim that they retained some of the broad concepts of the model. The faculty of the programs that have continued to use the model claim that they "think Neuman" and their graduates find the Neuman Systems Model useful as an organizing tool. The teaching strategies used to facilitate student learning are a tribute to faculty creativity. As nursing education in other countries moves from an apprentice style process to theory-based curricula, the Neuman Systems Model frequently is selected to guide curriculum development. The Neuman Systems Model–based programs that have been described in the literature serve as prototypes for programs throughout the world.

REFERENCES

Accreditation self-study report. (1990). Unpublished manuscript. Athens Area Technical Institute, School of Nursing, Athens, GA.
Accreditation self-study report. (1993). Unpublished manuscript. Central Florida Community College, College of Nursing, Lecanto, FL.

Accreditation self-study report. (1999). Unpublished manuscript. Southern Adventist University, College of Nursing, Collegedale, TN.

Arndt, C. (1982). Systems theory and educational programs for nursing service administration. In B. Neuman (Ed.), *The Neuman Systems Model: Application to nursing education and practice* (pp. 182–87). Norwalk, CT: Appleton-Century-Crofts.

Baker, N. A. (1982a). The Neuman systems model as a conceptual framework for continuing education in the work place. In B. Neuman (Ed.), *The Neuman Systems Model: Application to nursing education and practice* (pp. 260–64). Norwalk, CT: Appleton-Century-Crofts.

Baker, N. A. (1982b). Use of the Neuman model in planning for the psychological needs of the respiratory disease patient. In B. Neuman (Ed.), *The Neuman Systems Model: Application to nursing education and practice* (pp. 241–51). Norwalk, CT: Appleton-Century-Crofts.

Beckman, S. J., Boxley-Harges, S., Bruick-Sorge, C., & Eichenauer, J. (1998a). Critical thinking, The Neuman Systems Model, and associate degree education. In L. Lowry (Ed.), *The Neuman Systems Model and nursing education: Teaching strategies and outcomes* (pp. 53–58). Indianapolis: Sigma Theta Tau International Center Nursing Press.

Beckman, S. J., Boxley-Harges, S., Bruick-Sorge, C., & Eichenauer, J. (1998b). Evaluation modalities for assessing student and program outcomes. In L. Lowry (Ed.), *The Neuman Systems Model and nursing education: Teaching strategies and outcomes* (pp. 149–60). Indianapolis: Sigma Theta Tau International Center Nursing Press.

Beddome, G. (1995). Community-as-client assessment: A Neuman-based guide for education and practice. In B. Neuman (Ed.), *The Neuman Systems Model* (3rd ed., pp. 567–79). Norwalk, CT: Appleton & Lange.

Beyea, S., & Matzo, M. (1989). Assessing elders using the functional health pattern assessment model. *Nurse Educator, 14*(5), 32–37.

Bloch, C., & Bloch, C. (1995). Teaching content and process of the Neuman Systems Model. In B. Neuman (Ed.), *The Neuman Systems Model* (3rd ed., pp. 175–82). Norwalk, CT: Appleton & Lange.

Bower, F. L. (1982). Curriculum development and the Neuman Model. In B. Neuman (Ed.), *The Neuman Systems Model: Application to nursing education and practice* (pp. 94–99). Norwalk, CT: Appleton-Century-Crofts.

Bruton, M. R., & Matzo, M. (1989). Curriculum revisions at Saint Anselm College: Focus on the older adult. In B. Neuman (Ed.), *The Neuman Systems Model* (2nd ed., pp. 201–10). Norwalk, CT: Appleton & Lange.

Busch, P., & Lynch, M. H. (1998). Creative teaching strategies in a Neuman-based baccalaureate curriculum. In L. Lowry (Ed.), *The Neuman Systems Model and nursing education: Teaching strategies and outcomes* (pp. 59–69). Indianapolis: Sigma Theta Tau International Center Nursing Press.

Capers, C. F. (1986). Some basic facts about models, nursing conceptualizations, and nursing theories. *Journal of Continuing Education, 16,* 149–54.

Chang, N. J., & Freese, B. T. (1998). Teaching culturally competent care: A Korean–American experience. In L. Lowry (Ed.), *The Neuman Systems Model and nursing education: Teaching strategies and outcomes* (pp. 85–90). Indianapolis: Sigma Theta Tau International Center Nursing Press.

Conners, V. L. (1982). Teaching the Neuman Systems Model: An approach to student and faculty development. In B. Neuman (Ed.), *The Neuman Systems Model: Application to nursing education and practice* (pp. 176–81). Norwalk, CT: Appleton-Century-Crofts.

Conners, V. L. (1989). An empirical evaluation of the Neuman Systems Model: The University of Missouri–Kansas City. In B. Neuman (Ed.), *The Neuman Systems Model* (2nd ed., pp. 249–58). Norwalk, CT: Appleton & Lange.

Conners, V., Harmon, V. M., & Langford, R. W. (1982). Course development and implementation using the Neuman Systems Model as a framework: Texas Woman's University (Houston campus). In B. Neuman (Ed.), *The Neuman Systems Model: Application to nursing education and practice* (pp. 153–58). Norwalk, CT: Appleton-Century-Crofts.

Cooper, H. N. (1989). *Integrating research: A guide for literature reviews.* Newbury Park, CA: Sage.

Craig, D. M. (1995). The Neuman model: Examples of its use in Canadian educational programs. In B. Neuman (Ed.), *The Neuman Systems Model* (3rd ed., pp. 521–27). Norwalk, CT: Appleton & Lange.

Damant, M. (1995). Community nursing in the United Kingdom: A case for reconciliation using the Neuman Systems Model. In B. Neuman (Ed.), *The Neuman Systems Model* (3rd ed., pp. 607–20). Norwalk, CT: Appleton & Lange.

Dyck, S. M., Innes, J. E., Rae, D. I., & Sawatzky, J. E. (1989). The Neuman Systems Model in curriculum revision: A baccalaureate program, University of Saskatchewan. In B. Neuman (Ed.), *The Neuman Systems Model* (2nd ed., pp. 225–36). Norwalk, CT: Appleton & Lange.

Edwards, P. A., & Kittler, A. W. (1991). Integrating rehabilitation content in nursing curricula. *Rehabilitation Nursing, 16,* 70–73.

Engberg, I. B. (1995). Brief abstracts: Use of the Neuman Systems Model in Sweden. In B. Neuman (Ed.), *The Neuman Systems Model* (3rd ed., pp. 653–56). Norwalk, CT: Appleton & Lange.

Engberg, I. B., Bjälming, E., & Bertilson, B. (1995). A structure for documenting primary health care in Sweden using the Neuman Systems Model. In B. Neuman (Ed.), *The Neuman Systems Model* (3rd ed., pp. 637–51). Norwalk, CT: Appleton & Lange.

Evans, B. (1998). Fourth-generation evaluation and the Neuman Systems Model. In L. Lowry (Ed.), *The Neuman Systems Model and nursing education: Teaching strategies and outcomes* (pp. 117–27). Indianapolis: Sigma Theta Tau International Center Nursing Press.

Fawcett, J. (1989). *Analysis and evaluation of conceptual models of nursing* (2nd ed.). Philadelphia: Davis

Freese, B. T., & Scales, C. J. (1998). NSM-based care as an NLN program evaluation outcome. In L. Lowry (Ed.), *The Neuman Systems Model and nursing education: Teaching strategies and outcomes* (pp. 135–38). Indianapolis: Sigma Theta Tau International Center Nursing Press.

Freiburger, O. A. (1998a). the Neuman Systems Model, critical thinking, and cooperative learning in a nursing issues course. In L. Lowry (Ed.), *The Neuman Systems Model and nursing education: Teaching strategies and outcomes* (pp. 79–84). Indianapolis: Sigma Theta Tau International Center Nursing Press.

Freiburger, O. A. (1998b). Overview of strategies that integrate the Neuman Systems Model, critical thinking, and cooperative learning. In L. Lowry (Ed.), *The Neuman Systems Model and nursing education: Teaching strategies and outcomes* (pp. 31–36). Indianapolis: Sigma Theta Tau International Center Nursing Press.

Ganong, L. H. (1987). Integrative reviews of nursing research. *Research in Nursing and Health, 10*(1), 1–11.

Glazebrook, R. S. (1995). The Neuman Systems Model in cooperative baccalaureate nursing education: The Minnesota Intercollegiate Nursing Consortium experience. In B. Neuman (Ed.), *The Neuman Systems Model* (3rd ed., pp. 227–30). Norwalk, CT: Appleton & Lange.

Gunter, L. M. (1982). Application of the Neuman Systems Model to gerontic nursing. In B. Neuman (Ed.), *The Neuman Systems Model: Application to nursing education and practice* (pp. 196–210). Norwalk, CT: Appleton-Century-Crofts.

Harty, M. B. (1982). Continuing education in nursing and the Neuman model. In B. Neuman (Ed.), *The Neuman Systems Model: Application to nursing education and practice* (pp. 100–106). Norwalk, CT: Appleton-Century-Crofts.

Hassell, J. S. (1998). Critical thinking strategies for family and community client systems. In L. Lowry (Ed.), *The Neuman Systems Model and nursing education: Teaching strategies and outcomes* (pp. 71–77). Indianapolis: Sigma Theta Tau International Center Nursing Press.

Hilton, S. A., & Grafton, M. D. (1995). Curriculum transition based on the Neuman Systems Model: Los Angeles County Medical Center School of Nursing. In B. Neuman (Ed.), *The Neuman Systems Model* (3rd ed., pp. 163–74). Norwalk, CT: Appleton & Lange.

Johansen, H. (1989). Neuman model concepts in joint use—community health practice and student teaching—School of Advanced Nursing Education, Aarhus University, Aarhus, Denmark. In B. Neuman (Ed.), *The Neuman Systems Model* (2nd ed., pp. 334–62). Norwalk, CT: Appleton & Lange.

Johnson, M. N., Vaughn-Wrobel, B., Ziegler, S., et al. (1982). Use of the Neuman health-care systems model in the master's curriculum: Texas Woman's University. In B. Neuman (Ed.), *The Neuman Systems Model: Application to nursing education and practice* (pp. 130–52). Norwalk, CT: Appleton-Century-Crofts.

Johnson, S. E. (1989). A picture is worth a thousand words: Helping students visualize a conceptual model. *Nurse Educator, 14*(3), 21–24.

Karmels, P. (1993). Conundrum game for nursing theorists: Neuman, King, and Johnson. *Nurse Educator, 18*(6), 8–9.

Klotz, L. C. (1995). Integration of the Neuman Systems Model into the BSN curriculum at the University of Texas at Tyler. In B. Neuman (Ed.), *The Neuman Systems Model* (3rd ed., pp. 183–95). Norwalk, CT: Appleton & Lange.

Knox, J. E., Kilchenstein, L., & Yakulis, I. M. (1982). Utilization of the Neuman model in an integrated baccalaureate program: University of Pittsburgh. In B. Neuman (Ed.), *The Neuman Systems Model: Application to nursing education and practice* (pp. 117–23). Norwalk, CT: Appleton-Century-Crofts.

Laschinger, S. J., Maloney, R., & Tranmer, J. E. (1989). An evaluation of student use of the Neuman Systems Model: Queen's University, Canada. In B. Neuman (Ed.), *The Neuman Systems Model* (2nd ed., pp. 211–24). Norwalk, CT: Appleton & Lange.

Lebold, M. M., & Davis, L. H. (1982). A baccalaureate nursing curriculum based on the Neuman Systems Model: Saint Xavier College. In B. Neuman (Ed.), *The Neuman Systems Model: Application to nursing education and practice* (pp. 124–29). Norwalk, CT: Appleton-Century-Crofts.

Louis, M., Witt, R., & LaMancusa, M. (1989). The Neuman Systems Model in multilevel nurse education programs: University of Nevada, Las Vegas. In B. Neuman (Ed.), *The Neuman Systems Model* (2nd ed., pp. 237–48). Norwalk, CT: Appleton & Lange.

Lowry, L. (1988). Operationalizing the Neuman Systems Model: A course in concepts and process. *Nurse Educator, 13*(3), 19–22.

Lowry, L. W. (1998a). Creative teaching and effective evaluation. In L. Lowry (Ed.), *The Neuman Systems Model and nursing education: Teaching strategies and outcomes* (pp. 17–29). Indianapolis: Sigma Theta Tau International Center Nursing Press.

Lowry, L. (1998b). Efficacy of the Neuman Systems Model as a curriculum framework: A longitudinal study. In L. Lowry (Ed.), *The Neuman Systems Model and nursing education: Teaching strategies and outcomes* (pp. 139–47). Indianapolis: Sigma Theta Tau International Center Nursing Press.

Lowry, L. (1998c). *The Neuman Systems Model and nursing education: Teaching strategies and outcomes.* Indianapolis: Sigma Theta Tau International Center Nursing Press.

Lowry, L. W. (1998d). Vision, values, and verities. In L. Lowry (Ed.), *The Neuman Systems Model and nursing education: Teaching strategies and outcomes* (pp. 167–74). Indianapolis: Sigma Theta Tau International Center Nursing Press.

Lowry, L. W., Bruick-Sorge, C., Freese, B. T., & Sutherland, R. (1998). Development and renewal of faculty for Neuman-based teaching. In L. Lowry (Ed.), *The Neuman Systems Model and nursing education: Teaching strategies and outcomes* (pp. 161–66). Indianapolis: Sigma Theta Tau International Center Nursing Press.

Lowry, L. W., Burns, C. M., Smith, A. A., & Jacobson, H. (2000). An interdisciplinary approach to training health professionals. *Nursing & Health Care Perspectives, 21*(2), 76–80.

Lowry, L., & Green, G. H. (1989). Four Neuman-based associate degree programs: Brief description and evaluation. In B. Neuman (Ed.), *The Neuman Systems Model* (2nd ed., pp. 283–12). Norwalk, CT: Appleton & Lange.

Lowry, L. W., & Jopp, M. C. (1989). An evaluation instrument for assessing an associate degree nursing curriculum based on the Neuman Systems Model. In J. P. Riehl-Sisca (Ed.), *Conceptual models for nursing practice* (3rd ed., pp. 73–85). Norwalk, CT: Appleton & Lange.

Lowry, L. W., & Martin, K. (2000). Organizing frameworks applied to community health nursing. In M. Stanhope & J. Lancaster (Eds.), *Community and public health nursing* (5th ed., pp. 202–25). St Louis: Mosby.

Lowry, L. W., & Newsome, G. G. (1995). Neuman-based associate degree programs: Past, present, and future. In B. Neuman (Ed.), *The Neuman Systems Model* (3rd ed., pp. 197–214). Norwalk, CT: Appleton & Lange.

Major, S. (1989). Neuman's systems model and experiential taxonomy. *Senior Nurse, 9*(6), 25–27.

McCulloch, S. J. (1995). Utilization of the Neuman Systems Model: University of South Australia. In B. Neuman (Ed.), *The Neuman Systems Model* (3rd ed., pp. 591–97). Norwalk, CT: Appleton & Lange.

McHolm, F. A., & Geib, K. M. (1998). Application of the Neuman Systems Model to teaching health assessment and nursing process. *Nursing Diagnosis: The Journal of Nursing Language and Classification, 9,* 23–33.

Mirenda, R. (1986a). The Neuman Systems Model and its clinical utility in a baccalaureate nursing program. *Senior Nurse, 5*(3) 24–25.

Mirenda, R. M. (1986b). The Neuman Systems Model and nursing education for a new age: A ten-year journey. *Proceedings of the First International Nursing Symposium on the Neuman Systems Model* (pp. 2.1–2.6). Aston, PA: Neumann College.

Mirenda, R. M. (1986c). The Neuman Systems Model: Description and application. In P. Winstead-Fry (Ed.), *Case studies in nursing theory* (pp. 127–66). New York: NLN.

Mirenda, R. M., & Wright, C. (1987). Using a nursing model to affirm Catholic identity. *Health Progress. 68,* 63–67.

Moxley, P. A., & Allen, L. M. H. (1982). The Neuman Systems Model approach in a master's degree program: Northwestern State University. In B. Neuman (Ed.), *The Neuman Systems Model: Application to nursing education and practice* (pp. 168–75). Norwalk, CT: Appleton-Century-Crofts.

Mrkonich, D., Miller, M., & Hessian, M. (1989). Cooperative baccalaureate education: The Minnesota intercollegiate nursing consortium. In B. Neuman (Ed.), *The Neuman Systems Model* (2nd ed., pp. 175–82). Norwalk, CT: Appleton & Lange.

Nelson, L. F., Hansen, M., & McCullagh, M. (1989). A new baccalaureate North Dakota-Minnesota nursing education consortium. In B. Neuman (Ed.), *The Neuman Systems Model* (2nd ed., pp. 183–92). Norwalk, CT: Appleton & Lange.

Neuman, B., & Wyatt, M. (1980). The Neuman stress/adaptation systems approach to education for nurse administrators. In J. P. Riehl & C. Roy (Ed.), *Conceptual models for nursing practice* (2nd ed., pp. 142–50). New York: Appleton-Century-Crofts.

Neuman, B. (1995). In conclusion—toward new beginnings. In B. Neuman (Ed.), *The Neuman Systems Model* (3rd ed., pp. 671–703). Norwalk, CT: Appleton & Lange.

Neuman, B. (1998). NDs should be future coordinators of health care (letter to the editor). *Image: Journal of Nursing Scholarship, 30,* 106.

Newsome, G. G., & Lowry, L. (1998). Evaluation in nursing: History, models, and Neuman's framework. In L. Lowry (Ed.), *The Neuman Systems Model and nursing education: Teaching strategies and outcomes* (pp. 37–51). Indianapolis: Sigma Theta Tau International Center Nursing Press.

Nichols, E. G., Dale, M. L., & Turley, J. (1989). The University of Wyoming evaluation of a Neuman-based curriculum. In B. Neuman (Ed.), *The Neuman Systems Model* (2nd ed., pp. 259–82). Norwalk, CT: Appleton & Lange.

Nuttall, P., Stittich, E. M., & Flores, F. C. (1998). The Neuman Systems Model in advanced practice nursing. In L. Lowry (Ed.), *The Neuman Systems Model and nursing education: Teaching strategies and outcomes* (pp. 109–14). Indianapolis: Sigma Theta Tau International Center Nursing Press.

Peternelj-Taylor, C. A., & Johnson, R. (1996). Custody and caring: Clinical placement of student nurses in a forensic setting. *Perspectives in Psychiatric Care, 32*(4), 23–29.

Reed-Sorrow, K., Harmon, R. L., & Kitundu, M. E. (1989). Computer-assisted learning and the Neuman Systems Model. In B. Neuman (Ed.), *The Neuman Systems Model* (2nd ed., pp. 155–60). Norwalk, CT: Appleton & Lange.

Roberts, A. G. (1994). Effective inservice education process. *Oklahoma Nurse, 39*(4), 11.

Ross, M. M., Bourbonnais, F. F., & Carroll, G. (1987). Curricular design and the Betty Neuman systems model: A new approach to learning. *International Nursing Review, 34,* 75–79.

Sipple, J. A., & Freese, B. T. (1989). Transition from technical to professional-level nursing education. In B. Neuman (Ed.), *The Neuman Systems Model* (2nd ed., pp. 193–200). Norwalk, CT: Appleton & Lange.

Stittich, E. M., Avent, C. L., & Patterson, K. (1989). Neuman-based baccalaureate and graduate nursing programs, California State University, Fresno. In B. Neuman (Ed.), *The Neuman Systems Model* (2nd ed., pp. 163–74). Norwalk, CT: Appleton & Lange.

Stittich, E. M., Flores, F. C., & Nuttall, P. (1995). Cultural considerations in a Neuman-based curriculum. In B. Neuman (Ed.), *The Neuman Systems Model* (3rd ed., pp. 147–62). Norwalk, CT: Appleton & Lange.

Story, E. L., & DuGas, B. W. (1988). A teaching strategy to facilitate conceptual model implementation in practice. *Journal of Continuing Education in Nursing, 19,* 244–47.

Strickland-Seng, V. (1995). The Neuman Systems Model in clinical evaluation of students. In B. Neuman (Ed.), *The Neuman Systems Model* (3rd ed., pp. 215–25). Norwalk, CT: Appleton & Lange.

Strickland-Seng, V., Mirenda, R., & Lowry, L.W. (1996). The Neuman Systems Model in nursing education. In P. Hinton Walker & B. Neuman (Eds.), *Blueprint for use of nursing models* (pp. 91–140). New York: NLN Press.

Strickland-Seng, V. (1998). Clinical evaluation: The heart of clinical performance. In L. Lowry (Ed.), *The Neuman Systems Model and nursing education: Teaching strategies and outcomes* (pp. 129–34). Indianapolis: Sigma Theta Tau International Center Nursing Press.

Sutherland, R., & Forrest, D. L. (1998). Primary prevention in an associate of science curriculum. In L. Lowry (Ed.), *The Neuman Systems Model and nursing education: Teaching strategies and outcomes* (pp. 99–108). Indianapolis: Sigma Theta Tau International Center Nursing Press.

Tollett, S. M. (1982). Teaching geriatrics and gerontology: Use of the Neuman Systems Model. In B. Neuman (Ed.), *The Neuman Systems Model: Application to nursing education and practice* (pp. 159–64). Norwalk, CT: Appleton-Century-Crofts.

Toot, J. L., & Schmoll, B. J. (1995). The Neuman Systems Model and physical therapy educational curricula. In B. Neuman (Ed.), *The Neuman Systems Model* (3rd ed., pp. 231–46). Norwalk, CT: Appleton & Lange.

Weitzel, A., & Wood, K. (1998). Community health nursing: Keystone of baccalaureate education. In L. Lowry (Ed.), *The Neuman Systems Model and nursing education: Teaching strategies and outcomes* (pp. 91–98). Indianapolis: Sigma Theta Tau International Center Nursing Press.

Personal Communications

Name	College/University	Date
Gwen Alcorn, RN, PhD	Central Florida Community College	4/27/00
Patricia Aylward, RN, MSN	Santa Fe Community College	5/8/00
Patricia Aylward, RN, MSN	Gulf Coast Community College	8/21/00
Gloria Buck, RN, PhD	Athens Technical College	9/1/00
Barbara Cammuso, RN, MSN	Fitchburg State College	3/20/00
Phyllis Chelette, RN, PhD	Louisiana College	5/1/00
Elizabeth Clarke, RN, MSN	Methodist Hospital SON	4/14/00
Melinda Collins, RN, MSN	Milligan College	8/14/00
Linda Davidson, RN, PhD	University of Pittsburgh	4/20/00
Anita Fields, RN, PhD	McNeese University	3/14/00
Anne Filipsi, RN, PhD	St. Xavier College	3/28/00
Carol Frazier, RN, PhD	Simmons College	3/21/00
Barbara Freese, RN, EdD	Lander University	6/12/00
Rita Glazebrook, RNC, PhD	Minnesota Intercollegiate Consortium	3/20/00
Chris Hawkins, RN, PhD	Texas Woman's University	4/11/00
Emily Hitchens, MN, EdD	Seattle Pacific University	4/26/00
Phil Hunt, RN, PhD	Southern Adventist University	5/22/99
Helen King, RN, PhD	Loma Linda University	6/21/00
Connie Koch, RN, PhD	Barnes College of Nursing, University of Missouri	5/13/00
Martha Lynch, RN, EdD	St. Anselm's College	3/15/00
Marilyn McArthur	Union College	4/11/00
Rosalie Mirenda, RN, PhD	Neumann College	4/26/00
Maureen Probst, RN, PhD	Delta State University	3/24/00
Carol Roane, RN, MS	Cecil Community College	5/2/00
Mary Lou Rusin, RN, EdD	Daemen College	5/18/00
Victoria Seng RN, PhD	University of Tennessee at Martin	6/1/00
Janeen Sheehe, RN, DNS	Mansfield College	5/2/00
Diane Stefanson, RN, PhD	Holy Names College	7/9/00
Carol Sternbarger, RNC, PhD	Indiana University–Purdue University	6/2/00
Eleanor Stittich, RN, MLitt	California State University, Fresno	5/1/00
Pamela Stutz, RN, PhD	University of Texas at Tyler	4/11/00
Mike Tarko, RN, MSN	Douglas College	5/15/00
Winn Wagaman, RN, PhD	Los Angeles County Medical Center	6/15/00
Francene Weatherby, RNC, PhD	University of Oklahoma	5/9/00
Rosemary Witt, RN, PhD	University of Nevada	5/5/00

fourteen

The Neuman Systems Model and Educational Tools

Karen S. Reed

The link between educational tools and the Neuman Systems Model is perhaps the oldest and strongest bond. Indeed, the model initially was designed as an "educational tool" to help students organize the content of clinical nurse specialist courses at the University of California–Los Angeles (Neuman & Young, 1972). As Neuman (1995) explained:

> In 1970 I developed the Neuman Systems Model to provide unity, or a focal point, for student learning. . . . Since my major concern was how to provide structure to best integrate student learning in a wholistic manner, I personally developed the model design as it still exists today. . . . The model was developed strictly as a teaching aid. (p. 674)

Since 1970, the "teaching aid" has become one of the most widely used models in nursing education (Lowry, 1998a). The purpose of this chapter is to discuss educational tools that have been developed to guide students' learning regarding the Neuman Systems Model, or to examine students' progress, course material, or curricula based on the Neuman Systems Model. All educational tools are, in their broadest sense, teaching strategies. Therefore, it is possible that some educational tools may be used to help students organize and understand Neuman Systems Model terminology but may not be used to evaluate students' progression within the curriculum. Such tools are categorized as *nonevaluative*. The first section of the chapter focuses on nonevaluative educational tools. The second section of the chapter focuses on educational tools that are used to evaluate student progression or curricular design and programs of study. The various tools are listed in Table 14-1.

TABLE 14-1. Neuman Systems Model–Based Educational Tools

Educational Tool	Purpose of Tool	System of Focus	Citation
Variable and Intervention Tool	Nonevaluative—Student learning	Student	Tollet, 1982
The Assessment and Analysis Guideline Tool	Nonevaluative—Student learning	Student	McHolm & Geib, 1998
Nursing Assessment Guide	Nonevaluative—Student learning	Student	Beckman et al., 1998
Student Clinical Performance Evaluation	Evaluative—Student learning	Student	Beckman et al., 1998
Clinical Evaluation Instrument	Evaluative—Student clinical performance	Student	Strickland-Seng, 1998
Summary of Clinical Evaluation Tool	Evaluative—Cumulative summaries of student behaviors	Student	Strickland-Seng, 1998
Profile of Clinical Evaluation	Evaluative—Student's progression through program	Student	Strickland-Seng, 1998
Lowry–Jopp Neuman Model Evaluation Instrument	Evaluative—Course, Curriculum, End of Program, Employer Satisfaction	Curriculum, Program Evaluation	Lowry, 1998c

NONEVALUATIVE EDUCATIONAL TOOLS

In the 1970s and 1980s, accrediting bodies in the United States mandated the use of nursing conceptual frameworks for nursing curricula. The introduction of a conceptual framework requires students to become familiar with the nomenclature of the framework and to apply the framework concepts in written assignments and clinical practice. Various methods may be used to help students organize information. Different techniques help the students understand, categorize, and apply the linkages between the framework and the course material. Examples of teaching strategies using the Neuman Systems Model are readily available in the nursing literature (Dale & Savala, 1990; Edwards & Kittler, 1991; Lowry, 1988; Russell & Hezel, 1994; Story & DuGas, 1988). Some articles are descriptions of the use of known strategies, such as journaling or role analysis, to incorporate Neuman System Model concepts into an existing course. Other articles present explanations of a process to develop course material in a curriculum. Articles describing formalized teaching tools developed specifically to help students are less common.

Variable and Intervention Tool

One of the earliest published Neuman Systems Model–based teaching tools facilitates the organization of course content by client system variable areas and prevention interventions (Tollett, 1982). Initially used as a method to design the school's gerontology nursing curriculum, the tool is a general format for organizing class content by four client system variables—physiological, psychological, sociocultural, and developmental—at the three prevention intervention levels. (Note that the Neuman Systems Model did not include the spiritual client system variable when Tollett developed her tool.) Content within the three courses—Primary Care, Secondary Care, and Tertiary Care of Older Adults—is organized using the same format.

Nursing Assessment Guide

The Nursing Assessment Guide developed at Indiana University–Purdue University at Fort Wayne helps students to collect and organize client data (Beckman et al., 1998). The format includes a glossary of terms to promote consistency of language. The guide is an integral part of the school's evaluation process, but is not used as an evaluation tool. Rather, the guide serves as an interim assessment measure of students' knowledge and enables faculty to observe and record the students' ability to apply concepts of the Neuman Systems Model.

The Assessment and Analysis Guideline Tool

The Assessment and Analysis Guideline tool was developed by faculty at Malone College in Ohio (McHolm & Geib, 1998). In conjunction with a change in the nursing model used to guide the curriculum, the faculty developed an educational tool used to teach sophomore baccalaureate nursing students how to do a Neuman Systems Model–based assessment and analysis. Nursing diagnoses were reorganized to reflect the Neuman Systems Model, and guidelines were developed to connect the model to the nursing diagnostic labels. The tool includes a client profile; stressors as perceived by the client and the caregiver; and intrapersonal, interpersonal, and extrapersonal factors. McHolm and Geib noted that the tool was being evaluated for use as part of the student evaluation process.

USING EDUCATIONAL TOOLS TO EVALUATE PROGRESS

Many articles about educational tools include a notation that the tool could (or will) be further developed for use in the evaluation of students' progress. Lowry (1998b) defined evaluation as "a tool and means to determine merit or worth of progress, direction, effectiveness, and usefulness" (p. 26). Gronlund and Linn (1990) maintained that educational evaluation should be viewed as "an integrated process for determining the nature and extent of pupil learning and development" (p. 6). When using the Neuman Systems Model in practice, the first step is to identify the client system of interest. Similarly, the first step in educational evaluation is to identify which system is to be evaluated. Is the system a student, whose clinical progression or learning of certain material is to be evaluated? Is the system a course, to be evaluated as part of curricular planning? Or is the system the entire curriculum, to be evaluated as part of a systematic evaluation of the program?

Student Evaluation Tools

Given the extensive use of the Neuman Systems Model as a framework for nursing curricula in the United States and other countries, one might assume that Neuman Systems

Model–based student evaluation tools are quite common. Yet a search of the literature yielded only a few such tools.

Student Clinical Performance Evaluation. The faculty at Indiana University–Purdue University at Fort Wayne developed a Student Clinical Performance Evaluation Tool as part of their evaluation model. This tool was designed to "enhance evaluator objectivity while controlling evaluator subjectivity" (Beckman et al., 1998, p. 150). Student competencies are leveled and weighted so that as students progress through the program, their ability to function independently is evaluated accordingly. The tool includes behavioral objectives, which are used as the basis for measurement of student performance with clients and staff, as well as outcome criteria.

Clinical Evaluation Instruments. Strickland-Seng (1998) described the development of an evaluation package used at the University of Tennessee at Martin that includes three clinical evaluation forms. The Clinical Evaluation Form consists of 25 behaviors based on Neuman Systems Model terminology. Students are ranked from Intradependency (optimal) through Unsatisfactory on each item. Cumulative summaries of each student's behaviors are placed on the Summary of Clinical Evaluation Form. The third tool, the Profile of Clinical Evaluation, is used to document each student's progress throughout the program.

Curriculum and Program Evaluation Tools

Most evaluation models for curriculum and programs are developed using guidelines derived from education paradigms. It follows that nursing model–based tools for curriculum and program evaluation are rare. Indeed, even though evaluation of Neuman Systems Model–based curricula has been the topic of three doctoral dissertations (Fulton, 1992; Mirenda, 1995; Sipple, 1989), the investigators did not use evaluation tools derived from the Neuman Systems Model.

The Lowry–Jopp Neuman Model Evaluation Instrument (LJNMEI). Beginning in 1989, the faculty at the Cecil Community College developed a curriculum evaluation plan to "evaluate the efficacy of a model-based curriculum" (Lowry, 1998c, p. 139). They designed a study to "judge the educational effectiveness of using a nursing model, so that future curriculum decisions would be founded on sound data" (p. 139). Research questions focused on questions about internalization of the Neuman Systems Model, the use of the model in practice by program alumni, and changes that had occurred within the curriculum and the use of the model over time. Alumni were asked to complete the LJNMEI, which is a self-report questionnaire made up of 90 items that measure the graduates' incorporation of the Neuman Systems Model into their practice. The LJNMEI also has been used as the basis for curriculum evaluation in other programs, including Indiana University–Purdue University at Fort Wayne, where it was revised to meet the specific needs of that program (Beckman et al., 1998).

CONCLUSION

Given the widespread use of the Neuman Systems Model in educational settings, the apparent paucity of educational tools is surprising. One explanation for the small number of tools may be that faculty have developed tools but have not published their work. If that is the case, faculty are encouraged to make the time to write about their work and submit it for publication, so that other faculties and students can benefit.

An alternate explanation may be that the inherent complexity in transferring the abstractness of a conceptual model to a concrete measurement tool limits tool development. Newsome and Lowry (1998) discussed the difficulty they experienced developing a Neuman Systems Model–based evaluation tool that included measurable goals and objectives. They stated:

> Although the Neuman Systems Model presents a broad and comprehensive framework based on theories of holism, systems, and gestalt, when it is adopted by educators with a behaviorist bias [which requires measurable goals and objectives] much of the richness and creativity of the model is at risk of loss as faculty attempt to reduce the model propositions to fit specific objectives. (p. 45)

None of the descriptions of the educational tools discussed in this chapter included any information about validity and reliability testing. The development and testing of valid and reliable educational tools certainly requires considerable time. Given the many demands on faculty, tool development and psychometric testing rarely is a priority, unless linked to a research project. Yet educational tools are a valuable technique to help students to learn and faculty to evaluate the students' learning and the curriculum. Furthermore, lack of adequate psychometric properties severely limits any conclusions that may be drawn from administration of the tool. Educators are, therefore, encouraged to make the time for development and psychometric testing of educational tools that will provide meaningful information for evaluation of the students and the curriculum.

Furthermore, if nursing educators are willing to expend the time and effort to develop a curriculum that is based on a conceptual model of nursing, and if they expect students to use that model to guide practice, then evaluation of the students' knowledge and clinical skills should be based on the same conceptual model. More specifically, time and effort need to be devoted to development and psychometric testing of educational tools that are based on the same conceptual model as the curriculum. Attention to the details of educational tool development and testing certainly will increase the continuity and quality of the educational process, which is the ultimate goal of evaluation.

REFERENCES

Beckman, S., Boxley-Harges, S., Bruick-Sorge, C., & Eichenauer, J. (1998). Evaluation modalities for assessing student and program outcomes. In L. Lowry (Ed.), *The Neuman Systems Model and nursing education: Teaching strategies and outcomes* (pp. 149–60). Indianapolis: Sigma Theta Tau International Center Nursing Press.

Dale, M., & Savala, S. (1990). A new approach to the senior practicum. *Nursing Connections, 3*(1), 45–51.

Edwards, P., & Kittler, A. (1991). Integrating rehabilitation content in nursing curricula. *Rehabilitation Nursing, 16*(2), 70–73.

Fulton, B. J. (1992). Evaluation of the effectiveness of the Neuman Systems Model as a theoretical framework for baccalaureate nursing programs. Unpublished doctoral dissertation, University of Massachusetts.

Gronlund, N., & Linn, R. (1990). *Measurement and evaluation in teaching* (6th ed.). New York: Macmillan.

Lowry, L. (1988). Operationalizing the Neuman Systems Model: A course in concepts and process. *Nurse Educator, 13*(3), 19–22.

Lowry, L. (Ed.). (1998a). *The Neuman Systems Model and nursing education: Teaching strategies and outcomes.* Indianapolis: Sigma Theta Tau International Center Nursing Press.

Lowry, L. (1998b). Creative teaching and effective evaluation. In L. Lowry (Ed.), *The Neuman Systems Model and nursing education: Teaching strategies and outcomes* (pp. 17–30). Indianapolis: Sigma Theta Tau International Center Nursing Press.

Lowry, L. (1998c). Efficacy of the Neuman Systems Model as a curriculum framework: A longitudinal study. In L. Lowry (Ed.), *The Neuman Systems Model and nursing education: Teaching strategies and outcomes* (pp. 139–48). Indianapolis: Sigma Theta Tau International Center Nursing Press.

McHolm, F., & Geib, K. (1998). Application of the Neuman Systems Model to teaching health assessment and nursing process. *Nursing Diagnosis, 9*(1), 1–13.

Mirenda, R. (1995). A conceptual–theoretical strategy for curriculum development in baccalaureate nursing program. Unpublished doctoral dissertation. Widener University School of Nursing.

Neuman, B. (1995). In conclusion—Toward new beginnings. In B. Neuman (Ed.), *The Neuman Systems Model* (3rd ed., pp. 671–703). Norwalk, CT: Appleton & Lange.

Neuman, B. & Young, R. J. (1972). A model for teaching total person approach to patient problems. *Nursing Research, 21,* 264–69.

Newsome, G., & Lowry, L. (1998). Evaluation in nursing: History, models, and Neuman's framework. In L. Lowry (Ed.), *The Neuman Systems Model and nursing education: Teaching strategies and outcomes* (pp. 37–52). Indianapolis: Sigma Theta Tau International Center Nursing Press.

Russell, J., & Hezel, L. (1994). Role analysis of the advanced practice nurse using the Neuman health care systems model as a framework. *Clinical Nurse Specialist, 8,* 215–20.

Sipple, J. E. (1989). A model for curriculum change based on retrospective analysis. Unpublished doctoral dissertation. University of South Carolina.

Story, E., & DuGas, B. (1988). A teaching strategy to facilitate conceptual model implementation in practice. *The Journal of Continuing Education in Nursing, 19,* 244–47.

Strickland-Seng, V. (1998). Clinical evaluation: The heart of clinical performance. In L. Lowry (Ed.), *The Neuman Systems Model and nursing education: Teaching strategies and outcomes* (pp. 129–34). Indianapolis: Sigma Theta Tau International Center Nursing Press.

Tollet, S. (1982). Teaching geriatrics and gerontology: Use of the Neuman Systems Model. In B. Neuman (Ed.), *The Neuman Systems Model: Application to nursing education and practice.* Norwalk, CT: Appleton-Century-Crofts.

Using the Neuman Systems Model to Guide Nursing Education in the United States

Barbara Scott Cammuso, Andrea J. Wallen

The purpose of this chapter is to explain how the Neuman Systems Model can be used to guide nursing education. More specifically, this chapter focuses on the use of the Neuman Systems Model as a framework for teaching and learning in the undergraduate and graduate nursing programs at Fitchburg State College in Fitchburg, Massachusetts. The chapter content is directed to an audience of nurse educators, nursing students, nurse clinicians, and individuals in other health-related disciplines who practice in complex health care environments.

OVERVIEW OF THE FITCHBURG STATE COLLEGE NURSING PROGRAM

The purpose of the Fitchburg State College nursing program is to prepare professional nurses who can assume responsibility for planning and providing health care to individuals, families, groups, and communities in collaboration with other professionals. The college offers a nationally accredited baccalaureate degree nursing program, including a four-year generic program and an upper-division registered nurse program. In addition, the college recently began to offer a two-year post-baccalaureate degree program of study leading to a master of science degree, with the specialty focus of forensic nursing. Approximately 3,000 students have completed the baccalaureate degree program; almost 10 percent of those students already were registered nurses. To date, 20 students have completed the post-baccalaureate program.

BACCALAUREATE DEGREE NURSING CURRICULUM

The baccalaureate curriculum espouses a wholistic approach to nursing practice, with an emphasis on the integration of the care of the individual, family, group, and/or community. The nursing portion of the curriculum consists of 12 courses organized as levels based on liberal arts and science prerequisite and corequisite courses (Table 15-1). The Fitchburg State College nursing faculty use the Neuman System Model as a general guide to the organization and progression of nursing courses and as a specific guide for the content of one nursing course. Other nursing conceptual models and theories are used as guides for other nursing courses (Table 15-1). This approach has been used successfully at the University of Ottawa (Bourbonnais & Ross, 1985; Story & Ross, 1986). This approach also is in keeping with Meleis's (1997) position—she maintained that "curricula have become more coherent, systematic and theoretical, and therefore do not need to be limited to one framework" (p. 59).

The Neuman Systems Model concepts of primary, secondary, and tertiary prevention interventions and the five client system variables (physiological, psychological, sociocultural, developmental, and spiritual) pervade the curriculum in a general way. The courses gradually introduce information related to each client system variable through such foundational liberal arts and science prerequisite courses as psychology, sociology,

TABLE 15-1. Fitchburg State College Baccalaureate Program Nursing Courses

Course Number, Title, and Credits Nursing		Predominant Nursing Conceptual Model or Theory
NURS1010	Introduction to Nursing 1credit	
NURS2000	Scientific Foundations for Nursing Intervention I . . . . .2 credits	
NURS2200	Nutritional Foundations for Nursing Interventions . . . . .3 credits	
NURS2700	Nursing Process with the Well Client I .5 credits	Orlando's Theory Peplau's Theory
NURS2100	Scientific Foundations for Nursing Interventions II . . . . .2 credits	
NURS2800	Nursing Process with the Well Client II . . . . .5 credits	
NURS3100	Pharmacological Basis for Nursing Interventions . . . . .2 credits	
NURS3700	Nursing Process with Clients Experiencing Health Alterations I . . . . .10 credits	Roy's Model Orem's Model
NURS3800	Nursing Process with Clients Experiencing Health Alterations II . . . . .10 credits	
NURS4000	Nursing Research . . . . .2 credits	
NURS4700	Nursing Process with Families/Groups in Communities . . . . .6 credits	Neuman's Model
NURS4750	Nursing Process in Home Care . . . . .4 credits	
NURS4800	Nursing Process in a Selective Practicum . . . . .10 credits	
NURS4850	Nursing Leadership and Management Concepts for Nursing Practice . . . . .2 credits	

anatomy and physiology, microbiology, chemistry, and growth and development. The interactive nature of nursing with other sciences and arts is demonstrated throughout the curriculum as the knowledge gained from these basic courses is reinforced and progressively developed prior to the nursing courses. The nursing courses prepare students to focus on individual clients and the family unit as a client of increased care complexity. Nursing prevention interventions are taught sequentially in the various nursing courses, moving from primary prevention to secondary prevention to tertiary prevention intervention levels of care.

In the freshmen year, students take the one-credit course, "Introduction to Nursing," which focuses on the individual student. In this course, students apply concepts from concurrent arts and science courses to examine their own health beliefs, values, practices, and differing perceptions of health, wellness, and illness. The history of nursing theory is introduced in this course to help students appreciate nursing's proud professional heritage.

In the sophomore year, students integrate knowledge from previous courses as they focus on primary prevention intervention in the course, "Nursing Process with the Well Client I." Orlando's (1961) and Peplau's (1952) nursing theories are used in this course to explain the therapeutic relationship between the client and the nurse. A variety of clinical settings, including schools and day care centers, provide opportunities for students to carry out health promotion projects employing primary prevention interventions. Clinical experiences in outpatient wellness client settings and in maternal–newborn inpatient hospital units provide opportunities for exploration of the influences of developmental, sociocultural, and spiritual variables on wellness.

In the junior year, Roy's Adaptation Model (Roy & Andrews, 1999) and Orem's Self-Care Framework (1995) are introduced and concepts are applied as students study the application of the nursing process in the care of children, adolescents, and adults experiencing physical and/or mental health alterations. Secondary prevention intervention is the focus of learning as students provide wholistic nursing care to acutely ill clients. Both classroom content and clinical experiences are more complex with regard to use of theories, concepts, and skill development. Nursing research–related activities are emphasized to provide the scientific basis for nursing practice.

The senior year curriculum builds on and integrates all previous learning and broadens the students' application of the nursing process. Neuman Systems Model–based research reports are used as examples in the research course. The content of the course, "Nursing Process with Families/Groups in Communities," which is offered in the first semester of the senior year, is guided by the Neuman Systems Model. The five Neuman System Model client system variables are used to enhance understanding of families, groups, and communities as client systems. Primary, secondary, and tertiary prevention interventions are emphasized in the course.

The students also identify the intrapersonal, interpersonal, and extrapersonal stressors related to physiological, psychological, sociocultural, developmental, and spiritual variables during home visits with visiting nurses. Additional clinical experiences for this course include schools, senior centers, nursing homes, and occupational settings. Home visits, especially, afford the students opportunities to assess sociocultural variables and develop an understanding of the cultural aspects of care, as well as the financial constraints present within the community in which the client lives. Determination of individual, family, and group developmental history and current status facilitates the students' understanding of developmental variables. The spiritual variable is a difficult concept for students to fully integrate into assessments; indeed, many students view this variable as organized religion. Thus, clarification of focus of assessment of the spiritual variable often is required.

Within the framework of the Neuman Systems Model, students learn to integrate knowledge gained during previous courses, which strengthens the theoretical approach to practice. The Neuman Systems Model "provides a framework of structure and direction for information processing and goal directed activities within an increasing complex health care delivery system" (Klotz, 1995, p. 184). Thus, the Neuman Systems Model is conceptually congruent with the community focus of the first-semester senior nursing course. In particular, as a wholistic systems approach, the model provides an excellent framework for educating senior students during their broadly based community experience. The knowledge gained from this course is integrated into the students' professional practice as they consider case studies in weekly seminars. Two of those case studies illustrate use of the Neuman Systems Model in this senior year nursing course (P. Duynstee, personal communication, April 26, 2000) (Table 15-2).

During the final semester of the senior year, students are required to complete a 24-hour-per-week practicum, which focuses on clients with complex health problems. "To use all senses, experiences, and intuition requires involvement and immersion in situations as a whole, and to describe patterns of responses theoretically requires longer periods of engagement in situations where nursing phenomena occur" (Meleis, 1997, p. 65). During this extended clinical rotation, students are expected to wholistically understand and assess all client system variables and use all three types of prevention interventions.

The Neuman Systems Model gives direction for senior nursing students to provide comprehensive care using a nursing practice model. The richness of this experience is il-

TABLE 15-2. Case Studies

Impact of a Fire on Community System Stability

The assessment of a community in crisis occurred following a warehouse fire in Worcester, Massachusetts, in which six firefighters died. The intracommunity resources were other city departments including the police, city council, and city-paid counselors. In addition, volunteers cooked food and staffed tents, and schoolchildren offered comfort. The intercommunity resources included firefighters and policemen from other towns who worked to enable the Worcester firefighters to do the work of recovery. In addition, residents of surrounding communities sent funds to assist recovery efforts. The extracommunity resources were funds from the state and the federal government, including a Federal Emergency Management Agency (FEMA) grant.

Impact of Parental Variances from Wellness on Family System Stability

The assessment of a family in crisis involved a dysfunctional family secondary to the mother's uncontrolled bipolar illness and the father's history of pedophilia and incest. The intrafamily stressors were the adult roles adopted by the 15-year-old son and the 13-year-old daughter. Both children were acting out and had to rely on outsiders for their food and clothing. The interfamily stressors included isolation from the extended family and neighbors and lack of friends. The extrafamily stressors involved the children's reliance on public health nurses, school counselors, and the Department of Social Services to provide wholistic health care resources.

lustrated in the creative use of the Neuman Systems Model. Students are able to integrate clinical data to identify nursing needs and provide primary, secondary, and tertiary prevention interventions. When students complete the program, they have the ability to use the Neuman System Model to guide wholistic and comprehensive nursing practice.

MASTER'S DEGREE NURSING CURRICULUM

Fitchburg State College has a long history of providing education to baccalaureate nursing students. Over the past quarter century, many graduates have become leaders in nursing. A large number of these graduates, as well as community nurses and faculty, expressed interest in the establishment of a graduate program in nursing at Fitchburg State College. In response to these inquiries, the faculty of the Department of Nursing voted to establish an ad hoc committee to study the feasibility of beginning a master's degree program in nursing. At the conclusion of extensive preliminary work, the decision was made to offer a master's degree program in forensic nursing. The first class of students entered in summer 1997 and graduated in 1999. The Scope and Standards of Forensic Nursing Practice (American Nurses Association & International Association of Forensic Nurses, 1997) includes the following definition of forensic nursing: "The application of forensic science combined with the bio-psychological education of the Registered Nurse, in the scientific investigation, evidence collection and preservation, analysis, prevention and treatment of trauma and/or death related medical—legal issues" (p. v).

The Fitchburg State College master's degree program in forensic nursing encompasses the principles and philosophies of nursing science, forensic science, and criminal science. The program currently is offered on a part-time, two-calendar-year basis through evening, weekend, intersession, and summer courses. The nursing curriculum plan is presented in Table 15-3.

The Neuman Systems Model is used in the master's program curriculum as a conceptual base for care of individual clients and groups of clients. The model is presented

TABLE 15-3. Fitchburg State College Master of Science Program Nursing Courses

NURS7200	Nursing Theory	3 credits
NURS7500	Role Theory: Application to Advanced Practice	2 credits
NURS7400	Contexts for Advanced Practice	3 credits
NURS7300	Advanced Clinical Concepts	2 credits
NURS7000	Nursing with Diverse Populations	1 credit
NURS7900	Epidemiological & Experimental Nursing Research	2 credits
NURS7800	Qualitative Nursing Research	2 credits
NURS9000	Research Application	2 credits
NURS8000	Introduction to Forensic Nursing	2 credits
NURS8100	Scientific Foundations for Forensic Nursing Interventions	2 credits
NURS8200	Forensic Nursing: Victims and Perpetrators I	3 credits
NURS8300	Forensic Nursing: Victims and Perpetrators II	3 credits
NURS9500	Practicum in Forensic Nursing	2 credits

to graduate students in the initial course, "Nursing Theory." The faculty believe that the use and development of theory in nursing is necessary to provide guidelines for advanced practice, as well as to foster a deeper understanding of the discipline as a whole. In this course, the process of theory development is examined. The Neuman System Model is featured in this course because it presents a comprehensive, systems-based conceptual framework for nursing practice and because it facilitates the students' understanding of the client in a wholistic manner, in interaction with the environment, simultaneously integrating the interaction of physiological, psychological, sociological, developmental, and spiritual variables.

The Neuman Systems Model is introduced early in the course to provide a foundation for students as they explore other nursing theories throughout the course. The early introduction to the Neuman Systems Model helps students critically examine their practice early and to value conceptual thinking. The teaching strategies utilized in the presentation of the Neuman Systems Model include lecture, discussion, case studies, and group work.

·When a conceptual model is used to guide nursing education, the nursing metaparadigm concepts are reinterpreted. "Person becomes the student, and environment becomes the educational setting. Health refers to the student's state of wellness or illness, and nursing refers to the educational goals, outcomes, and processes" (Fawcett, 1995, p. 33). Therefore, the goal of the educator is to assist the student to attain and maintain health or optimal wellness. Accordingly, students are asked to use the Neuman Systems Model to assess their personal stressors. Each student is asked to answer the questions listed in Table 15-4. Students compile and analyze their answers to the questions using Johnson's (1989) visual representation of the Neuman Systems Model, which illustrates the pragmatic richness of the Neuman Systems Model (Figure 15-1). The students also are asked to identify primary, secondary, and tertiary preventions as interventions. This exercise clarifies use of the Neuman Systems Model in practical situations, and it fosters the students' personal and professional growth.

Furthermore, the students compare various nursing conceptual models and theories with regard to impact on diverse client populations and societal health needs. Although the Neuman Systems Model is the conceptual framework of the master's program, consideration of other relevant nursing models and theories provides students with the broadest possible theoretical background for advanced practice in forensic nursing. Guest speakers present their research, and students have the opportunity to evaluate

TABLE 15-4. Assessment of Students' Personal Stressors

1. What do you consider your major stressors, or areas of health concern?

2. How do present circumstances differ from usual patterns of living?

3. Have you ever experienced a similar problem? If so, what was the problem and how did you handle it? Were you successful?

4. What do you anticipate for yourself in the future as a consequence of your present situation?

5. What are you doing and what can you do to help yourself?

6. What would you like faculty, family, friends or others to do for you?

Adapted from Neuman, B. (1995). The Neuman Systems Model (3rd ed., pp 59–60). Norwalk, CT: Appleton & Lange.

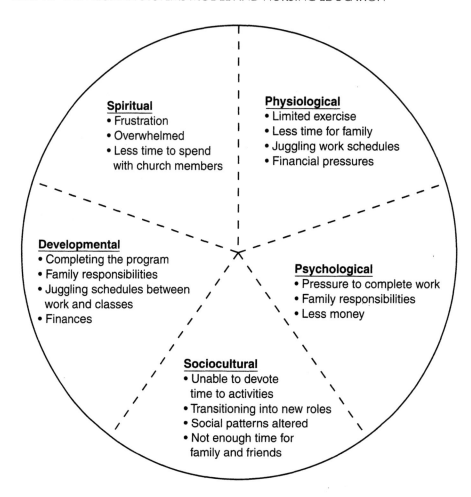

FIGURE 15-1. The Neuman Systems Model applied to graduate nursing students: wholistic stressors.

other nursing models and theories used in current research. Each student selects two nursing conceptual models or theories to study, analyze, and compare in a written assignment. Many students select the Neuman Systems Model to study in depth and to use to acquire new knowledge about a particular concept identified in their practice. Concepts include coping, homelessness, victimization, and loss. Recently, students were asked to discuss a nursing strike that had occurred at a clinical agency in Worcester, Massachusetts. The students then were asked to use a nursing model or theory to explain how they would conduct an assessment of the striking nurses and the nurses who crossed the picket lines, and to identify relevant nursing prevention interventions. This exercise helped the students to appreciate the application of a nursing model or theory in a contemporary clinical situation of considerable interest to them.

The Neuman Systems Model is reintroduced in the course, "Advanced Clinical Concepts." This course provides the opportunity for students to validate current clinical skills and to develop advanced professional decision-making skills. Clinical issues, such as performance evaluation, collaboration, and ethical considerations, are addressed. The Neuman

Systems Model provides an excellent framework for the course content, which includes interviewing techniques, advanced client system assessment, clinical and ethical decision making, and collaboration. Students use the Neuman Systems Model to analyze case studies each week. For each case study, two students participate in role-playing activities while the other students divide into small groups to identify and cluster client system stressors. They then determine what additional data are required to make a tentative nursing diagnosis for each client, select a specific nursing diagnosis, and identify relevant prevention interventions.

The Neuman Systems Model and the Integrated Practice Model of Forensic Nursing (Lynch, 1997) are presented in the course, "Forensic Nursing: Victims and Perpetrators I," to guide nursing practice. Clients of interest are those with such problems as psychiatric disorders resulting from forensic involvement, with a focus on individuals diagnosed with personality disorders, psychotic thinking, and drug addictions; violent behavior resulting in sexual assault, domestic violence, gang violence, and deviant cults; trauma and post-traumatic stress affecting victims of violence; and children in danger of becoming victims and/or perpetrators. The Neuman Systems Model is used in this course to explore the impact of trauma and violence on significant others, as well as the larger community and society. The model provides students with a purposeful guide for gaining professional knowledge in the theory and practice of forensic nursing. The usefulness of the model is particularly evident when the students comprehensively identify and categorize stressors that could possibly penetrate the victims' flexible and normal lines of defense (Figure 15-2). The students also develop primary, secondary, and tertiary prevention interventions for trauma victims and the community at large, and provide feedback about the effectiveness of those prevention interventions.

The Integrated Practice Model of Forensic Nursing (Lynch, 1997) complements the Neuman Systems Model in the course. Thus, the student is cross-trained in the principles and philosophies of nursing science, forensic science, and criminal justice. For example, when confronted with a victim of sexual assault, the student is able to base prevention interventions on findings of assessment using the five Neuman Systems Model client system variables. In addition, use of the Integrated Practice Model of Forensic Nursing enables the student to identify, collect, and preserve forensic evidence that may be admissible in a court of law.

Furthermore, the legal, ethical, clinical, and advocacy responsibilities of advanced practice nursing are emphasized throughout this course. Students are required to write a paper based on systems theory, with a major focus on a forensic topic related to course content. To date, 75 percent of the students have selected the Neumann Systems Model as the guiding framework for the written assignment.

CONCLUSION

The Fitchburg State College nursing faculty has used the Neuman Systems Model to conceptualize aspects of the curriculum in both the baccalaureate and master's degree nursing programs. Students value use of the Neuman Systems Model as a guide for comprehensive nursing practice with individuals, families, and groups. Furthermore, as an increasing array of multidisciplinary health professionals care for diverse groups of clients with complex health problems, the Neuman Systems Model offers direction for truly collaborative practice that can create a better world for clients and health professionals alike.

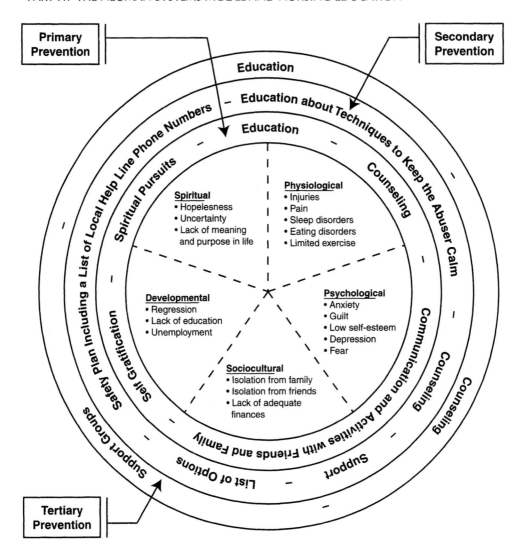

FIGURE 15-2.   The Neuman Systems Model applied to victims of domestic violence: wholistic variables and prevention interventions.

REFERENCES

American Nurses Association & International Association of Forensic Nurses. (1997). *Scope and standards of forensic nursing practice.* Washington, DC: American Nurses Publishing.

Bourbonnais, F. F., & Ross, M. M. (1985). The Neuman Systems Model in nursing education: Course development and implementation. *Journal of Advanced Nursing, 10,* 117–23.

Fawcett, J. (1995). *Analysis and evaluation of conceptual models of nursing* (3rd ed.). Philadelphia: Davis.

Johnson, S. E. (1989). A picture is worth a thousand words: Helping students visualize a conceptual model. *Nurse Educator, 13*(3), 21–24.

Klotz, L. C. (1995). Integration of the Neuman Systems Model into the BSN curriculum at the University of Texas at Tyler. In B. Neuman (Ed.), *The Neuman Systems Model* (3rd ed., pp. 147–62). Norwalk, CT: Appleton & Lange.

Lynch, V. (1997). *Clinical forensic nursing: A new perspective in trauma.* Fort Collins, CO: Bearhawk Consulting Group.

Meleis, A. I. (1997). *Theoretical nursing: Development and progress* (3rd ed.). Philadelphia: Lippincott.

Orem, D. E. (1995). *Nursing: Concepts of practice* (5th ed.). St. Louis: Mosby-Year Book.

Orlando, I. J. (1961). *The dynamic nurse–patient relationship: Function, process, and principles.* New York: G. P. Putnam's Sons (Reprinted 1990. New York: National League for Nursing).

Peplau, H. E. (1952). *Interpersonal relations in nursing: A conceptual frame of reference for psychodynamic nursing.* New York: G. P. Putnam's Sons (Reprinted 1991. New York: Springer).

Roy, C., & Andrews, H. A. (1999). *The Roy adaptation model* (2nd ed.). Stamford, CT: Appleton & Lange.

Story, E. L., & Ross, M. M. (1986). Family centered community health nursing and the Betty Neuman Systems Model. *Nursing Papers, 18,* 77–88.

sixteen

Using the Neuman Systems Model to Guide Nursing Education in Holland

Marlou de Kuiper

The purpose of this chapter is to describe the use of the Neuman Systems Model at a school of nursing in Holland. The chapter begins with a description of the educational system in Holland and continues with a discussion of the issues surrounding the selection and introduction of the Neuman Systems Model in nursing education programs in Holland.

NURSING EDUCATION IN HOLLAND

The educational system in Holland is a flexible system that permits students to follow different routes to the professions. After eight years of primary school, students are placed at four different levels of education (Figure 16-1).

A student can follow a route horizontally as well as vertically. For example, a student could go from middle preparation to higher preparation, then to higher professional education, and on to university. Nursing is taught at two levels: middle professional education and higher professional education.

Higher professional education is taught in institutes for higher professional education, which also are called universities. The level of teaching at the university level is comparable to a bachelor's degree, which can be followed by a master's degree. There are nine institutes of this type in Holland. Most serve a regional function, two have a Christian foundation, and all enroll students from throughout the country. The Visitation Committee, a council that is installed by the Ministry of Education, annually monitors the quality of all the Institutes for Higher Education. The Visitation Committee

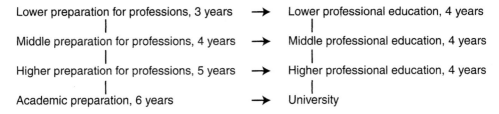

Lower preparation for professions, 3 years   →   Lower professional education, 4 years

Middle preparation for professions, 4 years   →   Middle professional education, 4 years

Higher preparation for professions, 5 years   →   Higher professional education, 4 years

Academic preparation, 6 years   →   University

FIGURE 16-1.   Levels of education in Holland.

members report their findings and state recommendations, which are binding advice to the institutes.

The Dutch Reformed Church has its own primary, secondary, and professional schools and a University. The Dutch Reformed University is in Zwolle, a town of 100,000 inhabitants in the eastern region of Holland.

SELECTION OF THE NEUMAN SYSTEMS MODEL

In 1991, the Visitation Committee came to the Dutch Reformed University and paid special attention to the Department of Nursing. The Visitation Committee gave the Department of Nursing a few compliments for the quality of nursing education and issued new challenges. The Committee members noted that the Department did not have a very clear philosophy of nursing, which resulted in an arbitrary curriculum that was not sufficiently clear to either the students or the institutes where the students did their internships. A new curriculum was needed, based on the combination of a clear philosophy of nursing and a clear statement about the Christian identity of the school.

The teaching staff studied the existing, published models in search of a philosophy that could meet their specific aims for a clear and Christian curriculum. They reviewed the works of Leininger (1991), Roy (Roy & Andrews, 1995), Orem (1995), Peplau (1952), and three models that had been developed in Holland and Belgium—the works of Grijpdonck (Koene et al., 1982), van der Brink-Tjebbes (1987), and De Jong (De Jong & Salentijn, 1993), using a questionnaire based on Fawcett's (1989) framework for the evaluation of conceptual models of nursing (Table 16-1).

TABLE 16-1. Questionnaire to Evaluate Nursing Models and Theories

- Are the assumptions in the model or theory explicated?
- Are the four elements of the metaparadigm (person, health, environment, and nursing) explicit and clearly defined?
- Have the relationships between the four elements been defined?
- Is the theory or model consistent and logical?
- Is there empirical evidence for the theory or model?
- Is the theory or model relevant and applicable to our society/culture?
- Can it be taught to students?
- Are the concepts of God and religion clearly addressed?

Each member of the teaching staff studied and then presented one theory or model to colleagues at special meetings. This approach provided an opportunity for very interesting and educational discussions among the members of the teaching staff, which enabled them to become increasingly clear about the specific aims for the new curriculum. However, a model that was suited to their needs was not yet identified.

The teaching staff identified several reasons that supported a change in the curriculum, beyond the need for a clear and Christian curriculum. One reason was that students' parents, institutes for internships, and the teaching staff all wanted a curriculum that would clearly state the school's identity as a Christian institute but at the same time, educate students as tolerant and respectful nurses. Another reason was that the teaching staff was not satisfied with the lack of integration of the subjects that were taught, including anatomy, physiology, psychology, sociology, and nursing. The lack of integration led to a view of people with health problems as first divided into many different aspects and then integrated into one person by the students.

The third reason for a curriculum change was that a new educational system for nursing and caring had been introduced in Holland. That system mandated that care is to be provided by individuals at five different levels: (1) Helper, (2) Assistant, (3) Caregiver, (4) Nursing Level four, and (5) Nursing Level five.

The fourth reason was a need for refinement in the nursing process, including Functional Health Patterns (Gordon, 1997), North American Nursing Diagnosis Association (NANDA) nursing diagnoses (Gordon, 1997), International Classification of Impairment, Disorders, and Handicaps (ICIDH), and Nursing Classification of Interventions (NIC) (McCloskey & Bulechek, 1997). The fifth reason was that students found a gap between theory and practice and also found no element of Christianity in the curriculum.

INTRODUCTION OF THE NEUMAN SYSTEMS MODEL TO HOLLAND

Frans Verberk became enthusiastic about the Neuman Systems Model when he was studying for his master's degree in nursing from 1988 to 1991. He introduced the model to the Institute for Ambulant Mental Health Care, where he was working at that time. Some of his colleagues also became enthusiastic, and they started studying the model. At the same time, Verberk introduced the model to several committees of which he was a member. As Verberk's enthusiasm spread, he gathered people around him and formed the Neuman Systems Model Study Group. This study group now is called the International Neuman Systems Model Association (INSMA), Department of Holland. People from all areas of health care participate in the INSMA. The goals of the INSMA are to promote the implementation of the Neuman Systems Model in Holland and to provide advice and assistance to individuals and institutes who request it. The INSMA organizes a yearly conference, at which two Neuman Systems Model Trustees from the United States lecture. The author of this chapter has been a member of this group since 1994 and is the secretary of the INSMA. There is, then, a group of health care professionals in Holland who are well acquainted with the Neuman Systems Model.

At about the same time, one member of the teaching staff at the Dutch Reformed University Department of Nursing discovered the Neuman Systems Model while studying for his master's degree. He introduced the model to his colleagues, who agreed that the concept of wholism was very well represented in the model, especially since the spiritual variable was included. Other reasons for selecting the Neuman Systems Model included its focus on health and well-being instead of illness and disease; the concept of negotiation with clients, which represents a basic attitude of equality; the opportunity for cooperation with other disciplines from the same basic general philosophy; and the concept of the client system as an individual, a group, or a community. Consequently, the teaching staff decided that the Neuman Systems Model offered a conceptual frame of reference that was congruent with all of the reasons for a new curriculum; they then agreed that their choice would not be discussed again to avoid delay in the development of the new curriculum.

Betty Neuman and Dorothy Craig visited Holland in 1995. They lectured to a large audience and presented a Master Class. Jan de Meij, Director of the Department of Nursing at the Dutch Reformed University, and Gert Westrik attended that lecture, where they met with Frans Verberk and Marlou de Kuiper, who had just published an introduction to the Neuman Systems Model for Holland (Verberk & de Kuiper, 1998). De Meij asked de Kuiper to be the external advisor for the development of the new curriculum, and she agreed, regarding this as an excellent opportunity to promote the application of the Neuman Systems Model in Holland.

From September 1995 to June 1996, the teaching staff, de Meij, and de Kuiper met every two weeks for two hours on Monday mornings to study the Neuman Systems Model extensively and to formulate the basic principles for the new curriculum. At the end of that year, all participants spoke "Neuman language" and felt confident that they knew the model very well, even though they still had to determine how to apply it to the new curriculum. From September 1996 to June 1997, the basis for the new curriculum was laid, based on the statements listed in Figure 16-2.

IMPLEMENTATION OF THE NEUMAN SYSTEMS MODEL AT THE DUTCH REFORMED UNIVERSITY DEPARTMENT OF NURSING

Teaching Staff

The teaching staff consisted of seven people with a nursing and teaching professional background. Most of the teaching staff worked part time and also were involved in supervising the internships, the organization of teaching, and mentoring students. Members of other disciplines also taught in the Department of Nursing—a physician taught

- Nursing is the core of the curriculum

- Teaching is done from a continuum for which the polarities are:

    Health (well-being) → Illness
    Primary prevention → Tertiary prevention
    Knowing self → Knowledge of other
    Simple → Complex
    Teaching → Problem-based learning
    Group → Individual learning

FIGURE 16-2.   Basis for the new curriculum.

anatomy and physiology and pathology, a sociologist taught sociology, and so on. Consequently, these professionals had to be convinced of the advantages of the Neuman Systems Model as the basis for the new curriculum. De Kuiper asked these individuals to study the biblical book of Job and to consider Job their client, to be diagnosed according to the Neuman Systems Model. The request appealed to them, and they found that the Christian foundation for nursing was well represented in the model. At the same time, it was not a dogmatic approach, allowing room for the students to develop a respectful and tolerant attitude toward clients of all religions and backgrounds.

Complicating Factors

The teaching staff developed a positive attitude toward the Neuman Systems Model even though the change in the curriculum meant that they would have to rewrite all of their lectures. Other complications included the introduction of problem-based learning in the second year; the application of scientific research and classifications to the nursing process; and the introduction of the five levels of caring, which meant that the students were to be educated for a higher level of competence.

In addition, the teaching staff and external advisor had to face the fact that they were to develop a new curriculum, based on four principles that were new to all of them and very different from what they had experienced themselves. They felt almost like amateurs faced with a very complicated professional challenge. Moreover, funds and expertise were limited, so that they had to deal with having both the old and the new curricula at the same time for a few years.

Internships

In Holland, nursing students do internships at institutes for health care, which provide the practical part of nursing education. The institutes have their own teaching staffs; the teaching staff from the nursing program remain in contact with the students and the institutes, but they do not provide any practical teaching. This means that very close collaboration is needed, and is stated in contracts between the nursing education programs and the institutes. The institutes stipulate their own demands for the level of competence of the students and their specific goals, as part of the overall guidelines provided by the Ministry of Education. The institutes may or may not have an explicit philosophy of health or nursing. Furthermore, nursing students from various nursing education programs typically are at the same institute at the same time. That means that the various nursing education programs cannot have too many differences in their teaching methods and philosophy of nursing and nursing education.

Therefore, to maintain good functional relationships, it was important that the institutes agree with the teaching staff's decision to use the Neuman Systems Model as the guide for the nursing curriculum, and agree that the students would speak the language of both the Neuman Systems Model and the institute where they do their internships. Toward that end, representatives from the affiliated institutes were invited to a conference at which the Neuman Systems Model, problem-based learning, the new level of competency, and the developments about the nursing process were introduced. The new levels of competence and the developments about the nursing process already had been introduced in all of the schools of nursing and the affiliated institutes throughout Holland. Furthermore, problem-based learning had become very popular, so these elements were being introduced nearly everywhere. However, the Neuman Systems Model was new to them.

The Culture of Holland

Holland is a small country, and probably because of its small size, it has business interests all over the world. It has become a multicultural society, more so because of the large number of fugitives and asylum seekers in recent years, combined with a colonial past and a history of immigrants from Morocco and Turkey. The people in Holland like to be thought of as tolerant to other cultures, religions, and ideas because they value the democratic history of their past. This means that the statement of a distinctive philosophy often is frowned upon; it is thought that if one makes distinctive choices, one might not be very tolerant of people who make different choices. That is probably the main reason why there are very few institutes and schools of nursing that use a particular nursing theory or model. The Dutch Reformed University distinguishes itself from other schools because of its specific Christian background and added the selection of the Neuman Systems Model. Such a choice could easily lead to estrangement from other institutes. Fortunately, the representatives from the institutes found that the Neuman Systems Model was a good choice, clear enough to understand and apply, and flexible in its philosophy about client systems and their needs. Thus, the Neuman Systems Model was accepted with some enthusiasm.

Support for Implementation of the Neuman Systems Model

The teaching staff was in dire need of support, which was provided through an external advisor on education from the University of Leiden, and through the Theological University of Kampen. The University of Leiden advisor was asked to give his opinion on two questions: (1) Can the new educational demands be combined with the Neuman Systems Model?, and (2) Is it wise to combine all four changes for a new curriculum at the same time, or should the changes be introduced gradually? The advisor was given background material and studied the questions intensively. He decided that the model was very well suited to combine all four demands for the new curriculum.

The Theological University faculty was asked to help the teaching staff to develop the spiritual variable further and to provide advice about the right match between the orthodox background of the school and the open and tolerant attitude toward other religions and spiritual needs that is needed for the education of nurses.

During this time, de Meij and Westrik wrote several articles about the introduction of the Neuman Systems Model in newspapers and magazines with the same Christian background. Those articles generated interest and support, which resulted in funds for the project. Two secretaries, who were former nursing students, were hired to support the new curriculum. They were asked to be secretaries for the project because they had a clear view about what students needed and how some fun and a lot of interest in studying nursing could be incorporated into the curriculum.

The New Curriculum

Nursing education for Level five takes four years. Each year of the new curriculum was developed and then implemented. The students are required to study 1,680 hours in each year of their education, which is accomplished in 40 hours each week for 42 weeks.

TABLE 16-2. First-Year Curriculum Objectives

Students gain knowledge, skills, and understanding in:

- The concept of health (well-being)
- Knowing self concerning the Functional Health Patterns and the five Neuman Systems Model client system variables
- Primary prevention interventions
- The concept of environment
- The relationships between these aspects of the curriculum

The First Year. The objectives for the first year curriculum are listed in Table 16-2. In the first year, the students have an introductory internship in one of the institutes for 4 weeks. The first week of the educational year is an introduction to the school and each other, and the last week is spent on different activities. The remaining weeks of the first year took shape as a combination of the Neuman Systems Model and Gordon's (1997) Functional Health Patterns. The introduction of the Functional Health Patterns was not a free choice; this perspective is part of all nursing education programs in Holland.

The first year was divided into 11 units of learning, called modules. Each module addresses one Functional Health Pattern. The weekly schedule is given in Table 16-3.

The teaching staff developed a new curriculum with new assignments and tests, which required a lot of work, but that work was coupled with inspiration. The first-year students not only seemed happy but also stated that the lessons were very interesting and that the program was stimulating and presented a clear view of nursing.

The Second Year. Problem-based learning was introduced in the second year. The units of learning were based on subjects as prescribed by the Ministry of Education and according to categories of illness—chronic, psychiatric, geriatric, surgical, mental handicap, and maternity and child health. The basic objectives for the content of the second year curriculum are listed in Table 16-4.

An internship of three months is included; this experience adds considerably to the students' skills in problem-based learning. The teaching staff found that students applied the Neuman Systems Model implicitly, both in school and during their internships. The institutes where the internships took place found that the students were well able to take care of clients, that they had a methodological approach to client problems, and that they were more autonomous than would have been expected for their level of education.

The Third Year. Most of the time in the third year is spent on two internships, each four months in length. The remaining time is spent on supportive teaching of clinical skills

TABLE 16-3. First-Year Curriculum Weekly Schedule

Monday	Introduction to the subjects and assignments of that week
Tuesday	Physiological variable and technical nursing skills
Wednesday	Psychological and developmental variable and communication skills
Thursday	Sociocultural variable and assignments
Friday	Spiritual variable and integration of all subjects by means of a nursing case history

TABLE 16-4. Second-Year Curriculum Objectives

Students gain knowledge, skills, and understanding of:

- Clinical skills
- Coordination of care
- Quality of care
- Secondary prevention interventions

and problem-based learning, in the form of supervision meetings. Here, the students discuss their experiences in a small group with a supervisor. The goal of the supervision meetings is to improve reflective learning so to enhance problem-solving skills.

The students and two members of the teaching staff also spend two weeks in Israel, where they visit institutes for health care and several holy places. The aim of this experience is to introduce the students to another culture and its system of health care. The trip to Israel is very much appreciated by the students. They have to pay their own way, and they find many creative ways to generate the money for the trip.

The Fourth Year. In the last year of their educational program, the students have to select a specific area of practice from among the following: intensive clinical care, psychiatry and care for the mentally handicapped, care for the chronically ill, geriatric care, or maternity and child health. This choice is called the differentiation of care. Students write a thesis about a theoretical aspect of the differentiation, and they gain specific theoretical and practical knowledge about their subject of choice at the level of tertiary prevention. At this stage of their education, they are able to manage the care situation at the level of the primary care process for complex patients. They contribute to the quality of nursing practice and can be role models for the Level four nurses.

EVALUATION OF THE CURRICULUM PROJECT

The implementation of the Neuman Systems Model will be completed in June 2001. To date, the project has been successful. It will be evaluated scientifically in the fall of 2001. The Neuman Systems Model has served as a framework and basis for the curriculum. It also has served as a framework for the determination of the conditions that were needed to make the project successful. The teaching staff and external advisor found that the model can be applied to many different situations to state a diagnosis for that situation and to select the prevention interventions that would best meet the needs of that situation. For example, when trying to create favorable conditions for the implementation of the Neuman Systems Model in the curriculum, it was applied to the present situation. Subsequently, the teaching staff found that they needed more support for the physical, developmental, and spiritual variables. The University of Leiden Faculty of Education, the Theological University of Kampen, and the two secretaries for the project provided that support. Applying the Neuman Systems Model also made the teaching staff aware of the external stressors encountered by the Department of Nursing and the project, as well as the created environment of each member of the teaching staff.

The effect of the Neuman Systems Model as the basis for the new curriculum on the student's level of performance will be measured in 2001. Success is evident at the present time—the students are happy, and the affiliated institutes are satisfied with the students' level of competence. Every year, the students and the Visitation Committee evaluate the schools for nursing education. The quality, clarity, and philosophy of the curriculum are evaluated and the students rate such topics as integration of subjects, quality of lectures, and professional skills. The findings of that evaluation are published in the larger newspapers in Holland. The 19 schools for nursing education are rated; a high place on this list represents a high quality of education. Four years ago, before the introduction of the Neuman Systems Model, the Dutch Reformed University took twelfth place. Since the introduction of the Neuman Systems Model, the University has been on the top of the list for three consecutive years. Clearly, the Neuman Systems Model has provided the teaching staff, students, affiliated institutes, and clients with a stimulating and professional basis for nursing and has improved the quality of teaching and practice.

ENDNOTES

Grateful appreciation is expressed to Dr. Jan de Meij, Director of the Dutch Reformed University Department of Nursing, for his steadfast support of the Neuman Systems Model and all that he continues to do to facilitate implementation of the model in the Department of Nursing.

REFERENCES

De Jong, J., & Salentijn, C. (1993). *Verpleegkunde in perspectief* [Nursing in perspective]. Zaventhem: Bohn, Stafleu Van Loghum, Houten.

Fawcett, J. (1989). *Analysis and evaluation of conceptual models of nursing* (2nd ed.). Philadelphia: Davis.

Gordon, M. (1997). Verpleegkundige diagnostiek: Process en toepassing [Dutch translation of Nursing diagnoses, process, and application]. Utrecht: Lemma.

Koene, G., Grijpdonck, M., Rodenbach, M.Th., & Windey, T. (1982). *Integrerende verpleegkunde: Wetenschap in praktijk* [Integrated nursing: Science in practice]. Lochem: De Tijdstroom.

Leininger, M. M. (Ed.). (1991). *Culture care diversity and universality: A theory of nursing.* New York: National League for Nursing Press.

McCloskey, J. C., & Bulechek, G. M. (1997). *Verpleegkundige interventies.* Utrecht: De Tijdstroom.

Orem, D. E. (1995). *Nursing: Concepts of practice* (5th ed.). St. Louis: Mosby-Year Book.

Peplau, H. E. (1952). *Interpersonal relations in nursing: A conceptual frame of reference for psychodynamic nursing.* New York: G. P. Putnam's Sons (Reprinted 1991. New York: Springer).

Roy, C., & Andrews, H. A. (1991). *The Roy adaptation model: The definitive statement.* Stamford, CT: Appleton & Lange.

van der Brink-Tjebbes, J. A. (1987). *Verplen naar de maat, een verplegingswetenschappelijke optiek* [A scientific approach to individual nursing]. Lochem: De Tijdstroom.

Verbek, F., & de Kuiper, M. (1998). *Verpleegkunde volgens het Neuman systems model.* Assen: Van Gorcum.

PART V

THE NEUMAN SYSTEMS MODEL AND NURSING ADMINISTRATION

seventeen

Guidelines for Neuman Systems Model–Based Administration of Health Care Services

Barbara F. Shambaugh, Betty Neuman, Jacqueline Fawcett

T   he Neuman Systems Model was developed as a way to organize clinical course content and wholistic nursing practice (Neuman, 1982; Neuman & Young, 1972). As a systems approach, the Neuman Systems Model is easily adapted by nurse administrators for the management of nursing services. The Neuman Systems Model also can be used by the administrators of the full array of other health care services, including medicine, physical therapy, occupational therapy, respiratory therapy, and so on. Consequently, both clinicians and administrators from all disciplines can use the same frame of reference for their activities, which strengthens interdisciplinary communication. Moreover, the use of a common conceptual framework, common language, and a common commitment to wholistic health care offer a unique opportunity for provision of the highest quality of health care, as well as for managerial excellence.

The application of the Neuman Systems Model for use in the administration of health care services requires a modification in the focus of the four nursing metaparadigm concepts. *Person* becomes the staff of a clinical agency, the department of nursing as a whole, and the entire clinical agency, as well as any larger health care organization with which the clinical agency is affiliated. *Environment* becomes the surroundings of the staff and the setting in which nursing administration occurs, as well as the relevant surroundings of the department, agency, and organization. *Health* becomes the wellness or illness state of the staff, as well as of the entire clinical agency and the larger health care organization. *Nursing* becomes the management strategies and the administrative policies used by nurse administrators on behalf of or in conjunction with the staff, the nursing department, the clinical agency, and the health care organization. Similar modifi-

265

cations are required for each discipline utilizing the Neuman Systems Model. These modifications will lead to a unified vision and interdisciplinary integration for any health care organization.

This chapter identifies guidelines for Neuman Systems Model–based administration of health care services. These guidelines are applicable to the administration of services in any health care discipline. The chapter includes a discussion of each guideline and an explanation of how the Neuman Systems Model facilitates wholistic administration of health care services.

THE NEUMAN SYSTEMS MODEL ADMINISTRATION GUIDELINES

Guidelines for Neuman Systems Model–based nursing practice were extracted from the content of the model several years ago (Fawcett et al., 1989). Those guidelines have been refined as the result of dialogue among the three authors of this chapter. Although the guidelines initially were targeted to nursing, our interest in the multidisciplinary use of the Neuman Systems Model called for the extrapolation of the guidelines for use by administrators of all health care services, regardless of disciplinary affiliation. Consequently, the guidelines listed in Table 17-1 have been written for the administrators of all health care services.

The first guideline stipulates that the focus of Neuman Systems Model–based health care services is the client system, which can be individuals, families, groups, and communities. The administrator regards the collective staff as a client system that is a composite of physiological, psychological, sociocultural, developmental, and spiritual variables. The administrator also may regard each department of a clinical agency or the larger health care institution as the client system. The client system is the focal point for the administrators' activities. Thus, the identification of a particular entity as the client system of interest to the administrator is a crucial first step in the use of the Neuman Systems Model as a guide for the administration of health care services. The client system most likely is identified by virtue of the administrator's particular role in the health care organization. For example, the chief executive officer most likely would identify all personnel in the entire health care organization as the client system, whereas a nurse manager most likely would identify the staff of a particular clinical unit in the organization as the client system. Regardless of the client system of interest, the administrator realizes that that system is made up of wholistic human beings and attends to the physiological, psychological, sociocultural, developmental, and spiritual aspects of that client system. In addition, the administrator always remembers that health care is directed to human beings, so that the services are for the sake of those human beings rather than for the organization per se.

The second guideline stipulates that the purpose of the administration of health care services is to facilitate the delivery of the primary, secondary, and tertiary prevention interventions that will best help client systems to retain, attain, and maintain optimal stability. This guideline focuses attention on the need to think within a prevention perspective. That is, all interventions are directed toward preventive practices that will foster optimal client system stability and prevent the occurrence or extension of stressor reactions. Moreover, this guideline focuses the administrator's attention on the management strategies and administrative policies that best facilitate the delivery of prevention interventions.

TABLE 17-1. Guidelines for Administration of Neuman Systems Model–Based Health Care Services

1. Focus of Health Care Services	The focus of Neuman Systems Model–based health care services is the client system, which can be individuals, families, groups, and communities. The administrator regards the collective staff as a client system that is a composite of physiological, psychological, sociocultural, developmental, and spiritual variables. The administrator also may regard each department of a clinical agency or the larger health care institution as the client system.
2. Purpose of Administration of Health Care Services	The purpose of the administration of health care services is to facilitate the delivery of the primary, secondary, and tertiary prevention interventions that will best help client systems to retain, attain, and maintain optimal stability.
3. Characteristics of Health Care Personnel	Health care personnel, including administrators and clinicians, must have knowledge of the content of the Neuman Systems Model, as well as the willingness to implement this conceptual model as a guide for administration and clinical practice. Personnel also must appreciate systems thinking.
4. Settings for Health Care Services	Health care services are located in settings in which primary, secondary, and tertiary prevention is appropriate, including but not limited to ambulatory clinics, acute care medical centers, community hospitals, rehabilitation units, elementary and secondary schools, colleges and universities, prisons, retirement communities, life care communities, assisted living facilities, nursing homes, hospices, clients' homes, community centers, and the streets and sidewalks of the community.
5. Management Strategies and Administrative Policies	Management strategies and administrative policies focus on the staff, the departments, or the total institution as the client system of the administrator, who uses management practices that promote optimal client system stability.

The third guideline stipulates that health care personnel, including administrators and clinicians, must have knowledge of the content of the Neuman Systems Model, as well as the willingness to implement this conceptual model as a guide for administration and clinical practice. Comprehensive understanding of the content of the Neuman Systems Model is, of course, mandatory for any application. Readers are referred to the primary source—Chapter 1 of this book—as well as to Fawcett's (2000) analysis and evaluation of the Neuman Systems Model. The willingness to implement the Neuman Systems Model as the guide for administration and clinical practice requires a commitment to a particular wholistic frame of reference and a particular way of thinking about the administration of health care services and the focus of those services. It follows, then, that the third guideline also stipulates that personnel also must appreciate systems thinking. Indeed, the key to successful Neuman Systems Model–based administration of health care services is comprehensive understanding of general system theory, as explained by von Bertalanffy (1968) in his landmark treatise on living open systems. Successful administration also is facilitated by understanding the knowledge from the various adjunctive disciplines that contributed to the development of the Neuman Systems Model, such as de Chardin's (1955) philosophical beliefs about the wholeness of life and various perspectives of stress (Lazarus, 1981; Selye, 1950).

The fourth guideline stipulates that health care services are located in settings in which primary, secondary, and tertiary prevention is appropriate, including but not limited to ambulatory clinics, acute care medical centers, community hospitals, rehabilitation units, elementary and secondary schools, colleges and universities, prisons, retirement communities, life care communities, assisted living facilities, nursing homes, hospices, clients' homes, community centers, and the streets and sidewalks of the community. This means that administration of health care services is not limited to designated clinical agencies and health care organizations but also is needed in any setting in which nurses and other members of the multidisciplinary health care team are engaged in helping clients to attain, retain, or maintain optimal system stability.

The fifth guideline stipulates that management strategies and administrative policies focus on the staff, the departments, or the total institution as the client system of the administrator, who uses management practices that promote optimal client system stability. Optimal stability means that there is harmony among the five client system variables—physiological, psychological, sociocultural, developmental, and spiritual. The client system's potential for optimal stability may vary with events that occur within a particular department or health care organization, as well as events and policies that affect the delivery and financing of all health care services. Thus, the administrator must devise and use dynamic management strategies and administrative policies that are sensitive to changes in the organization, the client system, and the larger health care arena.

IMPLEMENTING THE NEUMAN SYSTEMS MODEL IN HEALTH CARE ADMINISTRATION

A turbulent health care landscape provides both challenges and opportunities for the administration of health care services. Changes in practice sites, payment methods, insurance programs, and population demographics have upset the vision of established organizations and clinicians. New visions must be bold and progressive. The administration and delivery of health care services require a new web of relationships between and among multidisciplinary administrators and clinicians, new services to constituents, and a business environment focused on services to wholistic human beings. Use of the Neuman Systems Model by administrators can greatly facilitate the development of requisite relationships, services, and a humanistic business environment. In particular, the Neuman Systems Model guides identification of political, regulatory, and ethical stressors that affect the administration and delivery of health care services. The economic health of the health care organization is protected when such stressors are identified and appropriate prevention interventions are developed.

The Neuman Systems Model can guide articulation of the philosophy, vision, and mission statements of the health care organization and each unit of that organization. Management practices and administrative policies, which can be structured according to primary, secondary, and tertiary prevention interventions, follow from those statements. For example, primary prevention administrative interventions could include recruitment and retention of well-qualified personnel for all positions in the organization, in-depth education and a strong orientation program for all administrators and staff, promotion of ongoing professional development of all administrators and staff through attendance at local seminars and national and international conferences, clear lines of communication, promotion of effective interpersonal relations, and responsible and equitable use of economic resources. Secondary prevention administrative interventions could include clarification of communications to all client systems, early identification of noxious stressors, problem solving by individuals and groups within the organization, and use of economic and other resources to support the organization, the administrators, and the staff. Tertiary prevention administrative interventions could include articulation of a renewed commitment to the Neuman Systems Model and the promotion of optimal client system stability, use of negotiation as a management strategy, continued education of administrators and staff, and once again, clear communication. Many other examples of Neuman Systems Model–based management practices and administrative policies are cited in Chapter 18.

The cost containment measures undertaken in recent years by health care organizations have resulted in a flattening of organizational structures through removal of various layers of managers and supervisors. Consequently, there is considerable need for further development of the leadership capabilities of staff through continuing education, mentoring, and coaching. The Neuman Systems Model is an ideal conceptual frame of reference for such activities because its wholistic perspective fosters a broad view of situations, events, and services that can accommodate changes in policies, while at the same time informing policy.

Moreover, inasmuch as the systems perspective in which the Neuman Systems Model is grounded is prevalent in many contemporary health care organizations, it is easily understood and accepted by administrators and clinicians of all health care disciplines. Furthermore, the systems perspective of the Neuman Systems Model provides a context for processing the large amounts of critical and sometimes conflicting information that comes to the administrator. The Neuman Systems Model goal of optimal client system stability provides an additional and more specific context for information processing. Thus, the administrator does not have to wonder what to do with all the information—the goal of information processing is decisions that will promote optimal stability of the client system of interest. As Neuman (1982) pointed out many years ago, "We must emphatically refuse to deal with single components, but instead relate to the concept of wholeness. We need to think and act systematically. Systems thinking enables us to effectively handle all parts of a system simultaneously in an interrelated manner, thus avoiding the fragmented and isolated nature of past functioning in [health care]" (p. 1).

The strength of the Neuman Systems Model for administration of health care services is the organizing framework it provides for administrative activities. Paraphrasing Tyler's (1949) admonition to educators, administrators are encouraged "to recognize that [administrative] experiences need to be organized to achieve continuity, sequence, and integration, and that major elements must be identified to serve as organizing threads for these [administrative] experiences. It is also essential to identify the organizing principles by which these threads shall be woven together" (p. 95). Excellent organizing principles flow, of course, from the content of Neuman Systems Model.

CONCLUSION

Application of the guidelines for Neuman Systems Model–based administration of health care services that were presented in this chapter is evident in Chapters 19 and 20. An integrated review of the published reports dealing with administration of nursing services based on the Neuman Systems Model is the subject matter of Chapter 18. Tools that have been developed for Neuman Systems Model–based clinical practice are identified and discussed in Chapter 4.

REFERENCES

de Chardin, P. T. (1955). *The phenomenon of man.* London: Collins.

Fawcett, J. (2000). *Analysis and evaluation of contemporary nursing knowledge: Nursing models and theories.* Philadelphia: Davis.

Fawcett, J., Botter, M. L., Burritt, J., Crossley, J. D., & Fink, B. B. (1989). Conceptual models of nursing and organization theories. In B. Henry, M. DiVincenti, C. Arndt, & A. Marriner-Tomey (Eds.), *Dimensions of nursing administration: Theory, research, education, and practice* (pp. 143–54). Boston: Blackwell Scientific.

Lazarus, R. (1981). The stress and coping paradigm. In C. Eisdorfer, D. Cohen, A. Kleinman, & P. Maxim (Eds.), *Models for clinical psychopathology* (pp. 177–214). New York: SP Medical and Scientific Books.

Neuman, B. (1982). *The Neuman Systems Model: Application to nursing education and practice.* Norwalk, CT: Appleton-Century-Crofts.

Neuman, B., & Young, R. J. (1972). A model for teaching total person approach to patient problems. *Nursing Research, 21,* 264–69.

Selye, H. (1950). *The physiology and pathology of exposure to stress.* Montreal: ACTA.

Tyler, R. (1949). *Basic principles of curriculum and instruction.* Chicago: University of Chicago Press.

von Bertalanffy, L. (1968). *General system theory.* New York: George Braziller.

eighteen

The Neuman Systems Model and Administration of Nursing Services: An Integrative Review

Nena F. Sanders, Jean A. Kelley

Since the publication of our chapter, "A Systems Approach to Health and Health Care Organizations" in the third edition of *The Neuman Systems Model* (Kelley & Sanders, 1995), the administrative practice and work environment for nurses has changed dramatically, moving from being in a fee-for-service health care organizational structure to an integrated health care system in a managed care market. The managed care work environment provides a continuum of care, which may include primary, specialty, hospital, hospice, and home health care services across various health care facilities and clinical settings. The work environment in managed systems of care values efficiency and effectiveness in general, and cost containment, improved patient and consumer satisfaction, and documentation of health outcomes in particular. The managed care work environment expects nurses and administrators to continue to assess, plan, coordinate, and evaluate health care delivery services for individuals and populations but across a continuum of health care facilities and clinical settings.

In addition to the environmental change, expectations for health professionals have changed. The Pew Health Professions Commission produced several publications throughout the 1990s aimed at reforming and revitalizing the health professions. For example, a set of 17 clinical competencies expected of all health care professionals by the year 2005 (Shugars, O'Neil, & Bader, 1991), which was later expanded to 21 competencies (Bellack & O'Neil, 2000) was widely disseminated. Another publication offered a sample curriculum and guidelines for preparing health professionals to practice as members of interdisciplinary teams in primary care (Grant et al., 1995). Another Pew report called for a redesign of the health care workforce into a cadre of health care providers who are "able to bring a 'systems approach' to the way health care is organized and delivered, and able to work within collaborative practice models" (Pew Health Professions Commission, 1995, p. 17). By 1998, the Pew Health Professions Commission recognized that due to their experience with case management, nurses could assume a larger role as care managers within integrated health care delivery systems (O'Neil & Coffman, 1998). We believe that nurses and administrators with knowledge and use of the Neuman Systems Model can readily assume a leadership role in care management within current and future health care delivery organizations.

This chapter presents an integrative review of literature addressing the application of the Neuman Systems Model to administrative practice in a variety of health care delivery settings. The literature review was guided by our version of Neuman Systems Model–based rules for nursing administration, education, research, and practice, which were adapted from Fawcett's (2000) work (see Chapters 2, 7, 12, and 17 for other versions of these rules). The rules encompass six basic categories: purpose/focus, phenomena/characteristics of participant(s), participant/system, problem/issue, methods/strategies, and contributions (Table 18-1). The literature for the review includes published materials and dissertation research that address nursing administration and the implementation of the Neuman Systems Model in clinical agencies. The literature was organized into the following four categories: nurse administrator role and practice, nursing administration education, nursing administration research, and structuring nursing practice in various clinical agency settings.

NURSE ADMINISTRATOR ROLE AND PRACTICE

The utility of the Neuman Systems Model in nursing practice is well documented in the literature (see Chapter 3). The utility of the Neuman Systems Model as a guide for the role and practice of the nurse administrator, however, has been documented infrequently.

In two previous publications, we documented the value of the Neuman Systems Model in providing an integrated framework for organizing knowledge related to nursing administration and guiding the nurse's practice in an administrative role (Kelley & Sanders, 1995; Kelley, Sanders, & Pierce, 1989). The purpose of our earliest publication was to present a synthesized framework for use by nurse administrators to assess, plan, implement, direct, and evaluate the effectiveness and efficiency of their practice and to identify and implement interventions to maintain, adapt, or reconstitute themselves or a system to its environment (Kelley, Sanders, & Pierce, 1989). The four core concepts of the Neuman Systems Model (person, environment, health, and nursing) were operationalized for the nurse administrator role and integrated with the management process to establish a synthesized framework for nursing administration practice. We maintained that the primary role of the nurse administrator is to maintain system integrity by realigning the nursing or organizational system to its internal and external environment. We asserted that the nurse administrator should use an integrated framework that provides "a more comprehensive approach to assessing and resolving problems in nursing administration and to evaluate the total system's response to stressors" (Kelley, Sanders, & Pierce, 1989, p. 127). The complexity of the health care environment requires the nurse administrator to use systems thinking in assessing and resolving administrative and practice issues.

The Neuman Systems Model can be implemented by a nurse administrator in any management position, in any health care agency, regardless of size or complexity, and for all scopes of services provided. The integrated framework identified the potential for ad-

TABLE 18-1. Sanders and Kelley's Rules for Nursing Administration, Education, Research, and Practice Guided by the Neuman System Model

ADMINISTRATION		EDUCATION		RESEARCH		PRACTICE	
Element	**Descriptor**	**Element**	**Descriptor**	**Element**	**Descriptor**	**Element**	**Descriptor**
Focus of Nursing in an Agency	• Client/client system, nursing staff, nursing department, or health care agency	Focus of Curriculum Purpose of Nursing Education	• Client/client system's reaction to environmental stressors • Teach students to use prevention interventions to impact stability of client/client system	Purpose	• Effectiveness of interventions • Cost–benefit and utility of intervention	Purpose	• Assists client system to achieve stability
Purpose of Nursing Services	• Delivery of nursing practices that have an impact on the stability of the client/client system						
Characteristics of Nursing Personnel	• Use of Neuman Systems Model and systems thinking by nursing personnel	Nature and Sequence of Content	• Focuses on content and sequencing of curriculum and course content based on the Neuman Systems Model	Phenomena	• Focus on variables in client system	Characteristics of Participants	• Individuals, families, groups, and communities • Reaction to stressors
Administrative Problem/Issue	• Deals with impact of stressors on client system	Characteristics of Students	• Description of the intellectual and critical thinking abilities/capabilities of the students	Problem	• Deals with impact of stressors on client system stability	Clinical Problem of Interest	• Potential or actual reactions to stressors

TABLE 18-1. Sanders and Kelley's Rules for Nursing Administration, Education, Research and Practice Guided by the Neuman System Model *(continued)*

ADMINISTRATION		EDUCATION		RESEARCH		PRACTICE	
Element	**Descriptor**	**Element**	**Descriptor**	**Element**	**Descriptor**	**Element**	**Descriptor**
Setting or System	• Agency focus, scope or level of services provided	Program Focus or Level of Academic Program	• Target system—level of academic preparation and focus of the academic program—generic, nursing administration, nurse practitioner, clinical nurse specialist, etc.	Client System	• Target system—individual, families, groups, communities, organizations	Practice Setting	• Any health care or community-based setting
Management Strategies and Administrative Practices	• Focus on nursing staff, department of nursing, or organizational system	Teaching Learning Strategies and Methods	• Design and selection of teaching/learning strategies and methodologies	Research Methods	• Design and Instrumentation • Analysis of Data	Nursing Process	• Uses the Neuman Systems Model Nursing Process Format
Contributions	• To nursing administration practice • Impact of interventions on client/organizational system stability	Contributions	• To nursing education • To accomplish the desired outcomes of nursing educational programs	Contributions	• Influence of interventions on the relation between stressors and client system	Contributions	• To nursing practice • To patient care outcomes

ministrative issues/problems to arise at intra-, inter-, and extraorganizational levels; at first, middle, and top levels of management; and to be due to penetration of the primary, secondary, or tertiary levels of prevention. Similarly, the management strategies and practices selected to serve as interventions can be focused on the individual, the nursing staff, the department of nursing, or the organizational system as a whole. The major contributions of the integrated framework for the nurse administrator include its applicability to the role of nurse administrator in both practice and educational settings; ability to address the role of nurse administrator at all levels of management; utility in any size or type of health care entity or system; usefulness in assessing and evaluating management situations, diagnosing issues/problems, determining appropriate interventions, and evaluating resulting outcomes; and ability to direct and guide nursing and organizational research related to the impact–reaction–response of the nurse administrator, nursing system, and the organization to environmental factors that are reshaping the delivery of health care.

Whereas we initially focused on the personal client system or the personal role of the nurse administrator (Kelley, Sanders, & Pierce, 1989), our second publication (Kelley & Sanders, 1995) focused on the nursing and organizational system levels. We explained how the Neuman Systems Model can be applied at the nursing and organizational levels and presented a synthesized assessment tool that combined the management process, the Neuman Systems Model, and five environmental dimensions (human resources, culture, socio/technical, structure/function, and decision making) that provided the nurse administrator with a more comprehensive approach to prioritizing needed organizational interventions. Numerous applications of the Neuman Systems Model have been made to the personal client system; however, limited application at the nursing system or organizational levels has been noted in the literature. The significance of application at these levels relates to the impact of the complex environmental stressors that have an impact on the organization and nursing department. The four core concepts of the Neuman Systems Model (person, environment, health, nursing) were operationally defined as they apply to the nursing department and the organization as a system. By operationalizing the concepts more broadly, the Neuman Systems Model became a framework for administrators in all health care disciplines, not just for nurse administrators. For example, instead of the nurse administrator being identified as the core structure, a manager of a service, a product line, or a business entity could be identified as the core entity. This conceptualization of the Neuman Systems Model significantly expands its utility for the health care system as a whole, and collaboration and a more global systems view of the organization and its environment are facilitated.

The administrative problems/issues addressed in this focused application of the Neuman Systems Model are complex and global in nature; they generally are systemic in nature and originate from the wider health care environment and forces within the global environment that have an impact on health and health care delivery. It follows that the problems and issues identified at this complex system level require multidimensional, comprehensive, and collaborative interventions to maintain, restore, or revive the health of complex systems. The contributions of applying the Neuman Systems Model at a complex system level resulted in a framework that can guide the management of complex health care organizations by providing structure for mission, goals, and objectives; direction for administrative decision making; improvements in nursing practice, patient care outcomes, and organizational performance; and application across disciplines and levels of management.

Fawcett and colleagues (1989) supported the need to apply a conceptual framework to the practice of nursing administration. The purpose of their work was to define, describe, and explain how conceptual models, including the Neuman Systems Model, and theories can be operationalized and applied to nursing administration. Although Fawcett and colleagues focused on the nurse administrator, they noted that the Neuman Systems Model could be applied more broadly to include a nursing department or a health care organization as a whole. Indeed, virtually any type or size of clinical agency could utilize the model as a basis for structuring and delivering nursing services. Fawcett and colleagues pointed out that any setting where primary, secondary, or tertiary nursing care is provided would be an appropriate setting for implementation of the Neuman Systems Model. They identified the staff, the department of nursing, or the total institution as the focus of management strategies. They pointed out that the nurse administrator can implement management strategies or administrative practices that restabilize the individual, departmental, or organizational system. Fawcett and colleagues did not discuss the impact of stressors on the client system (administrative problem/issue) or the contribution of applying the Neuman Systems Model to nursing administration. Noteworthy, however, is their linkage between the Neuman Systems Model and contingency theory, role theory, and marketing theory. The theoretical constructs inherent in these three organizational theories augment the operationalization of the Neuman Systems Model for the practice of the nurse administrator.

In an earlier publication, Arndt (1982a) discussed the value of applying system concepts as an intervention or management strategy to reduce stress in complex health care organizations. She likened organizations to organisms and the administration of nursing services to biology. Arndt compared organizations in general, and health care organizations in particular, to living systems. She proposed that nursing administration is "concerned with growth and decline, with mutual relationships between organ systems and their environment, and with the cultural environment that supports life" (p. 107). In addition, she acknowledged that the environment extends far beyond an individual and deals with the individual's reaction to and interaction with the environment. Consistent with this holistic view, Arndt proposed that the Neuman Systems Model describes organizations as systems of interdependent parts within the larger context of society. One of the strongest principles pervading Arndt's paper concerns the complex and multidisciplinary nature of health care organizations and the necessity of these organizations to be integrated to function effectively. She identified the Neuman Systems Model as a framework for addressing these complex problems and issues. Arndt's purpose was not to apply the Neuman Systems Model to nursing administration or nursing practice but rather to apply general systems concepts to manage stressors confronting complex health care organizations. However, she clearly acknowledged the utility of the Neuman Systems Model as an effective framework to address the multiplicity of issues faced by administrators in complex health care organizations.

EDUCATION FOR NURSING ADMINISTRATION

The use of the Neuman Systems Model as an effective framework for educating nursing students is extensively documented in the literature; indeed, the model has served as the guiding framework for structuring nursing curricula in a variety of degree programs throughout the United States and other countries (see Chapter 13). In addition, the model has served as a basis for developing educational tools, documentation tools, and evaluation tools for students and nursing programs (see Chapter 14). The success and acceptance of the Neuman Systems Model by the nursing academic community is overwhelming. It was, therefore, a logical next step to adopt the Neuman Systems Model as a guide for graduate programs in nursing administration.

Neuman and Wyatt (1980) published one of the earliest works describing the use of the Neuman Systems Model as a framework for educational preparation of nurse administrators. They documented the critical need to prepare nurse administrators at the graduate level, as well as the need to synthesize the domains of nursing and management to provide the nurse administrator with the knowledge and skills necessary for leadership in nursing and health care organizations. In recognition of these needs, the Ohio University School of Nursing, in the College of Education, at Athens, Ohio, developed a master's program in nursing administration, utilizing the Neuman Systems Model as the foundation of the program. The Neuman Systems Model served as a general guide for curriculum planning, course development, and program implementation. Neuman and Wyatt identified and described five dimensions of nursing administration as the overarching framework for the curriculum model—stress/adaptation intervention, nurse administrator/health manager role, applied research or inquiry, "a total view of man," and interaction between nursing theory and practice. The five dimensions provided the major organizing themes for five modules comprising the program curriculum model. The five modules, which contained courses built around the these themes and related principles, were sequenced to provide a progressive understanding of nursing and management content and skills requisite to the effective practice of nursing administration.

The major contribution of Neuman and Wyatt's publication is the conceptualization of the curriculum design and the organization of program content according to the five dimensions of nursing administration, guided by the Neuman Systems Model. Although some content areas would need to be updated, the simplicity and generalizability of the proposed integrated framework is relevant even in today's complex and integrated world of nursing and health care management.

Graduate programs in nursing administration were proliferating during the 1980s. In an attempt to develop curricular models that integrated the domains of organization, management, and nursing theory and practice, a number of publications documented the utility of the Neuman Systems Model as a framework for graduate programs in nursing administration. Arndt (1982b) discussed the need for nurse administrators of the future to function in less structured, more complex, and dynamic organizational structures. She stated, "The authority of future managers will not be viewed purely in traditional hierarchical terms, but will stem from abilities to influence others, from the ability to elicit interest and enthusiasm in problems and programs and from the skill to generate among members of a group a sense of identification and commitment to program goals" (p. 182). These words continue to be true for the practice of nursing administration even in today's health care environment. Arndt focused on the importance of adopting a theoretical framework for the practice of nursing administration and maintained that a systems approach to nursing administration is preferred to other approaches. Her assessment of the nursing, organization, and management literature led her to conclude that systems theory provided a new framework for examining the structure, process, and outcomes of organizations. She did not present a clearly defined curriculum model or plan for graduate programs in nursing administration. Instead, she described a general overview of the systems-based literature, research, and practice utilized in various nursing administration programs.

Although Arndt did not identify specific teaching strategies based on systems thinking, she referred to the need to utilize system principles when establishing course content and teaching strategies for master's level programs in nursing administration. In addition, she suggested that traditional pedagogical teaching strategies be replaced with more contemporary strategies, including case studies and problem-based learning principles. Arndt's major contribution is her further documentation of the utility of systems theory in general, and the Neuman Systems Model in particular, as a dynamic and comprehensive framework for guiding the development of graduate programs in nursing administration and the practice of nursing administration.

In a more recent work, Hinton-Walker (1995b) blended the concepts and principles associated with total quality management (TQM) and continuous quality improvement (CQI) into a framework for teaching health care administrators. She used the term *health care administrator* rather than *nurse administrator* to underscore the multidisciplinary nature of the Neuman Systems Model. She described an interdisciplinary health care administration program that allows medical fellows to attend selected courses to gain basic administrative skills. She pointed out that the faculty wanted to prepare nurse administrators for health care management roles that would be effective across delivery settings and would be consistent with the knowledge, skills, and philosophies required of administrators in the twenty-first century. Walker did not explain how the curriculum was structured or the specific content included in the courses. She did, however, note that teaching strategies were significantly influenced by the Neuman Systems Model, and that the model was used to guide major course assignments, including assignments requiring an organizational or person-level assessment, and as a framework for addressing external environmental stressors. Walker included a diagram of the blended Neuman Systems Model and TQM framework that more clearly depicted the concepts and content areas included in the program of studies. The description of the curriculum content clearly addresses the role of the nurse administrator and the impact of the nurse administrator on stabilizing the client system or organization. Specific attention is placed on the need for the nurse administrator to make "shifts" in their role. This focus on shift in role is consistent with the lines of defense and prevention-as-intervention strategies outlined in the Neuman Systems Model. Walker identified three categories of roles the nurse administrator must assume and be able to make shifts in focus: patient/client as consumer, organization as consumer, and employee/staff as consumer. The primary contribution of Walker's paper is the broadening of the Neuman Systems Model to include such contemporary concepts as TQM to strengthen the collaboration between the health care provider and the client system to achieve mutual goals. Another contribution is the evidence that a nursing framework is effective in guiding an interdisciplinary approach to preparing nurse and non-nurse health care administrators.

Lowry and colleagues (2000) described an externally funded demonstration project designed to develop interdisciplinary collaborative teams for delivery of health care across a continuum of nine agencies, settings, and a hospital that serves a predominantly rural population with seasonal farm workers, in one south Florida county, that used the Neuman Systems Model as the clinical practice model. The focus of the project was to develop a collaborative practice model and an interdisciplinary curriculum to guide education for collaborative practice in four health professional disciplines (nursing, medicine, social work, and public health) for collaborative practice. Although only the first phase of the project was described, the practice model mirrors the essential elements in the rules for nursing practice guided by the Neuman Systems Model (Table 18-1). First, the project's practice model encompassed three modes of health care delivery: health promotion (primary prevention), health maintenance (tertiary prevention), and illness care (secondary prevention) to a designated rural community. Members of the four collaborating disciplines, along with personnel from the county's Health Resource Alliance, AHEC units, and nine clinical sites, viewed the core of their collaboration as the client system, which could be individuals, families, groups, or the rural community. The internal environment of a client system was regarded as health status and lines of defense capabilities, and the external environment was seen as the rural community and its unique culture. Anticipated practice outcomes from the model resemble the values of a managed system of care—cost effectiveness, client satisfaction, and documentation of health outcomes. The project makes a major contribution to the Neuman Systems Model by not only operationalizing the philosophic basis of the model, but more importantly educating personnel in nine agencies, clinical settings, and one rural hospital about "systems thinking" based on the Neuman Systems Model, which may have an effect long after the demonstration project is completed.

RESEARCH IN NURSING ADMINISTRATION

The Neuman Systems Model has been used extensively to guide nursing research (see Chapter 8). In general, the studies conducted are descriptive, correlational, and experimental in design and have focused on such Neuman Systems Model phenomena as perception of stressors, stressor reaction, interventions, nursing process, and selected client system outcomes. Although much Neuman Systems Model–based research has been conducted, minimal Neuman Systems Model–based nursing administration research has been conducted. The published reports of administrative research focus on examination of the effects of environmental stressors on autonomy, stress, and burnout of staff nurses, and the effect of an educational program on nurses' attitudes.

Because of its simplicity and generalizability, the Neuman Systems Model is a preferred framework for master's theses and doctoral dissertations (Appendix E). Although a multitude of doctoral dissertations and master's theses have been guided by the Neuman Systems Model, very few of those dissertations or theses have focused on nursing administration. The paucity of Neuman Systems Model–based nursing administration research is due to several factors. First, the number of graduate programs in nursing administration has declined over the last decade, and most master's degree programs no longer require a thesis for degree completion. Second, few doctoral programs in nursing include a nursing administration track or concentration. Third, the nurse administrator's practice environment, especially during the past five years, has been chaotic and not conducive to the conduct of research. The Neuman Systems Model–based nursing administration doctoral dissertations that have been conducted are limited to studies of congestive heart failure patients' satisfaction with nursing care related to case management (Bittinger, 1996); the effects of social support on the relation between job stress, satisfaction, and performance among registered nurses (Burritt, 1988); the relations between selected client, provider, and agency variables and the utilization of resources of home health care services (Peoples, 1991); and the relation of selected personal and organizational variables to the tenure of directors of nursing in nursing homes (Rowles, 1993).

The number of published reports of nursing administrative research guided by the Neuman Systems Model is even lower than the number of dissertations. Just two journal articles were located; both reported correlational studies focusing on staff nurses in acute care facilities. The first study, conducted by George (1997), examined the relation between demographic variables and perceived autonomy. The study participants were registered nurses working in a clinical agency with shared governance. The second study was conducted by Collins (1996), who addressed the relation of personality hardiness to job stress and burnout. The study participants were hospital staff nurses.

The Neuman Systems Model is an excellent framework to guide nursing administration research focused on the client, staff nurse, nurse administrator, nursing department, organization, or community. As the health care environment continues to evolve, the future demands that many more studies be conducted to examine the impact of the multitude of environmental stressors on the practice of nursing and nursing administration, the effectiveness and efficiency of organizational performance, and resulting patient care outcomes. We anticipate that an increase in the number of nursing administration studies will occur as more graduate programs in nursing revitalize their nursing administration programs. The contributions of the existing research to the advancement and further development of the Neuman Systems Model have been minimal. However, future Neuman Systems Model–based nursing administration research could contribute not only to the development of the model, but also to the practice of nursing administration and the academic preparation of these practitioners.

IMPLEMENTATION OF THE NEUMAN SYSTEMS MODEL IN CLINICAL AGENCIES

The literature is replete with documented use of the Neuman Systems Model as the conceptual model for nursing practice (see Chapters 3, 5, and 6). The Neuman Systems Model has been used for nursing practice targeted to a variety of patients/patient population groups, the family, community, and nurse as the client system. The scope of the Neuman Systems Model in practice encompasses inpatient and outpatient settings; clients from neonates to the elderly; acute and chronic illnesses; health on a wellness and illness continuum; and various disease-based clinical conditions. The literature reviewed in this section is representative of the published reports documenting the use of the Neuman Systems Model as the organizing framework for structuring the practice of nursing in a variety of health care agencies. The review of literature presented is from an administrative perspective. The works reviewed and presented will be organized according to country of origin.

The United States

The clarity, simplicity, and generalizability of the Neuman Systems Model is demonstrated by the frequency with which it has been implemented in clinical agencies as a framework for both administrative and clinical practice. The use of the Neuman Systems Model as a framework for practice in clinical agencies is clearly documented in the literature. The Neuman Systems Model has been implemented as the basis for nursing practice targeting acute care organizations, public health services, psychiatric facilities, occupational health nursing, primary care clinics, and retirement communities. This review of literature is representative of the total body of publications documenting the implementation of the Neuman Systems Model in clinical agencies. A more detailed and comprehensive list of published reports of the Neuman Systems Model in clinical agencies can be found in Appendix B.

During the last two decades, the Neuman Systems Model has served as a framework for designing and delivering nursing and health care services in a variety of health care agencies. The types of settings serving as the site of implementation encompass acute care organizations, psychiatric facilities, public health services, occupational health settings, community nursing centers, and retirement centers. The Neuman Systems Model has been used most frequently in acute care organizations. Our experiences and observations suggest that many more clinical agencies have adopted the Neuman Systems Model as a framework for practice than is evident in the literature. A representative selection of the published reports is presented here.

In 1980, the Mercy Catholic Medical Center implemented the Neuman Systems Model as the conceptual model for professional nursing practice. A number of journal articles have documented this organization's experience with adopting and implementing the Neuman Systems Model (Capers et al., 1985; Burke et al., 1989). The primary goals of the nursing department were to promote high-quality care; facilitate a unified, goal-directed approach to care; increase professionalism among the nursing staff; provide a rewarding practice environment; and give purpose, direction, and organization to the nursing department. An overview of the planning and implementation process was outlined as a guide for other nursing organizations contemplating such an initiative. An evaluation of the project revealed several significant findings. First, a tool was developed to measure the outcomes related to the formulation of the nursing care plan, increase attention to the patient's physical and nonphysical needs, and achievement of client goals. Additional anticipated outcomes included increased job satisfaction, decreased nursing turnover, more cost-effective care, and increased professionalism among the nursing staff. The issues related to the process of implementing the Neuman Systems Model included the need to consider all levels of nursing, allow an appropriate time frame for implementation, gain support for the initiative, prepare the organization for the change, identify key individuals to serve as project leaders, and include an educational phase, which is critical to the success of the implementation process. The issues identified are consistent with any large organizational change initiative and should be anticipated.

Hinton-Walker and Raborn (1989) documented the value of the Neuman Systems Model as an organizing framework for the structure and function of nursing administration and the practice of clinical nursing in a variety of health care agencies. In 1984, Jefferson Davis Memorial Hospital used the Neuman Systems Model as a framework to reorganize its nursing department. The impetus for adopting a conceptual model was multidimensional; however, the major driver was to establish a focus for nursing practice. An additional aim of the initiative was to provide a common language and conceptual frame of reference for data collection and documentation purposes. The nursing staff recognized the need to adopt a more global and systematic approach to nursing practice. The nursing organization went through a very organized and systematic process to evaluate and select the Neuman Systems Model as the model that would best fit the organization. The model allowed implementation at the patient, nurse, nursing organization, and health care entity levels. A significant and unique feature of this project was that the Neuman Systems Model not only served as the framework selected to guide the planned change within the nursing organization, but also as the conceptual basis for nursing practice. Applying the Neuman Systems Model, the nursing organization implemented a major change process that included revisions in all aspects of nursing practice within the organization. Changes included revisions in nursing process, data collection and documentation, job descriptions, organizational structure, staffing methodologies, and patient classification. All nursing interventions were driven by the Neuman Systems Model Nursing Process Format (Appendix C, Table C-1). The outcomes of this initiative contributed to improved patient care outcomes, increased staff satisfaction, a more comprehensive and consistent data collection and documentation system, a significant change in attitude and professional growth of nurses, and improved communication. Hinton-Walker and Raborn (1989) identified several issues inherent in any organizational change of this magnitude that would need to be addressed by others exploring such a restructure, including costs associated with implementing significant change, the need for a conducive organizational climate, ability to sustain the change process over time, impact on the budget, the scope and intensity of educational support, and the impact on other non-nursing clinical departments.

The second most frequently targeted site for implementing the Neuman Systems Model as a basis for practice is public health nursing. Benedict and Sproles (1982) provided one of the earliest examples of the application of the Neuman Systems Model to public health nursing practice. They described the usefulness and appropriateness of adapting the Neuman Systems Model to nursing practice at the community level and outlined the similarities and differences among public health, community health nursing, and other community nursing specialized functions. In addition, they identified environmental forces that have an impact on the health care delivery system in general, and public health in particular. Benedict and Sproles also presented a detailed description of the major concepts in community health systems as applied to the Neuman Systems Model. The operationalization of the Neuman Systems Model is presented at both a client and health care delivery system level. Furthermore, the Neuman Systems Model provided a framework and guide for the development of the agency's or department's philosophy, program goals, objectives, job descriptions, and a structure for data gathering, organizing, analysis, and reporting.

After revising job descriptions and attempting to develop a job performance tool, the leadership of the Oklahoma State Department of Health identified the need to adopt and implement a nursing theory-based framework for organizing nursing practice in public health (Frioux, Roberts, & Butler, 1995). The health department was involved in an initiative to revise and restructure the organizational dimensions of the public health services provided, from both clinical and administrative perspectives. The objectives of the change effort were to implement an organizing framework to integrate all service program standards under an umbrella, establish a collaborative decision-making and participatory management approach within the department, increase the focus placed on health promotion and disease prevention, and establish a framework that facilitated a comprehensive, wholistic, systematic approach to client care, while maintaining efficiency and a high quality of care. Frioux and colleagues did not identify the actual contributions or the significance of adopting the Neuman Systems Model as a framework for practice.

In addition to its use in traditional acute care facilities, the Neuman Systems Model has been implemented in a variety of nontraditional settings. Implementation of the model in a psychiatric hospital was documented by Scicchitani and colleagues (1995). The outcomes of this organization's implementation of the Neuman Systems Model included an increase in attention focused on the client's perceptions, a more wholistic view of the patient's state of health/wellness, and a more comprehensive and fluid conceptualization of nursing and associated nursing interventions.

Occupational health nursing is another nontraditional setting where the Neuman Systems Model has been implemented. McGee (1995) identified and discussed the congruence between the principles underlying occupational health nursing and the Neuman Systems Model. The major areas of congruence between the two orientations to practice include the alignment of the Neuman Systems Model with the imperatives of public health science (primary, secondary, and tertiary prevention), the emphasis placed on problem prevention and health promotion, and the interaction among the client, nurse, and environment.

Hinton-Walker (1995a) documented the implementation of the Neuman Systems Model in a community nursing center. The Community Nursing Center of the University of Rochester School of Nursing was the site selected for implementation. Hinton-Walker described the need for the center, along with the goals and expected scope of center services. In addition, Walker presented a detailed description of the Neuman Systems Model and its operationalization as a framework for the center. She anticipated conducting research to document the value of the Neuman Systems Model as a framework for practice in this setting and to evaluate the cost effectiveness of care.

As the population of the United States ages, the implementation of the Neuman Systems Model in retirement community settings will increase in significance. Rodriguez (1995) described an application of the Neuman Systems Model in a continuing care retirement community. In this setting, the Neuman Systems Model served as the conceptual basis for both the organizing structure and the care/interventions provided by health personnel in the clinic. Rodriguez presented a rationale for adopting theory-based practice in long-term care, along with an adaptation of the Neuman Systems Model for long-term care nursing practice. The application was at two levels—the resident level and the clinic level. Although a number of benefits resulted from the utilization of the model, the most significant contribution was to establish and strengthen an interdisciplinary team approach to care planning and continuous quality improvement.

Other Countries

The use of the Neuman Systems Model in clinical practice agencies has been as pervasive in other countries as in the United States. Second only to the United States, Canada has adopted the Neuman Systems Model as the nursing model of choice for guiding nursing practice in a variety of health care agencies. During the late 1980s and early 1990s, public/community health nursing in Canada underwent a major change in organizational structure, service delivery, and roles for nurses. Drew and colleagues (1989) documented the impact of using the Neuman Systems Model to systematically examine three critical issues confronting the efficient and effective delivery of community health services in Manitoba and Ontario. They provided a comprehensive description of how the Neuman Systems Model was applied to three organizational issues to establish a matrix for integrating community health programs into a global framework, provide a conceptual basis for developing provincial standards for community health nursing practice, and adopt a theoretical framework for planning and providing care to clients and families. In addition, they documented the versatility and generalizability of the Neuman Systems Model in a variety of health care settings and the ability of the model to provide guidance to the administrative and clinical practice dimensions of community health programs.

Craig (1995) presented abstracts of the numerous examples of clinical agencies adapting and implementing the Neuman Systems Model as the framework for nursing practice in Canada. The examples included the following initiatives: the Public Health Nursing Division of the Elgin–St. Thomas Health Unit in St. Thomas, Ontario; the Public Health Nursing Division of the Middlesex–London Health Unit in Ontario; and an adolescent psychiatric unit in Calgary, Alberta. These overviews underscored the usefulness of implementing the Neuman Systems Model as an administrative and clinical framework for practice and the resulting contributions to nursing practice and client outcomes.

In a more detailed report, Beynon (1995) documented the experiences of the Middlesex–London Health Unit related to the adoption and implementation of the Neuman Systems Model as a framework for public health services. Her account of the experience followed the implementation of the planned change and presented the outcomes and recommendations generated as a result of the initiative. In addition, Beynon presented preliminary work focused on application of the Neuman Systems Model to the community as client.

In addition to its use in public health nursing settings, the Neuman Systems Model has been successfully and effectively implemented in a Canadian psychiatric facility (Craig & Morris-Coulter, 1995) and in a chronic care facility (Felix et al., 1995). In both of these facilities, the aim of the organization was to adapt and implement a conceptual base for nursing practice. In the instance of the psychiatric facility, the desired outcomes included more complete and comprehensive client assessments, an organizing guide for client data collection, more involvement of clients in care, and a clearer definition and articulation of nursing roles. The impetus for implementing the Neuman Systems Model in the chronic care facility included the desire to provide a high level of care, from a wholistic perspective, within an interdisciplinary framework. Both reports documented the usefulness and effectiveness of the Neuman Systems Model in accomplishing the desired outcomes. Moreover, Echlin (1982) described the use of the Neuman Systems Model in palliative care at the Hospice of Windsor, in Ontario.

In addition to Canada, a growing number of nurses in other countries now have documented evidence of the use of the Neuman Systems Model in their clinical agencies. Examples of the use of the Neuman Systems Model, from an administrative perspective, in other countries include:

- Primary Health Care, University College in Health and Caring Sciences, Eskilstuna, Sweden (Engberg, 1995)
- University College of Health Sciences, Jönköping, Sweden (Engberg, 1995)
- Psychiatric Nursing, University of Limburg in Maastricht, Netherlands (Verberk, 1995)
- Community Mental Health Nursing, Wales (Davies, 1989; Davies & Proctor, 1995).

Other worldwide uses of the Neuman Systems Model are listed in Appendix B.

CONCLUSION

Nursing administrative practice is critical for the future of health care delivery systems. Expansion of demonstration projects should be continued, and research and instrument development related to nursing administration should be increased. These initiatives would contribute greatly to further knowledge development and advance the understanding of the Nueman Systems Model.

REFERENCES

Arndt, C. (1982a). Systems concepts for management of stress in complex health-care organizations. In B. Neuman (Ed.), *Neuman Systems Model: Application to nursing education and practice* (pp. 97–114). Norwalk, CT: Appleton-Century-Crofts.

Arndt, C. (1982b). Systems theory and educational programs for nursing service administration. In B. Neuman (Ed.), *The Neuman Systems Model* (2nd ed., pp. 182–89). Norwalk, CT: Appleton & Lange.

Bellack, J. P., & O'Neil, E. H. (2000). Recreating nursing practice for a new century. *Nursing and Health Care Perspectives, 21*(1), 14–21.

Benedict, M. B., & Sproles, J. B. (1982). Application of the Neuman model to public health nursing practice. In B. Neuman (Ed.), *The Neuman Systems Model: Application to nursing education and practice* (pp. 223–37). Norwalk, CT: Appleton-Century-Crofts.

Beynon, C. E. (1995). Neuman-based experiences of the Middlesex–London health unit. In B. Neuman (Ed.), *The Neuman Systems Model* (3rd ed., pp. 537–47). Norwalk, CT: Appleton & Lange.

Bittinger, J. P. (1996). Case management and satisfaction with nursing care of patients hospitalized with congestive heart failure. *Dissertation Abstracts International, 56,* 3866B.

Burke, M. E. Sr., Capers, C. F., O'Connell, R. K., Quinn, R. M., & Sinnott, M. (1989). Neuman-based nursing practice in a hospital setting. In B. Neuman (Ed.), *The Neuman Systems Model* (2nd ed., pp. 423–44). Norwalk, CT: Appleton & Lange.

Burritt, J. E. (1988). The effect of perceived social support on the relationship between job stress and job satisfaction and job performance among registered nurses employed in acute care facilities. *Dissertation Abstracts International, 49,* 2123B.

Capers, C. F., O'Brien, C., Quinn, R., Kelley, R., & Fenerty, A. (1985). The Neuman Systems Model in practice: Planning phase. *Journal of Nursing Administration, 15*(5), 29–39.

Collins, M. A. (1996). The relation of work stress, hardiness, and burnout among full-time hospital staff nurses. *Journal of Nursing Staff Development, 12,* 81–85.

Craig, D. M. (1995). Community/public health nursig in Canada. Use of the Neuman Systems Model in a new paradigm. In B. Neuman (Ed.), *The Neuman Systems Model* (3rd ed., pp. 529–35). Norwalk, CT: Appleton & Lange.

Craig, D. M., & Morris-Coulter, C. (1995). Neuman implementation in a Canadian psychiatric facility. In B. Neuman (Ed.), *The Neuman Systems Model* (3rd ed., pp. 397–406). Norwalk, CT: Appleton & Lange.

Davies, P. (1989). In Wales: Use of the Neuman Systems Model by community psychiatric nurses. In B. Neuman (Ed.), *The Neuman Systems Model* (2nd ed., pp. 375–84). Norwalk, CT: Appleton & Lange.

Davies, P. & Proctor, H. (1995). In Wales: Using the model in community mental health nursing. In B. Neuman (Ed.), *The Neuman Systems Model* (3rd ed., pp. 621–27). Norwalk, CT: Appleton & Lange.

Drew, L. L., Craig, D. M., & Beynon, C. E. (1989). The Neuman Systems Model for community health administration and practice: Provinces of Manitoba and Ontario, Canada. In B. Neuman (Ed.), *The Neuman Systems Model* (2nd ed., pp. 315–42). Norwalk, CT: Appleton & Lange.

Echlin, D. J. (1982). Palliative care and the Neuman model. In B. Neuman (Ed.), *The Neuman Systems Model: Application to nursing education and practice* (pp. 257–59). Norwalk, CT: Appleton-Century-Crofts.

Engberg, I. B. (1995). Brief abstracts: Use of the Neuman Systems Model in Sweden. In B. Neuman (Ed.), *The Neuman Systems Model* (3rd ed., pp. 653–56). Norwalk, CT: Appleton & Lange.

Fawcett, J. (2000). *Analysis and evaluation of contemporary nursing knowledge: Nursing models and theories.* Philadelphia: Davis.

Fawcett, J., Botter, M. L., Burritt, J., Crossley, J. D., & Fink, B. B. (1989). Conceptual models of nursing and organization theories. In B. Henry, M. DiVincenti, C. Arndt, & A. Marriner (Eds.), *Dimensions of nursing administration: Theory, research, education, and practice* (pp. 143–54). Boston: Blackwell Scientific.

Felix, M., Hinds, C., Wolfe, S. C., & Martin, A. (1995). The Neuman Systems Model in a chronic care facility: A Canadian experience. In B. Neuman (Ed.), *The Neuman Systems Model* (3rd ed., pp. 549–65). Norwalk, CT: Appleton & Lange.

Frioux, T. D., Roberts, A. G., & Butler, S. J. (1995). Oklahoma state public health nursing: Neuman-based. In B. Neuman (Ed.), *The Neuman Systems Model* (3rd ed., pp. 407–14). Norwalk, CT: Appleton & Lange.

George, J. (1997). Nurses' perceived autonomy in a shared governance setting. *Journal of Shared Governance, 3*(2), 17–21.

Grant, R. W., Finocchio, L. J., et al. (1995). *Interdisciplinary collaborative teams in primary care: A model curriculum and resource guide.* San Francisco: Pew Health Professions Commission.

Hinton-Walker, P. (1995a). Neuman-based education, practice, and research in a community nursing center. In B. Neuman (Ed.), *The Neuman Systems Model* (3rd ed., pp. 415–30). Norwalk, CT: Appleton & Lange.

Hinton-Walker, P. (1995b). TQM and the Neuman Systems Model: Education for health care administration. In B. Neuman (Ed.), *The Neuman Systems Model* (3rd ed., pp. 365–76). Norwalk, CT: Appleton & Lange.

Hinton-Walker, P., & Raborn, M. (1989). Application of the Neuman model in nursing administration and practice. In B. Henry, C. Arndt, M. DiVincenti, & A. Marriner-Tomey (Eds.), *Dimensions of nursing administration: Theory, research, education, and practice* (pp. 711–23). Boston: Blackwell Scientific.

Kelley, J. A., & Sanders, N. F. (1995). A systems approach to the health of nursing and health care organizations. In B. Neuman (Ed.), *The Neuman Systems Model* (3rd ed., pp. 347–64). Norwalk, CT: Appleton & Lange.

Kelley, J. A., Sanders, N. F., & Pierce, J. D. (1989). A systems approach to the role of the nurse administrator in education and practice. In B. Neuman (Ed.), *The Neuman Systems Model* (2nd ed., pp. 115–38). Norwalk, CT: Appleton & Lange.

Lowry, L. W., Burns, C. M., Smith, A. A., & Jacobson, H. (2000). An interdisciplinary approach to training health professionals. *Nursing and Health Care Perspectives, 21*(2), 76–80.

McGee, M. (1995). Implications for use of the Neuman Systems Model in occupational health nursing. In B. Neuman (Ed.), *The Neuman Systems Model* (3rd ed., pp. 657–67). Norwalk, CT: Appleton & Lange.

Neuman, B. & Wyatt, M. (1980). The Neuman stress/adaptation systems approach to education for nurse administrators. In J. Riehl & C. Roy (Eds.), *Conceptual models for nursing practice* (2nd ed., pp. 142–50). New York: Appleton-Century-Crofts.

O'Neil, E. H., & Coffman, J. (Eds.) (1998). *Strategies for the future of nursing: Changing roles, responsibilities and employment patterns for registered nurses.* San Francisco: Jossey-Bass.

Peoples, L. (1991). The relationship between selected client, provider, and agency variables and the utilization of home care services. *Dissertation Abstracts International, 51,* 3782B.

Pew Health Professions Commission. (1995). *Critical challenges: Revitalizing the health professions for the twenty-first century.* San Francisco: UCSF Center for the Health Professions.

Rodriguez, M. L. (1995). The Neuman Systems Model adapted to a continuing care retirement community. In B. Neuman (Ed.), *The Neuman Systems Model* (3rd ed., pp. 431–42). Norwalk, CT: Appleton & Lange.

Rowles, C. (1993). The relationship of selected personal and organizational variables and the tenure of directors of nursing in nursing homes. *Dissertation Abstracts International, 53,* 4593B.

Scicchitani, B., Cox, J. G., Heyduk, L. J., Maglicco, P. A., & Sargent, N. A. (1995). Implementing the Neuman model in a psychiatric hospital. In B. Neuman (Ed.), *The Neuman Systems Model* (3rd ed., pp. 387–95). Norwalk, CT: Appleton & Lange.

Shugars, D. A., O'Neil, E. M., & Bader, J. D. (Eds.). (1991). *Healthy America: Practitioners for 2005: An agenda for action for US health professions.* Durham, NC: Pew Health Professions Commission, Duke University.

Verberk, F. (1995). In Holland: Application of the Neuman model in psychiatric nursing. In B. Neuman (Ed.), *The Neuman Systems Model* (3rd ed., pp. 629–36). Norwalk, CT: Appleton & Lange.

nineteen

Using the Neuman Systems Model to Guide Administration of Nursing Services in the United States: Redirecting Nursing Practice in a Freestanding Pediatric Hospital

Madelyn L. Torakis

Children's Hospital of Michigan is the only exclusively pediatric institution within the eight-hospital Detroit Medical Center and the only freestanding pediatric hospital in Michigan. It is a 228-bed facility that services children from the Detroit metropolitan area, as well the state of Michigan. In addition, patients are referred from other states and countries. The hospital houses a pediatric intensive care unit, a neonatal intensive care unit, and a Level I trauma center. The hospital first opened its doors in 1886 as Children's Free Hospital. Since that time, Children's Hospital of Michigan has serviced thousands of children and their families, offering more than 30 subspecialties and services.

Children's Hospital employs 530 nursing staff, encompassing registered nurses, licensed practical nurses, nurse educators, advanced practice nurses, nursing managers, and nursing administrators. The nurses have preparation at the diploma, associate, bachelor's, master's, and doctoral levels of nursing. Prior to the introduction of the Neuman Systems Model, no well-defined nursing conceptual model was utilized to guide nursing practice.

The process of redirecting nursing practice requires understanding of the progression from model selection through implementation. The development of nursing practice is closely meshed with the entire implementation process and, therefore, warrants simultaneous discussion throughout this chapter. The purpose of this chapter is to describe the impact of the implementation of the Neuman Systems Model on the nursing staff, from its earliest conception to the most recent challenges.[1,2]

SELECTION OF THE MODEL

Conceptual models of nursing provide an efficient and well-organized approach to nursing practice, research, education, and administration (Fawcett, 1995). Oliver (1991) commented that "true believers" have found that nursing models help to explain human behaviors, relationships, and experiences. Conceptual models of nursing enable nurses to gather a detailed database that, in turn, identifies actual or potential health care problems. In addition, Fawcett (1995) regards conceptual models of nursing as a beneficial way to recognize the purpose and define the scope of nursing practice. Neuman (1995) views models as directives for organizing nursing activities. Conceptual models provide frameworks for objective records of the effects of nursing care. Undoubtedly, the importance of nursing models lies in the fact that their use improves communication among health care professionals. Additionally, Kozier and colleagues (1992) suggested that clear and explicit communication styles created by using nursing conceptual frameworks establish the unique and important contributions nursing makes to the multidisciplinary health care team.

   With this orientation as a basis, the Department of Nursing closely examined the direction of nursing practice and professionalism at Children's Hospital. In January 1994, the department formed a Professional Nursing Practice Model project team. The team was composed of 51 percent staff nurses, with the remaining 49 percent nurse educators, advanced practice nurses, and nurse managers. The goal of the team was to develop a professional nursing practice model that would meet the needs of its clients and compliment the unique and diverse culture of the hospital. The Professional Nursing Practice Model team addressed several areas, including standards of care, registered nurse role definition, professional development, and nursing practice. The group agreed that a conceptual framework was essential to guide nursing practice. The team as a whole conducted a careful examination of several conceptual models of nursing. After detailed review, the Neuman Systems Model was selected as the foundation for the Professional Nursing Practice Model (unpublished report, Children's Hospital of Michigan, 1994). The components of the model were found to be congruent with the underlying assumptions and beliefs proposed by the Professional Nursing Practice Model project team and the Department of Nursing. The model also was viewed as an excellent framework for pediatric nursing practice in a setting dedicated to a family-centered care philosophy.

MODEL DEVELOPMENT AND REFINEMENT

Although the Neuman Systems Model has much to offer nursing practice, there has been very little development and use within a pediatric institution. It was challenging to develop and implement the model with no examples, references, or prototypes from similar institutions. It was obvious that in order to implement the model, nursing staff needed to acquire the knowledge necessary to begin placing components of the model into practice. Upon initial model development, however, the work group was unable to adequately discuss the details of the model. Model development and education could not commence without an opportunity to meet and discuss components of the model with Dr. Neuman. Consequently, a day-long "kick-off" conference was held for the nursing staff, with Betty Neuman as the keynote speaker. Following this conference, the work group was better educated and subsequently began the complicated process of dissecting and analyzing the model to facilitate the educational process for the nursing staff.

The Model as Stressor

Neuman (1995) describes environmental stressors as internal and external stimuli or forces that may produce a positive or negative reaction. With this definition in mind, it was recognized early on that adopting a more conceptually based and structured approach to nursing practice would be identified by many staff as a stressor. Although stressors have the potential for a reaction within the client or client system (i.e., the nursing staff), many factors influence the outcome. Response to the process may be influenced by the timing of the implementation process, the nursing staff's past experience, if any, with a nursing model or theory, the experience level of the staff (novice vs. expert), and individual staff members' willingness to change.

The type of environmental stressor associated with implementation of the model could vary depending on the individual nurse's perception. For many, implementation of the model may be viewed as an extrapersonal stressor, occurring outside of the nurses' personal boundaries and one in which they have little or no control. To some, the decision to redirect nursing practice was viewed as a decision made exclusively by administration and thus an extrapersonal stressor. For others, the stressor was viewed as interpersonal in nature. In this case, the stressor reflects a conflict between nursing administration's desire to format nursing practice in one direction and the staff wishing to resist the impending changes. The stressor also may be evident as a result of staff not understanding the need for a conceptual basis for nursing practice. Finally, some staff found the adoption of the Neuman Systems Model in conflict with their own views, values, and beliefs associated with their personal nursing practice. This internal discord created a sense of intrapersonal stress for some staff. In contrast, a small percentage of the client system perceived the implementation of the model as a positive, exciting, and challenging stressor, thus creating a beneficial personal and professional outcome. These nurses' perception was that the introduction of a conceptual framework, specifically the Neuman Systems Model, was both personally advantageous and an asset for the entire nursing department.

PREVENTION AS INTERVENTION

Neuman (1995) proposes that nursing interventions focus on retaining, attaining, or maintaining the best possible health state of the client system. The three levels of prevention—primary, secondary, and tertiary—are vital in preserving client system stability.

Primary Prevention Prior to Model Implementation

Primary prevention was one of the strategies utilized with staff prior to implementation of the model. Neuman describes primary prevention efforts as necessary to help strengthen the flexible line of defense, as well as to reduce the possibility of encounters with stressors. Because of the stress associated with the impending model implementation, various educational tools were developed to strengthen the nursing staff's flexible line of defense and retain client system stability.

The first intervention provided was a biweekly publication entitled *Neuman Notes* (Figure 19-1). *Neuman Notes* enabled the work group to slowly and methodically introduce model content to the nursing staff in a less threatening manner. The model was discussed in its entirety in manageable sections over a number of weeks. The publication was distributed with paychecks and posted on the individual units. Feedback was positive and most nursing staff found the content easy to absorb and comprehend.

Although *Neuman Notes* proved to be an excellent introduction to the Neuman Systems Model, a more thorough educational tool needed to be developed. The work group created a self-directed learning module entitled "The Neuman Systems Model: Application to Clinical Practice." The module begins with a review of the metaparadigm of nursing; reviews the concepts of the Neuman Systems Model, including the nursing process; and concludes with the application of the model through a case presentation. Modules were distributed to all staff through numerous in-services and unit meetings. Follow-up sessions were held to discuss module content and review the case presentation. Educational contact hours were awarded at these sessions as incentive for attendance. Again, staff acknowledged the usefulness of the self-directed learning module as a means to increase knowledge.

MODEL IMPLEMENTATION

Successful implementation of the Neuman Systems Model required review and analysis of nursing documentation for congruency with the model components. As anticipated, several documents needed to be revised or developed in order to solidify model use. An examination of the nursing process according to the Neuman Systems Model proved helpful in this task (see Figure 19-1).

The Neuman Systems Model Nursing Process

The Neuman Systems Model nursing process format consists of three steps: nursing diagnosis, nursing goals, and nursing outcomes. This format differs slightly from the more traditional and familiar steps in the nursing process, which consists of assessment, diagnosis, intervention, and evaluation. Nursing diagnosis consists of both assessment and diagnosis of needs, stressors, and strengths. Nursing goals are the implementation of nursing prevention interventions intended to stabilize the client system through stressor reduction or elimination. In the final step, nursing outcomes, the effectiveness of the prevention interventions is evaluated and the client's status on the health–illness continuum can be determined and necessary changes made.

The assessment process begins at the time the client is admitted to the hospital unit. The nursing staff utilizes a newly revised pediatric admission database to gather appropriate information from both the child and family. The database questions are categorized into the five client system variables (physiological, psychological, sociocultural, developmental, spiritual). A sample of content areas assessed within each variable can be found in Table 19-1.

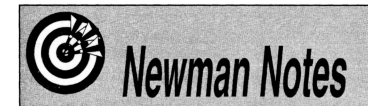

May 10, 1996

Children's Hospital of Michigan

"Obstacles are what you see when you take your eyes off the goal"

Nursing Process According to Neuman ☺

The Neuman Systems Model is an effective framework for unique and comprehensive approaches to the child or the family as the client. It is the goal of nursing in the Neuman Model to assist the child and family to attain, maintain, or retain a maximum level of wellness. The nurse uses specific interventions based on the degree of reaction to the stressor. The Neuman Nursing Process consists of three steps: nursing diagnosis, nursing goals, and nursing outcomes.

Assessment	Diagnosis	Planning	Implementation	Evaluation
Corresponds to Neuman's nursing diagnosis step.	Corresponds to Neuman's nursing diagnosis step.	Corresponds to Neuman's nursing diagnosis and her nursing goals step.	Corresponds to Neuman's nursing outcome step.	Corresponds to Neuman's nursing outcome step.
Gather information related to the five variables.	Identify needs and problems by analyzing client information.	Develop interventions to help the client retain, attain, or maintain stability.	Nursing intervention is accomplished through use of one of the three prevention modes: primary, secondary, or tertiary.	Determine if the goal or outcome has been achieved. If not, nursing goals are revised.
Identify and evaluate potential or actual stressors.		Negotiate interventions with the client for desired outcome goals to correct variances from wellness.		Client outcome validates the nursing goals and acts as feedback for further system input.
Collect data on how stressors effect the flexible line of defense, normal line of defense, lines of resistance, and basic structure.				
Assessing the client's past, present, and future coping patterns.				
(Nursing H & P)	*(Problem List)*	*(Standards of Care)*	*(Clinical Pathways)*	*(Nursing Focus Notes)*

FIGURE 19-1.   *Neuman Notes* [Sources: *Adapted from Wendy, R. L. (1995). Nursing theories and models (2nd ed.). Springhouse. Neuman, B. (1995). The Neuman Systems Model (3rd ed.). East Norwalk, CT: Appleton & Lange.*].

TABLE 19-1. Sample of Content Assessed Within the Pediatric Admission Database

Client System Variable	Sample Areas of Assessment
Physiological	Nutrition
	Elimination
	Pain
Psychological	Illness adjustment
	Participation in care
	Comfort measures
Sociocultural	Safety in the home
	Community assistance
	Car seat use
Developmental	Milestone attainment
	Delays
	School
Spiritual	Faith tradition
	Religious practices
	Chaplain support

The Neuman Process Summary (NPS) (Figure 19-2) was developed to further incorporate the Neuman Systems Model nursing process into nursing documentation. The goal of the NPS is to help the nurse synthesize the information obtained from each variable in the pediatric admission database. In addition, information may be obtained from the ongoing assessment of the client and family throughout the hospitalization. Client and family stressors (positive and negative) and strengths are documented under the appropriate variable. The NPS serves as the basis for making, revising, and resolving nursing diagnoses. The Children's Hospital nursing department uses the North American Nursing Diagnosis Association (NANDA)-approved nursing diagnoses to guide the development of the nursing plan of care. The NANDA (1990) definition of nursing diagnosis includes reference to the individual, family, or community's response to actual or potential health problems. The inclusion of individuals, families, and communities in this definition is congruent with the definition of the client system by Neuman (1995). NANDA-approved nursing diagnoses are indicated in the Patient Needs/Outcome Record (Figure 19-3).

Nursing Documentation

Nursing documentation within the client's medical record is integrated with documentation by all other health care professionals. The specific nursing documentation is called Focus Charting® (Lampe, 1986). Focus Charting uses the traditional nursing process as the method for organizing the documentation of patient care (Lampe, 1985). A specific NANDA nursing diagnosis (e.g., impaired physical mobility) guides the content of the note. The nursing diagnosis may address a current patient concern, a significant change in the patient's status, or a significant event in the patient's therapy. Three sections are addressed in each note—data, action, and response. The data section describes the nurse's assessment of the client based on the nursing diagnosis. The action step then addresses the planning and implementation of nursing care based on client data and nurs-

	Wayne State University		☐ Children's Hospital of Michigan
DMC	The Detroit		☐ Grace-Sinai
	Medical Center		☐ Huron Valley-Sinai
			☐ Other _____

NEUMAN PROCESS SUMMARY

Nursing Assessment of the five variables:
Data obtained from admission assessment as well as ongoing assessment

Indicate all appropriate variables: Include intrapersonal, interpersonal, and extrapersonal stressors*

PHYSIOLOGICAL	DATE	INITIALS	SOCIOCULTURAL	DATE	INITIALS
PSYCHOLOGICAL	DATE	INITIALS	DEVELOPMENTAL	DATE	INITIALS
SPIRITUAL	DATE	INITIALS	*Note: Stressors may be positive or negative		

FIGURE 19-2.   Neuman process summary.

ing model integration. In other words, the action step reflects nursing prevention interventions. The response section serves as the evaluation of the effectiveness of the nursing prevention interventions addressed in the action step. Because the action step is a description of immediate or future nursing interventions, this section most closely correlates with the Neuman Systems Model levels of prevention. Nursing staff were educated on how to categorize their interventions within the action step into the suitable level of prevention as described by Neuman. This modification was most logical and required the least amount of disruption to the current documentation method. Use of the Neuman Systems Model, however, required the nursing staff to realize the value of their nursing interventions. In addition, they had to acquire a clear understanding of the purpose of their interventions. For example, did their interventions help to strengthen the child's/family's flexible line of defense or was it aimed at reducing or eliminating a stressor? Educational efforts were aimed at improving nurses' overall understanding and description of nursing interventions. Examples of Focus Charting utilizing the levels of prevention are found in Figure 19-4.

PATIENT NEEDS / OUTCOME RECORD

Goals/outcome criteria are incorporated into the plan of care in
conjunction with the established standard of care for this diagnosis

DATE	PATIENT FOCUS / NURSING DIAGNOSIS	INITIALS	OUTCOMES			INITIALS
			DATE	MET	ONGOING*	
	Knowledge deficit / patient and parent education					

Note: Outcome remains unmet at time of patient discharge

SIGNATURE	INITIALS	SIGNATURE	INITIALS
SIGNATURE	INITIALS	SIGNATURE	INITIALS

322570AHHPK (9/98)

FIGURE 19-3.   Patient needs/outcome record.

Secondary Prevention as Intervention During Model Implementation

Despite numerous primary prevention interventions, the stressor of model implementation penetrated the flexible line of defense of many staff members. Nursing staff displayed confusion regarding appropriate use of levels of prevention and their placement within the Focus Note. As a result, model terminology was used inconsistently and documentation often was incomplete.

The goal of secondary prevention is to reduce or eliminate the stressor and thus maintain optimal client system stability. The model work group created a variety of interventions aimed at reachieving client system stability. Resource books were developed for each nursing unit with samples of a completed pediatric admission database, Neuman Process Summary, and Focus Notes utilizing the appropriate levels of prevention. Each book used a patient example common to that unit (e.g., cardiovascular surgery, chemotherapy administration, diabetic ketoacidosis). Nursing staff also were asked to supply ideas and examples of specific client case scenarios so that additional examples could be provided.

Positive reinforcement also was used as an intervention, again intended to decrease the stressor of model implementation. Charts were audited and assessed for appropriate use of model components and documentation. Nursing staff members were "rewarded" for accurate completion of the Neuman Process Summary and/or inclusion of appropriate levels of prevention in the Focus Note. The model work group chose a Tootsie® Pop

Focus: Ineffective Breathing Pattern

Data: BBSH w/GAE. Exp steth wheeze. Congested cough. Mild nasal flaring. No retracting. Pt complaining that "its sometimes hard to breathe." Color pink. Skin warm and dry. O_2 sats 90–94% on RA.

Action: II° *Prevention:* Resp assessment q 2 hrs and prn. Resp treatments q 3 hrs as ordered. Meds as ordered. ↑ HOB 45°. Encouraged clear liquids. Encouraged ambulation.

Response: ↓ exp wheeze following treatment. BS remain harsh/congested. Pt stated easier to breathe with ↑ 'd HOB. O_2 sats 92–96%. Drank 120 cc juice. Refused to ambulate.

Focus: Altered Nutrition, < body requirements

Data: Took bites of eggs for breakfast and macaroni and cheese for lunch. Bag of chips at 12:30. Lemonade x2 (240 cc). Asking for food from home. HAL/Lipids infusing as ordered. No stools. 350 cc urine output. Current weight: 19.7 kg.

Action: II° *prevention:* Encouraged oral intake. Offered variety of foods from tray. Monitored output. Contacted volunteer services to provide companionship during meals. Mother encouraged to bring favorite foods from home.
III° *prevention:* Dietitian consulted to review home dietary intake and provide education to parents for changes as necessary.

Response: Adequate urine output. No stools. Volunteer will be available for breakfast and lunch daily; if available will come for dinner. Mother states will bring in chicken fingers with next visit. Dietitian will contact family to address home diet.

Focus: Fear

Data: Continuously putting on call light asking to call his father. Crying and saying he was afraid to be alone.

Action: II° *prevention:* Writer attempted to calm Buddy—sat with him for 1/2 hour, provided diversional activities and play. Called father to tell him of current episode. Paged chaplain on call.
I^o *prevention:* Child life and Psychology will be notified in AM to to discuss plan to prevent future episodes as well as possible behavior modification plan.

Response: Father stated he would come to the hospital and bring Buddy his pizza. Chaplain spent time with Buddy. Quieted after 45 mins and fell asleep.

FIGURE 19-4.   Examples of focus charting using levels of prevention.

sucker as the reward given to nursing staff. The use of a Tootsie Pop was found to be quite suitable due to its similarities to the Neuman Systems Model. The group visualized the Tootsie Roll center as being synonymous with the basic structure. The candy surrounding the Tootsie Roll center therefore was thought to be similar to the lines of resistance described in the model. The Tootsie Pop in its usual state without the wrapper represents the normal line of defense. Finally, the outside wrapper is equated to the flexible line of defense that protects the sucker. The Tootsie Pops were attached to a recognition flag and posted in a prominent location on the unit. Staff found this analogy very helpful and an amusing way to reinforce components of the model.

According to Neuman, reconstitution describes a return of the client system to a stable state following treatment of a stressor or stressors. Nursing staff have demonstrated marked evidence of reconstitution following model implementation. Some examples include the increased use of model terminology when discussing various client/family situations, the inclusion of the model in such presentations as nursing grand rounds, and the increased use by nursing graduate students for projects and research. At the time this chapter was written, a formal reevaluation of the impact of model usage on practice had not been conducted. However, the perception of nursing staff in management, education, and administration positions is that adoption of the model has been favorable. Nursing staff appear much more eager to embrace the model in a variety of situations and settings. As hoped, reconstitution has progressed the client system (nursing staff) beyond the previously determined normal line of defense. The results are congruent with the original goal of the Professional Nursing Practice Model task force—to increase the professionalism of pediatric nurses within our institution.

Tertiary Prevention: Continuing Toward Model Wellness

Following successful model implementation on all inpatient units, the use of tertiary prevention as intervention facilitated stability of the nursing staff. The goals of tertiary prevention are to maintain wellness by supporting existing client system strengths and to provide reeducation to prevent any further stressor reaction or regression. Consequently, the work group developed a variety of methods to ensure this outcome.

One example of tertiary prevention is concurrent chart reviews to monitor appropriate and accurate usage of all forms of nursing documentation relevant to the model. Monthly reports are generated and shared with each unit nursing manager, nurse educator, and nursing staff. These reports facilitate identification of weak areas that require additional educational sessions with nursing staff through specially arranged unit inservices. Chart audits also facilitate identification of minor isolated problem areas in model use. Targeted reminders or clarification statements then are posted on the unit "Neuman" board to be shared by all nursing staff. Formal monthly audits of the Neuman Systems Model also have been included as a hospital performance improvement strategic initiative, as defined by the Joint Commission on Accreditation of Healthcare Organizations (1996).

Individual units also have incorporated the Neuman Systems Model as an essential component of yearly registered nurse (RN) competency assessments and as a vital inclusion in hospitalwide mandatory education sessions. In addition, unit nursing managers have customized methods of evaluating each nursing staff member's use and knowledge of the model. Professional accountability of model knowledge and usage serves as a useful tool for yearly performance review. Measurement criteria are directly related to practice standards. A thorough education session also is included in the new RN orientation program.

IMPLICATIONS FOR THE FUTURE OF THE NEUMAN SYSTEMS MODEL

Ambulatory Settings

At the present time, only the inpatient units have adopted the Neuman Systems Model. The next goal is to incorporate its use in all ambulatory care settings, including the emergency department. The implementation process will require a similar approach, beginning with a thorough assessment of nursing practice standards and documentation, followed by the use of all three levels of prevention as intervention before, during, and after model implementation.

Beyond Children's Hospital

One other hospital within the Detroit Medical Center houses a small pediatric unit and three house neonatal intensive care units. Strategic plans are in progress to implement the Neuman Systems Model in all of these child and family care areas. The vision is to utilize the Neuman Systems Model in all hospitals of the medical center. That vision may not be attained for several years. In anticipation of medical center–wide use of the Neuman Systems Model, the Children's Hospital Web page now appears on the Detroit Medical Center Intraweb, making it accessible to staff at all of the hospitals. The Web page has information about the Neuman Systems Model, as well as examples of documentation.

CONCLUSION

The implementation process has been lengthy and often tiresome. The stressor associated with change often is difficult to manage, but the positive outcome is proof of a newly created healthy and stable professional environment. The use of the Neuman Systems Model in a pediatric hospital setting has many benefits. The Neuman Systems Model systems perspective provides an ideal framework for working closely with families. Therefore, the unique needs of children and their families together can be assessed by nurses; the illness episode as well as the hospitalization may only partially represent the stressors experienced by the child and family. Through the use of the Neuman Systems Model, nursing staff have greatly improved their ability to recognize and wholistically assess and care for the entire client system while greatly increasing their professionalism.

ENDNOTES

1. Grateful appreciation is expressed to Constance Smigielski, RN, BSN, MSA, for her helpful comments on an earlier version of this chapter.
2. In 2000, the nurses of Children's Hospital of Michigan received the first Excellence in Clinical Scholarship Award from the Society of Pediatric Nurses for the adoption and implementation of the Neuman Systems Model as the framework for nursing practice.

REFERENCES

Fawcett, J. (1995). *Analysis and evaluation of conceptual models of nursing* (3rd ed.). Philadelphia: Davis.

Joint Commission on Accreditation of Healthcare Organizations. (1996). *Comprehensive accreditation manual for hospitals.* Oakbrook Terrace, IL: Author.

Kozier, B., Blais, K., & Erb, G. (1992). *Concepts and issues in nursing practice.* Redwood City, CA: Addison-Wesley Nursing.

Lampe, S. (1985). Focus Charting: Streamlining documentation. *Nursing Management, 16*(7), 44–46.

Lampe, S. (1986). *Focus Charting: A patient-centered approach.* Minneapolis: Creative Nursing Management.

Neuman, B. (1995). *The Neuman Systems Model* (3rd ed.). Norwalk, CT: Appleton & Lange.

North American Nursing Diagnosis Association. (1990). *Taxonomy of nursing diagnosis.* St. Louis: Author.

Oliver, N. R. (1991). True believers: A case for model-based nursing practice. *Nursing Administration Quarterly, 15*(3), 37–43.

twenty

Using the Neuman Systems Model to Guide Administration of Nursing Services in Holland: The Case of Emergis, Institute for Mental Health Care

Ruud de Munck, André Merks

O ffering mental health care, close to home throughout Zeeland, Holland. Searching together for the best answer to everyone's personal question. Treating, supporting, and attending to people. Expert and reliable practice. All of that is what Emergis does, every day.

The Institute for Mental Health Care, Emergis, is of service to all inhabitants of Zeeland, regardless of their age or culture, close to home. Emergis puts the human being asking for help in the spotlight and looks for the best solution, together with the client. Most importantly, clients stay in their own environment for as long as possible and lead a life as independent as possible. Emergis treats, supports, and attends to people. The starting point is optimal quality, not only in a sense of expertise, but also in the interaction with clients and their environments. The purpose of this chapter is to describe the way in which the Neuman Systems Model is being used to guide the administration of nursing services at Emergis.

BACKGROUND OF EMERGIS

Emergis came into existence in January 1996, as the result of a merger of the Psychiatric Hospital Zeeland, the Institute for Outpatient Mental Health Care Zeeland, and the Institute for Community Residences. The organization has six divisions: Mental Health Care for Adults, Long-Term Care and Housing, Psychiatric Care for the Elderly, Child and Adolescent Psychiatric Care (Ithaca), Addiction Care (Reilof), and Social Care. Although the six divisions focus on different clients, they cooperate. The overall aim of all Emergis divisions is to be attainable and approachable for those who need mental health care. Emergis does not only want to help people to live their lives in a better way, but also wants to support people in their effort to regain and maintain a valued place in society.

The province of Zeeland is divided into three regions. In the Zeeuwsch-Vlaanderen, Walcheren, and Oosterschelde regions, there are basic facilities; treatment and support are available for people with problems that are not very complex. Emergis provides specialist treatment for people with complex problems at the basic facility, a clinic in Goes. Emergency services for Zeeuwsch-Vlaanderen and the region north of the Westerschelde are available if people need immediate help. There is close cooperation between Emergis and other institutions, such as the psychiatric wards of general hospitals.

DEVELOPMENT OF NURSING PRACTICE IN HOLLAND AND AT EMERGIS

Until the 1980s, nursing practice in Holland was not guided by nursing theories or models. The nursing process had been introduced in the 1970s, and some of the developments in nursing that were initiated in the United States also were introduced in Holland. In 1980, the first master's degree in nursing program was started at the University of Maastricht. Soon after, Holland had its own nursing models and theories, including the works by van der Brink-Tjebbes (1987), van Bergen (van Bergen, Hollands, & Nijhuis, 1980), and Grijpdonck (Koene et al., 1982). Publications slowly changed in perspective, from writing about nursing practice to the development of a philosophy about nursing practice, questions about the domain of nursing, and the meaning of the profession. Professionalization was initiated. At Emergis, which still was a general psychiatric hospital, the changes were experienced through the start of a new school for nursing. The new school educated nurses at the bachelor's level, which is called higher education for nurses (HBO-V) in Holland.

Since 1983, the students at the Emergis school have had clinical internships at various institutes in Holland. The feedback from the institutes indicated that the students had been trained at a higher level than in the past. This was particularly evident in that the students proposed improvements in nursing care plans and expressed innovative ideas about working with the nursing process. However, these ideas did not lead to actual changes on the wards until almost 10 years later.

In the 1990s, some of the ideas from nursing models and theories found their way to the wards. Nurses who had some influence in their team introduced some of the models. The ideas that were introduced initially were restricted to such elements of the models and theories as organizational ideas about nursing that are part of Grijpdonck's Integrated Nursing Care Model. Although the organizational ideas were implemented, the other elements of model were not even tested in practice. Each ward selected its own working model and developed its own files and forms. At the present time, this approach seems confusing but clearly was needed to develop nursing practice partly through trial and error.

DIFFERENTIATION OF NURSING FUNCTIONS

In the 1990s, the concept of quality of care became very popular. In 1993, that concept led to the question: "What is it that we do, and is it done by the right people?" Answers to the question were sought through a project designed to differentiate nursing functions for all nursing wards.

Emergis implemented differentiation of nursing functions in 1995, by means of an organizational structure for each ward (Figure 20-1). Differentiation of functions was implemented both horizontally and vertically. The deputy team leader's function disappeared. Vertical differentiation was achieved by introducing two levels of functions for nurses—nurses and attendants. There is a clear difference between these functions with regard to tasks and responsibilities. Nurses are responsible for the coordination of care for those patients to whom they are assigned; attendants contribute toward patient care but are not accountable. The nurses, who had new functions, received specific training.

Horizontal differentiation was achieved by introducing the function of senior nurse, which was new to the hospital. Senior nurses are part of each team; they do not have a hierarchically different position. This function is the most noticeable change on the wards. Senior nurses' responsibilities focus on quality development. Senior nurses are required to have been educated at the bachelor's level, with continuing education in a certain area of nursing. Education for clinical nurse specialists was started in 1999 at the Emergis school; this area is especially compatible with the senior nurse function and responsibilities.

Furthermore, the senior nurse function requires training in nursing diagnoses and nursing interventions and the ability to apply this knowledge in daily practice to contribute to the development of nursing practice at Emergis. Moreover, senior nurses have both specific and nonspecific professional knowledge, including analytical, problem-solving, and communication skills. Senior nurses monitor the quality of nursing care and

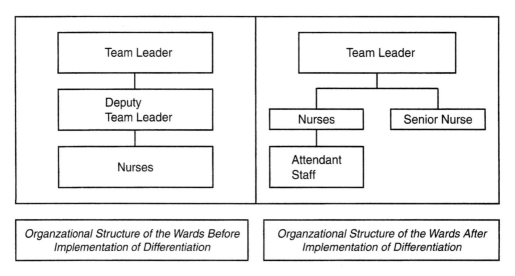

FIGURE 20-1.   Organization scheme of the wards before and after implementation of function differentiation.

contribute to the development and monitoring of the policies for the quality of nursing practice, the interpretation of the findings, and the implementation of strategies to improve nursing practice. In addition, senior nurses carry out complex interventions through a combination of new procedures and strategic and intelligent practice.

Especially important for senior nurses' tasks in the implementation of the Neuman Systems Model was their skill in applying principles of scientific research and their participation in and contributions to new projects and research on the ward. Indeed, senior nurses are increasingly involved in projects at Emergis. Involvement in the projects requires characteristics that are best compared to those of innovators—daring, prepared to take risks, and interested in new developments. Furthermore, innovators have their own networks, even if they do not meet very often (van Linge, 1998). In addition, innovators typically have charisma, which supports innovation and reduces resistance to change. They use several methods to influence their environment—they engage in coalitions, try to convince through using series of arguments, use their formal authority, and are self-assured. As they gain experience, these innovator characteristics become stronger.

SELECTION OF THE NEUMAN SYSTEMS MODEL AT EMERGIS

Implementation of differentiation of functions was followed by consideration of a nursing model to guide nursing practice. At Emergis, it was decided that a study group was needed to find out whether the implementation of a theoretical model for nursing practice would contribute to enhancement of the quality of nursing practice. The board of directors agreed that if a model were selected, it would have to be used through the entire institute. The model then would be used as a guideline for the practical activities of all nurses.

The study group meetings began with the study of present developments in nursing, an inventory of all the models that the nurses were using at the time, and a questionnaire that was used to evaluate the use of the different models. Several wards had already selected a model as a guideline. Those models, which had been selected as a result of publications in the nursing literature in which specific approaches to client situations were described, included Grijpdonck's Integrated Nursing Care Model (Koene et al., 1982), the Boston Rehabilitation Model, Gordon's Functional Health Patterns (Gordon, 1994), and the Neuman Systems Model (Neuman, 1982, 1995). Grijpdonck's model (Koene et al., 1982) emphasizes the responsibility of all those who participate in care. The Boston Rehabilitation Model focuses on helping the client to make his or her own decisions concerning housing, working, and leisure time. Gordon's (1994) work is a taxonomy of functional health patterns. The models were studied in small groups and then presented to the larger group. The last day was spent evaluating the models by using the questionnaire (Table 20-1).

Analysis of the questionnaire data revealed that the Neuman Systems Model had the highest mean score. More specifically, the Neuman Systems Model had high scores for questions 1 through 4, 8 through 10, and 12 through 16 (90 to 100 percent). The Rehabilitation Model also had high scores, although a little lower than the Neuman Systems Model (70 to 90 percent) for questions 1 through 4 and 8 through 10. But the Rehabilitation Model had low scores for questions 12 through 16 (15 to 40 percent). The Integrated Nursing Model scored high for questions 1 through 5 (80 to 100 percent) but only 50 percent for the remaining questions. Gordon's Functional Health Patterns had a high

TABLE 20-1. Nursing Theories Questionnaire

	Yes	No	Do not know
The model:			
1. Includes a holistic philosophy			
2. Is aimed at the client's responses to illness and the (remaining) resources of the client; is aimed at the client's environment			
3. Provides clarity for the client concerning the nursing care and offers the client (or his legal guardian) opportunities for negotiation and agreement on the nursing care plan			
4. Relates nursing care to the client's history, his uniqueness and his self-care pattern			
5. Provides transparency of the nursing care for other disciplines			
6. Contributes to cooperation of different disciplines			
7. Provides the domain for nursing care			
8. Provides an opportunity for supportive care in collaboration with other disciplines			
9. Is aimed toward prevention, recovery, and/or adaptation of the client's responses to illness and/or remaining resources and provides concrete guidelines for nursing interventions			
10. Agrees with the nursing care plan as provided by the faculty of nursing			
11. Agrees with present organization of the nursing discipline			
12. Offers the main wards room for their own philosophy			
13. Offers guidelines for reports and briefing			
14. Offers opportunities for monitoring the quality of the nursing care			
15. Offers opportunities for nursing research into nursing care and integration of evidence-based practice			

mean score but was rejected because it was considered neither a model nor a philosophy. Furthermore, although the representatives of the different sectors at Emergis wanted to use the model of their own choice, all found the Neuman Systems Model acceptable.

The study group's conclusion was presented to the board of directors: The Neuman Systems Model should be the model for nursing in Emergis. The philosophical claims undergirding the Neuman Systems Model correspond with the ideas that Emergis nurses have about nursing practice, and the model can accommodate the possibility of using the Rehabilitation Model as a guideline for tertiary prevention interventions. The Neuman Systems Model also fosters cooperation of different disciplines in patient care because it focuses on caregiving that extends beyond nursing practice. Furthermore, the Neuman Systems Model is client centered, which fits current developments in society, the basis for the quality-of-care laws. The study group recognized that the use of the model has to be accompanied by a system for applying nursing diagnoses in the future.

IMPLEMENTATION OF THE NEUMAN SYSTEMS MODEL AT EMERGIS

The implementation of the Neuman Systems Model was delayed because of the merger between the General Psychiatric Hospital, the Regional Institute for Mental Health Care, and the Zeeland Institutes for Protected Living, which became Emergis. Sooner than expected, however, Emergis was created on January 1, 1996. The creation of Emergis from the merger of the three clinical agencies meant that the findings of the study group were less relevant because only the nurses from the General Psychiatric Hospital had been involved. Social psychiatric nurses, social workers, and members of other disciplines now were part of the new institute, and their ideas had to be taken into account. Thus, although the implementation project proposal had been written, it was not moved forward immediately. Rather, following the merger, the individuals who had initiated the project met and decided to introduce the project partly through information disseminated throughout the institute and partly through a study conference, at which Frans Verberk (1995), who introduced the Neuman Systems Model in Holland, was invited to speak. These strategies led to wide support for the project. The project initiators became project leaders, and a project leader for the Regional Institute for Protected Housing was selected.

The implementation project began in 1997. The project was introduced in the first year, during which time the implementation plan was developed. The actual implementation of the model began in 1999. Very few examples of implementation plans and comparable methods were available, which meant that a lot of time was spent on developing the step-by-step plan for a practical implementation of the Neuman Systems Model. The plan was developed in close cooperation with the wards, to incorporate the nurses' ideas. The major guideline for this phase of the project was the literature, though limited, concerning comparable implementation projects of nursing models or theories (Antoni, 1995; Bekkers, van Dijk, & van Roekel, 1994; van Bergen, Hollands, & Nijhuis, 1980; Berkhout, Boumans, & Landeweerd, 1998).

It is anticipated that the implementation of the Neuman Systems Model at Emergis will take 3 years (Figure 20-2). One of the first activities of the Working Committee for Methodology is to identify the success factors. Once the implementation of the Neuman Systems Model is completed, the success factors will be evaluated. Another activity in the first year is the collection of the basic data, which provide the information that is needed to design the definitive implementation plan for each ward.

The implementation project includes two very important activities—education and coaching of the caregivers on the wards.

Education

Education on the wards begins after collection of basic data. The senior nurses are very important contributors to the educational program. They have an opportunity to carry out their new roles as senior nurses by functioning as trainers and coaches for the caregivers on their own and other wards. The involvement of the senior nurses in educational activities provided the time project leaders needed to spend on other activities.

The senior nurses were, therefore, trained first. A course was given by a senior nurse who had started his education as a clinical nurse specialist; he was assisted by one of the nursing students who had been involved in the collection of the basic data. In addition, several experts from within and outside Emergis contributed to the course. The course content focused on: (1) the connection between the Neuman Systems Model and recent developments in society and how the developments affect care; (2) the philosophical claims on which the Neuman Systems Model is based; (3) the concepts of the Neuman Systems

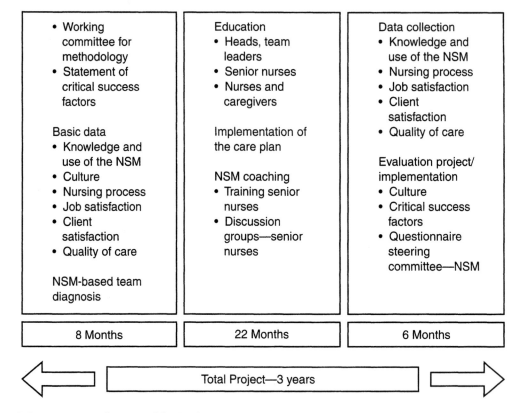

• Working committee for methodology • Statement of critical success factors Basic data • Knowledge and use of the NSM • Culture • Nursing process • Job satisfaction • Client satisfaction • Quality of care NSM-based team diagnosis	Education • Heads, team leaders • Senior nurses • Nurses and caregivers Implementation of the care plan NSM coaching • Training senior nurses • Discussion groups—senior nurses	Data collection • Knowledge and use of the NSM • Nursing process • Job satisfaction • Client satisfaction • Quality of care Evaluation project/ implementation • Culture • Critical success factors • Questionnaire steering committee—NSM
8 Months	22 Months	6 Months

Total Project—3 years

FIGURE 20-2.   Planning of the implementation.

Model; (4) the concept of negotiation; (5) how to make a Neuman Systems Model–based care plan; and (6) how to educate and coach the nurses. The concept of negotiation and its place in the Neuman Systems Model were depicted as an hourglass (Figure 20-3).

The senior nurses then gave a similar course to the nurses. The course for the nurses placed more emphasis on the care plan and the concept of negotiation and less emphasis on recent developments.

Coaching

The educational program includes coaching of team members in use of the Neuman Systems Model. The senior nurses had had very little experience with coaching. Therefore, a decision was made to begin the implementation project with a small number of coaches, who received additional training. The coaches train the senior nurses as coaches and hold discussion groups with the senior nurses to facilitate greater understanding of the issues involved in implementation of the Neuman Systems Model. The coaches also monitor the quality of the implementation project and provide reports to the management and the Steering Committee.

The admission ward within the adult care section was selected as the pilot ward. The findings from this ward have contributed to the implementation plan. The plan con-

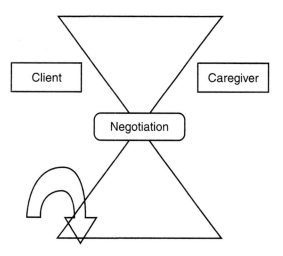

FIGURE 20-3.   Hourglass.

sists of a description of the starting situation on a ward, the team diagnosis, and the success factors. These data influence the specific implementation project plan for each ward.

The method for stating the starting situation of the ward is part of the research project, which accompanies the implementation of the Neuman Systems Model, and which will be discussed later in this chapter. The team diagnosis is an important aspect of the preparation for implementation of the Neuman Systems Model; Frans Verberk developed the guideline for this aspect of the project. The team is diagnosed according to the concepts of the Neuman Systems Model. The internal environment (intrapersonal) is mapped using a questionnaire for each client system variable. The physiological variable concerns the size, composition, and "physical" condition of the team. The psychological variable concerns the educational level, the perception of emotional safety and trust, and the psychological condition of the team. The sociocultural variable concerns the extent of the team's interactions with the environment, how the team members interact, and the sociocultural nature of the team. The developmental variable includes questions concerning recent changes in the team, the changes that can be expected in the (near) future, the ages of the team members, and the innovations and/or traumas recently experienced by the team. The spiritual variable includes questions about the team's values and ideas concerning the team. The answers to these questions come from the measurements taken as part of the research project, especially the investigation of the ward culture, the stated success factors, and the working committee for methodology. The team diagnosis and the diagnosis of the ward is the basis for the implementation of the Neuman Systems Model on that ward.

The project organizational structure is depicted in Figure 20-4. The project is structured around an advisory committee, which coordinates the project. The advisory committee includes a member of the board of directors and the section directors. They discuss all current matters, including the implementation of the Neuman Systems Model. The implementation of the model is being done by the steering committee, which includes a chairperson, the managers of the basic facilities, two project leaders, and a secretary. For

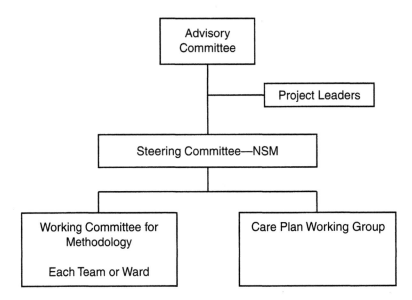

FIGURE 20-4.   Organizational structure of the Neuman Systems Model implementation project.

each ward on which the Neuman Systems Model is introduced, a Working Committee for Methodology is installed. The working committees include the manager of the basic facility, the team leader of the ward, the senior nurse, a project leader, and, if necessary, a secretary. In 1999, the Committee for Care Plans developed a new care plan based on the content of the Neuman Systems Model as part of the implementation project.

Several elements were taken into account as the implementation project went forward: data collection of the present situation, statement of final goal, selection of outcomes, statement concerning the client's needs, the professional statement, and the negotiation between client and caregiver.

Data Collection of the Present Situation

Soon after the merger, the staff who were not part of the former general psychiatric hospital were asked to respond to an inventory containing items that asked whether they used a model for practice and whether they thought that a model was needed. In general, responses were positive.

Collection of the data for the present situation was carried out by the seering committee at the start of the project. An inventory was used again, this time focusing on the client's needs.

Statement of Final Goal

A final goal for the project was stated, as follows: The implementation of the Neuman Systems Model as the working model for the nursing discipline, first for the clinical area, and complemented with nursing diagnoses will occur within three years following the formal start of the project for each section.

Selection of Outcomes

Statements about outcomes were developed as a collaborative activity of the advisory committee and the steering committee. The outcomes were formalized in a research proposal and critical success factors as stated by the advisory committee.

Statement Concerning the Client's Needs

Each time the project starts in a certain section, the needs of the clients are stated. This is done through the section director and the project leader. The sections are regarded as clients, who will have stated an interest in the project. The clients can adapt the project to meet their specific needs.

The Professional Statement

The project leaders considered the structure of the project extensively before it started. Management participation is not negotiable but there must be clear proof of commitment through a professional statement, so that the stated final goal cannot be compromised.

The Negotiation

The actual project plan is negotiable for each section. The client's needs and the professional statement of the project leader are stated in a consistent manner.

EVALUATING THE IMPLEMENTATION OF THE NEUMAN SYSTEMS MODEL AT EMERGIS: THE RESEARCH PROJECT

Research activities are an important part of the implementation plan (Figure 20-5). The first aim of the research project is to determine to what extent the components of the Neuman Systems Model that the steering committee considers to be characteristic for the model actually have been implemented on the wards. The second aim is to identify the effects of the implementation. The implementation of the Neuman Systems Model at Emergis is guided by the research project. This means that basic data must be obtained and analyzed before the implementation project can begin. After collecting the basic data, the plan for implementation activities, such as additional training, introduction of the new care plan, and coaching of the team, is written. It also is important to determine to what extent the elements of the implementation of the Neuman Systems Model influence the extent of the use of the nursing process. The research project largely determines the time management of the implementation project.

The implementation variables are those variables that are used for the evaluation of the project on the wards. The implementation project is being evaluated, in part, by studying the culture of the ward before and after the implementation of the Neuman Systems Model. The methodology team (including the head of basic provisions, the team leader of the ward on which the Neuman Systems Model is implemented, the senior nurse, and the project leader) states the critical success factors that are used to evaluate the project on the ward. Critical success factors are the factors that determine that the project has been successful when they have been achieved. The steering committee also has developed an instrument for measuring the success of the implementation on the wards.

The variables for the research project have been derived from the hypothesized effects as found in the literature concerning the implementation of the Neuman Systems Model, and from the variables that the steering committee stated as improvements that can be expected. The list of variables can be extended, but in order to manage the research project, the list has been restricted to those variables that are essential: knowledge of the Neuman Systems Model, extent of implementation of the nursing process, client satisfaction, caregiver satisfaction, culture of the ward, and the quality of the care (see Figure 20-5).

The research project concerns two Neuman Systems Model implementation variables: implementation of the nursing process and the extent to which nurses know and apply the Neuman Systems Model in daily practice (see Figure 20-5). It is hypothesized that there are several groups and individuals who benefit from working according to the model and that the implementation of the nursing process is a result of that. It also is hy-

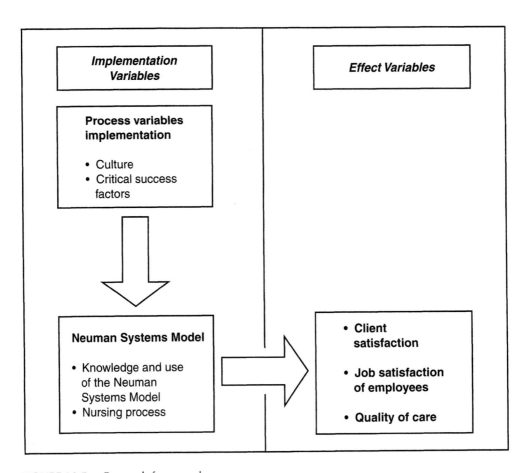

FIGURE 20-5.   Research framework.

pothesized that the nursing process has a positive effect on the quality of care; the client will have better quality of care because the quality and continuity of the care are improved. Furthermore, it is hypothesized that the nurses will have increased job satisfaction and more responsibility, which will improve the quality of care. The institute will benefit because the quality of care is operationalized. The nursing profession may benefit because autonomy and professional care are improved.

The variables included in the research project are being measured with existing instruments. The instruments share the common characteristic of having been developed elsewhere and are considered valid and reliable. Although further development of the instruments is beyond the scope of the research project, they are being evaluated for their applicability for the project of implementing the Neuman Systems Model. The instruments are used to collect basic data before the implementation of the model and after. Those data will be compared to determine to what extent the implementation of the model has affected the variables. Moreover, measurement of the variables should provide outcomes concerning the project, to what extent the nursing process has been implemented, and to what extent the nurses are familiar with the Neuman Systems Model and how it is being used in daily practice. The research project results also may reveal whether the implementation of the Neuman Systems Model has a positive effect on the variables.

Data about quality of care and application of the nursing process are being collected by interns from the Faculty of Nursing Education at Emergis. The students collect and analyze the data for the research reports for the wards. The findings then are presented to the steering committee. This has been a positive experience for both the interns and the project staff.

The research framework is based on three implementation variables and three effect variables for which a change is expected. The implementation variables are culture, knowledge and use of the Neuman Systems Model, and nursing process. The effect variables are quality of care, employee job satisfaction, and client satisfaction.

Culture

An important innovation such as the implementation of the Neuman Systems Model requires specific attention to the influence of the culture of the ward. The culture is a determining factor for the implementation of a nursing or caregiver method. A diagnosis of the culture may be the most important condition for successful implementation. For this project, it is important that the basic philosophy of the Neuman Systems Model can be combined with the existing culture of the organization or ward culture. The philosophy of the Neuman Systems Model is best combined with a ward culture that can be described as innovative. An innovative culture is strongly geared toward developments and changes outside the organization, such as the social aspects of illness and changes in the professions, insurance companies, and other health care organizations. The equality of people is strongly expressed. The senior nurse's function has been derived from this characterization. A good senior nurse is externally oriented and innovative by nature, which is a major reason to place these nurses in front positions for the implementation of the model on the wards and to include them in the project.

The cultural variable had a more prominent place in the first design of the project than in the definitive design. Research into the culture of the pilot ward appeared to generate high expectations among the nurses. For example, if questions were asked about the leadership style on the ward, it was assumed that the implementation of the Neuman Systems Model would automatically mean that the present team leader was to leave. The cultural variable was, therefore, placed in a less prominent position. It is no longer an effect variable but a process variable. The culture now is part of the research framework, so that a statement of the culture of the ward is made before implementation of the Neuman Systems Model and the extent to which this has changed can be determined afterward. Thus, culture not only is an interesting variable but also is part of the evaluation of the entire project.

Knowledge and Use of the Neuman Systems Model

Research about the extent to which individuals have knowledge of the Neuman Systems Model and how the knowledge of the different aspects of the model are applied to daily practice is an implementation variable in the research design. This variable will provide an answer to the question to what extent knowledge of the model has increased. It also is important to find out whether the knowledge actually is applied in practice. Here, the Lowry–Jopp Neuman Evaluation Instrument (LJNEI) (Lowry, 1998) was used. The LJNEI initially was developed to measure the effects of educating nurses in a Neuman Systems Model–based curriculum. Consultation with Dr. Lowry indicated that the instrument is suitable for the evaluation of the effects of the implementation of the Neuman Systems Model with regard to knowledge of the model and the application of this knowledge in practice. An important question about the use of the LJNEI is whether it can be used for the implementation of the Neuman Systems Model in practice. The first basic data collected on the wards have provided a detailed representation of the existing knowledge concerning the Neuman Systems Model and the practical application of the model. These data also are used to identify the content of continuing education programs on the wards.

Nursing Process

One of the hypotheses of the project was that the implementation of the Neuman Systems Model would affect the extent to which the nurses apply the nursing process. The extent to which the nursing process is applied at the start of the project was part of the basic data collection. The nursing process is applied with the aim of reaching the goals that the client and the nurse have stated as efficiently and effectively as possible. This variable is included to find out to what extent the nursing process is applied on wards where the Neuman Systems Model is being implemented.

Quality of Care

Quality of care is one of the effect variables that are included in the research project. The research question is to determine what the quality of care was before the implementation of the Neuman Systems Model and after. The quality of nursing care is defined as the characteristics of a product, process, or service that are important to meet stated or implicit needs. The basis for the instrument used to measure quality of care is a document that was developed at Emergis, which states the general requirements for quality of care.

The document is based on the philosophy of nursing articulated by van Bergen and colleagues (1980), and states the desired tasks for professionals at Emergis. The document contains only process variables, which are those variables that actually are connected to the professional's practice. The quality-of-care instrument is used to compare the desired quality of care (criterion) and the actual (measured) quality of care. The criteria reflect van Bergen and colleagues' (1980) focus on continuity of client-oriented care through management of the nursing process and use of technical skills. A disadvantage of the instrument is that it is not based on criteria that have been derived from the Neuman Systems Model.

Employee Job Satisfaction

Another hypothesis of the implementation project was that the nursing process would be applied more thoroughly; still another hypothesis was that implementation of the nursing process also improves the quality of the care. It was thought that quality of care would be relevant to both clients and nurses; the nursing process affects commitment and accountability. Thus, an effect variable is job satisfaction. The aim is to determine whether nurses' job satisfaction changes on the wards on which the Neuman Systems Model is implemented.

Client Satisfaction

The application of the Neuman Systems Model is hypothesized to positively affect client-centered nursing and the application of the nursing process. In turn, this is hypothesized to positively affect client satisfaction because the client can negotiate the care, which also will improve communication between client and caregiver. The instrument to measure client satisfaction provides data about the client's satisfaction with information concerning the treatment, the influence the client has on the treatment, and relationships between clients and caregivers, as well as data about the way clients spend their time and the extent to which they can influence this themselves.

CURRENT AND FUTURE WORK

Nursing Diagnosis Taxonomy

The decision to implement the Neuman Systems Model at Emergis was accompanied by a recommendation to implement nursing diagnosis at the same time. At that time, another institute in Holland had started an experiment using a matrix of Gordon's Functional Health Patterns and the five Neuman Systems Model client system variables. However, the Emergis project leaders found the classification of particular health patterns as particular Neuman Systems Model variables to be forced rather than logical.

Dissatisfaction with the matrix led to discovery of Ziegler's (1982) Neuman Systems Model–based taxonomy of nursing diagnoses. Ziegler's taxonomy was better suited to the needs of the project leaders because it provides more opportunity to work, think, and reason within the context of the Neuman Systems Model. The Emergis plan calls for documentation of the Ziegler taxonomy numerical code, as well as a narrative descriptive diagnosis. In the future, the Ziegler taxonomy will have to be combined or reconciled with Gordon's Functional Health Patterns classification. That work, which will begin in 2001, will provide the connection between the Neuman Systems Model as implemented in Emergis and developments in nursing diagnosis for the rest of Holland and in other countries.

Multidisciplinary Educational Program

During 2000, collection of basic data was completed. The implementation project now is focusing on the education program. The team leaders of the wards have started their education, which is being given by Frans Verberk. The Geriatric Care and Adult Care sections have started the implementation of the Neuman Systems Model for both clinical and ambulatory care. Inasmuch as caregivers from non-nursing disciplines indicated interest in participation, the implementation project has become multidisciplinary. Other sections of Emergis, including Child and Youth Psychiatry and Addict Care, will begin the implementation of the model in the near future.

Research Design Issues

The initial research project design called for exclusion of one ward from the implementation project, so that a control condition would be available. The ward that was selected was especially suitable because there are no student nurses, which meant that the influence of the project would hardly be felt. Emergis management, however, decided that the project should include all wards. Therefore, the project leaders decided to contact colleague psychiatric hospitals to request a control ward. To date, a specific control ward has not been located, although two colleague hospitals are considering participation in the project.

Maintaining the Project

The project will have to be maintained following the completion of the implementation project. Maintenance activities must include continuing education for all current and new employees. Variables that are to be expected to change very slowly, such as culture, may have to be studied again after a longer period of time.

CONCLUSION

A long process already has taken place. The nurses requested the implementation of the nursing process and deliberately selected the Neuman Systems Model. The actual start of the implementation of the model began recently, after much careful and systematic planning. The Neuman Systems Model has served not only as a model for practice but also guided the design of the implementation and research projects. Complete implementation of the model will continue to require much time and energy but a solid base already has been laid at Emergis.

REFERENCES

Antoni, M. (1995). *Introductieverslag the Neuman Systems Model* [Report about introducing the Neuman Systems Model]. Santpoort: Dr. B. H. Evertsenkliniek.

Bekkers, F., van Dijk, A., & van Roekel, W. (1994). *Kwaliteitsverbetering door patiëntgericht verplegen, theorie en praktijk van de implementatie van patiëntgericht verplegen* [Patient-oriented nursing as a means for upgrading quality of care, theory and practice of implementation]. Utrecht: Lemma.

Berkhout, A. J. M. B., Boumans, N. P. G., & Landeweerd, A. (1998). *Evaluatie van bewonergericht verplegen en verzorgen in verpleeghuizen* [Evaluation of resident-oriented care in nurisng homes]. Maastricht: Universiteit Maastricht.

Gordon, M. (1994). *Nurisng diagnoses, process and application.* St. Louis: Mosby.

Koene, G., Grijpdonck, M., Rodenbach, M.Th., & Windey, T. (1982). *Integrerende verpleegkunde: Wetenschap in praktijk* [Integrated nursing: Science in practice]. Lochem: De Tijdstroom.

Lowry, L. (1998). *The Neuman Systems Model and nursing education: Teaching, strategies and outcomes.* Indianapolis: Sigma Theta Tau International.

Neuman, B. (1982). *The Neuman Systems Model: Application to nursing education and practice.* Norwalk, CT: Appleton-Century-Crofts.

Neuman, B. (1995). *The Neuman Systems Model* (3rd ed.). Norwalk, CT: Appleton & Lange.

van Bergen, B., Hollands, L., & Nijhuis, H. (1980). *De ontwikkeling van een kwaliteitsprofiel* [Creating a profile for quality of care] (2nd ed.). Lochem-Poperinge: De Tijdstroom.

van der Brink-Tjebbes, J. A. (1987). *Verpleging naar de Maat, een verplegingswetenschappelijke optiek* [Nursing according to the standard, viewing nursing through science]. Lochem: De Tijdstroom.

van Linge, R. (1998). *Innoveren in de gezondheidszorg* [Innovations in healthcare]. Maarssen: Elesvier/De Tijdstroom.

Verberk, F. (1995). In Holland: Application of the Neuman model in psychiatric nursing. In B. Neuman (Ed.), *The Neuman Systems Model* (3rd ed., pp. 629–36). Norwalk, CT: Appleton & Lange.

Ziegler, S. M. (1982). Taxonomy for nursing diagnosis derived from the Numan Systems Model. In B. Neuman (Ed.), *The Neuman Systems Model: Application to nursing education and practice* (pp. 55–68). Norwalk, CT: Appleton-Century-Crofts.

PART VI

THE NEUMAN SYSTEMS MODEL AND THE FUTURE

twenty-one

The Future and the Neuman Systems Model

Betty Neuman

ased on past patterns of escalation in utilization of the Neuman Systems Model and current use of the model throughout the world, I foresee increasing utilization of systems models in general, and the Neuman Systems Model in particular, well into the twenty-first century, particularly in large-scale (state, regional, and global) programming. As catastrophic sociopolitical events affect health care, multidisciplinary involvement related to the human condition often will be required. The comprehensive and flexible structure of the Neuman Systems Model for assessment and intervention increases its relevancy for members of all health care disciplines. Indeed, since its inception, the model has both preceded and complemented changing trends in nursing in particular and health care in general. For example, the trend toward an eclectic approach has, paradoxically, given the Neuman Systems Model considerable exposure as an excellent representative of systems frameworks. Moreover, application of the model is virtually unlimited because of its wholistic systemic base and perspective.

I predict continued expansion of the utility of the Neuman Systems Model based on the following factors:

- With the increased trend toward home-based and community care, the wholistic concepts of the Neuman Systems Model will have continuing relevancy for both nursing education and practice within an expanding nursing domain. The model fits well with the continuing evolution of health care reform proposals that focus on primary and tertiary prevention for optimal wellness.
- Inasmuch as the adaptability and utility of the Neuman Systems Model has been documented in many countries, its use certainly can resolve cross-cultural differences and improve health care.
- The rigorous research that has been based on the Neuman Systems Model has contributed greatly to the growth of nursing science.

- The comprehensiveness of the Neuman Systems Model facilitates greater understanding of areas of nursing concern as well as areas of interdisciplinary and international concern. The model clearly supports interdisciplinary and multidisciplinary cooperation and collaboration, which are major health care trends.
- The Neuman Systems Model provides a viable structure for organizing, processing, and retrieving massive amounts of health information, which decreases the information overload that has become a major social issue.
- The continued evolution and visibility of the Neuman Systems Model are assured through the competent and dedicated membership of the Neuman Systems Model Trustees Group, including trustees and associate members, and the many fine Neuman Systems Model–based programs that have been implemented throughout the world.
- The Neuman Systems Model Trustees Group has sponsored the biennial International Neuman Systems Model symposia since 1986. The symposia continue to foster greater visibility and understanding of the Neuman Systems Model, as well as to facilitate networking among nurses and members of other health care disciplines worldwide.
- College, in Aston, Pennsylvania, now houses the Neuman Systems Model Archives.
- Neuman Systems Model Internet sites are in place: *http://www.neumann.edu* (click on nursing, click on Neuman Systems Model); *http://www.lemmus.demon.co.uk/neuman1.html* (link to this site through: *http://www.ualberta.ca/~jrnorris/nt/theory.html*)
- Annual Neuman newsletters keep subscribers informed about evolving Neuman Systems Model events and progress.
- The Neuman Systems Model is made up of concepts that support future changes in client care, such as issues within family and community systems. The model will serve evolving twenty-first century health care needs, easily adapting to interdisciplinary and multidisciplinary partnerships and crossing of cultural barriers.

THE NEUMAN SYSTEMS MODEL TRUSTEES SPEAK OUT ABOUT THE NEUMAN SYSTEMS MODEL AND THE FUTURE

The Neuman Systems Model trustees (Appendix E) highlighted several developments that are advancing the model:

- Traditional management models emphasizing power and control now require a different paradigm for shared governance, partnerships, and empowerment. The Neuman Systems Model readily incorporates concepts from other disciplines, such as learning organization, environmental scanning, and scenario planning. The model concepts and processes are relevant to twenty-first century changing health care horizons.
- Educators are developing curricula that promote critical thinking and accountability; the Neuman Systems Model components facilitate strategic planning and evidence-based decision making for relevant client care within any environment.
- The worldwide applicability of the Neuman Systems Model has been documented.

By 1995, 175 education and practice facilities throughout the world were identified as using the Neuman Systems Model. The model is well suited for community health and the increasing emphasis on health promotion in both retention and maintenance of optimal-level wellness. The model connects the universal aspects of society while advancing nursing knowledge globally through Neuman Systems Model–based international program implementations, studies, and special projects.

- The systemic perspective of the model encourages creativity for a new health care vision within changing forms of technology, communication, and intervention protocols for catastrophic and complex health situations.

- The model has been used as a standard for determining the wholistic nature of existing health care programs. It has facilitated team building and shared partnerships for health care services. The comprehensive nature of the model will continue to increase its value.

- Using the model as an international health care directive will move nursing closer to professionalism through a common philosophy, language, goals, and processes unifying interdisciplinary approaches to health care for a cost containment outcome and optimal client system wellness.

- Neuman Systems Model trustees report that students easily articulate and integrate the model concepts and processes, thereby enhancing their own personal and professional identity and development. Students find that the Neuman Systems Model Process Format provides a clear direction for practical application of the model concepts and processes.

- The model encompasses both knowledge concepts and processes to meet current and future health care challenges. It provides an orderly way of thinking about nursing activities, which will enhance cooperation and role definition in nursing practice. It provides an ideal multidimensional paradigm for proactively seeking new knowledge for providing optimal client care; it is a vital tool for shaping the future of nursing.

- The model has documented value for outcome-based studies and middle-range theory development. The model has the potential to guide research methodologies that capture the richness of the model and the Neuman Systems Model Process Format, including documentation of the perceptions of both caregiver and client, as well as the integration of practice and research. The model is viewed as a crucial guide for outcomes studies.

- One trustee stated: "The future of the Neuman Systems Model will be in its ability to define nursing education, practice, and research as a universal voice to better clarify the nursing profession throughout the world. Nursing practice will be more explicitly defined through further research in qualitative and quantitative paradigms to generate middle-range theories derived from the model."

- Another trustee stated: "I believe the nursing profession would be well advised to maintain the 20-year thrust of model-based inquiry in building the science of nursing."

Appendix A:
The Neuman Systems Model Definitions

Betty Neuman

Basic structure: The basic structure or central core consists of common client survival factors related to system variables as well as unique individual characteristics. It represents the basic system energy resources.

Boundary lines: The flexible line of defense is the outer boundary of the client system. All relevant variables must be taken into account, as the whole is greater than the sum of the parts; a change in one part affects all other system parts.

Client/client system: A total system in interaction with the internal and external environment. A composite of variables (physiological, psychological, sociocultural, developmental, and spiritual), each of which is a subpart of all parts, forms the whole of the client. The client as a system is composed of a core or basic structure of survival factors and surrounding protective concentric rings. The concentric rings are composed of similar factors, yet serve varied and different purposes in retention, attainment, or maintenance of system stability and integrity or a combination of these. The client is considered an open system in total interface and exchange of matter and information with the environment. The client is viewed as a system, and the term can be used interchangeably with the client/client system; that is, individual, family, community, and social issues are considered a system with boundaries and identifiable interacting parts.

Content: The five variables of person in interaction with the internal and external environment comprise the whole client system.

Degree of reaction: The degree of reaction is the degree of system instability resulting from stressor invasion of the normal line of defense.

Environment: The environment consists of both internal and external forces surrounding the client, influencing and being influenced by the client, at any point in time, as an open system. The created environment is an unconsciously developed protective environment that binds system energy and encompasses both the internal and external client environments; it acts as a perceptual safety mechanism to maintain system stability.

Feedback: The process within which matter, energy, and information, as system output, provide feedback for corrective action to change, enhance, or stabilize the system.

Flexible line of defense: The flexible line of defense is a protective, accordionlike mechanism that surrounds and protects the normal line of defense from invasion by stressors. The greater the expansiveness of this line from the normal line of defense, the greater the degree of protectiveness. Examples are situational, such as recently altered sleep patterns or immune functions that could threaten system stability and lessen the potential for survival and optimal wellness.

Health: A continuum of wellness to illness, dynamic in nature, that is constantly subject to change. Optimal wellness or stability indicates that total system needs are being met. A reduced state of wellness is the result of unmet systemic needs. The client is in a dynamic state of either wellness or illness, in varying degrees, at any given point in time. Health is related to available energy to support the system.

Input/output: The matter, energy, and information exchanged between client and environment that is entering or leaving the system at any point in time.

Lines of resistance: Protection factors activated when stressors have penetrated the normal line of defense, causing the reaction symptomatology. The resistance lines ideally protect the basic structure and facilitate reconstitution toward wellness during and following treatment, as the stressor reaction is decreased and client resistance is increased. All lines of defense and resistance are considered to contain both internal and external resources.

Negentropy: A process of energy conservation that increases organization and complexity, moving the system toward stability or a higher degree of wellness. Stability and degree of wellness have a direct relationship.

Normal line of defense: An adaptational level of health developed over time and considered normal for a particular individual client or system; it becomes a standard for wellness deviance determination.

Nursing: A unique profession concerned with all variables affecting clients in their environment. Nursing is preventive intervention.

Open system: A system in which there is a continuous flow of input and process, output and feedback. It is a system of organized complexity, where all elements are in interaction. Stress and reaction to stress are basic components.

Prevention as intervention: Intervention typology or modes for nursing action and determinants for entry of both client and caregiver into the health care system. *Primary prevention:* before a reaction to stressors occurs. *Secondary prevention:* treatment of symptoms following a reaction to stressors. *Tertiary prevention:* maintenance of optimal wellness following treatment.

Process/function: The function or process of the system is the exchange of matter, energy, and information with the environment and the interaction of the parts and subparts of the client system. A living system tends to move toward wholeness, stability, wellness, and negentropy based on effective use of available energy resources.

Reconstitution: Represents the return and maintenance of system stability, following treatment of a stressor reaction, which may result in a higher or lower level of wellness than previously. It represents successful mobilization of energy resources.

Stability: A desired state of balance or harmony while system energy exchanges take place without disrupting the character of the system. The dynamic nature of stability is seen as the client, as a system, adequately copes with stressors to retain, attain, or maintain optimal health and integrity.

Stressors: Environmental factors that are intra-, inter-, and extrapersonal in nature and have the potential for disrupting system stability by penetrating the system lines of defense and resistance. Their outcome may be either positive or negative; client perception and coping ability are major considerations for caregivers and clients.

Wellness/illness: Wellness is a stable condition in which system subparts are in harmony with the whole system. Wholeness is based on the interrelationships of variables, which determine the amount of resistance to stressors. Illness is on the opposite continuum from wellness and represents instability and energy depletion among the system parts or subparts affecting the whole.

Wholistic: A system is considered wholistic when its parts or subparts can be organized into an interrelating whole. The ideal is one of keeping parts stable within their intimate relationships with the whole system; that is, individuals are viewed as wholes whose component parts are in dynamic interdependent interaction while adjusting to environmental stressors.

Appendix B:
Betty Neuman's Autobiography and Chronology of the Development and Utilization of the Neuman Systems Model

Betty Neuman

I was born in southeastern Ohio on September 11, 1924, on our 100-acre family farm. My father, a farmer, died at age 37 when I was 11 years old and my brothers were ages 5 and 16. My mother was a hard-working, enterprising housewife, managing well our limited financial resources.

My older brother, mother, and I engaged in several summers of hard physical labor to keep the family and farm intact. My younger brother escaped most of the labors, because my mother moved us to a nearby town, Marietta, Ohio, where I completed my final year of high school. My older brother married and continued to maintain the family farm. For many years I have been proud of my early farming heritage, because it taught me the important values of simplicity, humility, and self-reliance.

Because my father had always praised his nurses during six years of intermittent hospitalizations prior to his death from chronic kidney disease, early in life I began to idealize the nursing profession. I developed a strong commitment to become an excellent bedside nurse to repay society a debt of gratitude. Another very important influence was the shared stories of my mother's charity experiences as a self-taught rural midwife. She was often called at night and rode by horse and buggy to perform home deliveries; a favorite memory is stealing away to read her battered general medical book.

When I graduated from high school in the summer of 1942, our country was six months into World War II. Local employment opportunities were limited. Being financially unable to attend nearby Marietta College as I had always wanted, I obtained a position at Wright Air Force Base in Dayton, Ohio, as an aircraft instrument repair technician. It was particularly exciting to install instruments in fighter warplanes following their repair. I recall refusing an offer of transfer to the New York–based Sperry Rand Company upon receiving the highest test results in this specialty area. Deciding factors were continuing homesickness, desire to accumulate money toward a nursing education, and charity involvement in the Dayton YWCA as a recreation hostess for servicemen.

Later, during evening school classes, I was chosen as a draftsperson by an aircraft contracting agency, where I worked for one year at a higher salary. Concurrent with this position, I often worked evenings as a short-order cook to supplement my income and contribute to my mother and younger brother's needs.

By the time that I had nearly accumulated the necessary funds for entrance into nurse's training, the Cadet Nurse Corps Program became available, expediting my entrance into the three-year diploma nurse program at People Hospital, Akron, Ohio, now renamed General Hospital Medical Center. My goal of becoming an excellent bedside nurse was accomplished as I graduated with honors for two combined graduating classes in the fall of 1947.

Although the diploma program followed the medical model, since the hospital was private in nature and had established a fine reputation, students were required to give excellent total care to clients.

During these years I had saved enough money to purchase from a family friend a 1935 Ford Coupe for $275. Taking our mother with us, my younger brother and I drove south to Florida then west to Los Angeles, where an uncle lived. Three months after arriving, my mother and brother drove back home to Ohio, and I began a position at the Los Angeles General Hospital as a staff communicable disease nurse. At the end of six months, I accepted a promotion to head nurse and remained there another year. Since I was eager to explore other areas of nursing, I assumed a one-year school nurse position followed by a one-year industrial nurse position, both in the greater Los Angeles area.

In 1950, I returned to the Los Angeles General Hospital as a private duty nurse and remained until 1956. During that time I developed broadly based knowledge and skill in critical care for medical, surgical, pediatrics, and many other specialty areas, such as burns, polio, and head injuries. This was long before the development of critical care units. A variety of shift work accommodated the evening classes I was taking preparatory to a one-year, full-time residency to complete the baccalaureate degree in nursing at UCLA. In 1954, I married a beginning resident obstetrician of the Good Samaritan Hospital, helping facilitate both our educational programs. I graduated from UCLA in June 1957 with a major in public health nursing and scholastic honors. My degree was the first from a large extended family of 125 first cousins; to travel so far from home was considered wayward. After helping initiate my husband's private practice, I worked as an office manager and nurse until the birth of a beautiful daughter, Nancy, in 1959.

Between 1964 and 1966, during my UCLA master's program, weekend, evening, and summer nursing activities included special education projects for the Glendale Memorial Hospital, acting as relief psychiatric head nurse at the Queen of Angels Hospital, and volunteer crisis counseling at the Benjamin Rush Clinic, Venice Clinic, and Los Angeles Suicide Prevention Center. Donna Aquilera and I were chosen by UCLA faculty to represent the school of nursing at these clinic facilities to determine the efficacy and relevancy of the nurse role as counselor within early community psychiatric settings. We were fortunate to be the first nurses to validate the nurse counselor role within such setting, as we received excellent supervision from agency directors well known in subsequent psychiatric literature. As a result of this experience, I continued to accumulate volunteer counseling hours to become one of the first California Nurse Licensed Clinical Fellows of the American Association of Marriage and Family Therapy.

My master's program was completed in June 1966. It was a federal grant–funded specialty program to prepare public health/mental health nurse consultants to pioneer nurse role development within newly emerging community mental health centers, for which no specific functions or processes were yet developed. In January 1967, I became a UCLA faculty member, assuming chairmanship of the program from which I graduated, though I had no previous teaching or curriculum preparation. Initial activities included grant writing to secure funds for expanding the program to become the first in community mental health nurse education. It became a two-quarter postgraduate optional program offering for completed nurse psychiatric master's students. It included one semester each in community organization and planning and mental health consultation. This program, which began in the fall of 1967, pioneered the first postmaster-level nurse involvement in role definition with interdisciplinary groups that were beginning to function in the newly emerging community mental health centers in the greater Los Angeles area. Early in the teaching program, an explicit teaching and practice model for mental health consultation was developed by me, validated by students, and published in 1971 in a first coauthored mental health textbook for nurses entitled *Consultation and Community Organization in Community Mental Health Nursing.* It has long been out of print; little interest existed in the area of community mental health for nursing during the late 1960s and very early 1970s. I am indeed grateful for the vital feedback and extraordinary pioneering and cooperative spirit of my students, particularly during the earliest period of this program implementation. They both reinforced and helped me expand my own knowledge and skill as I role-modeled for them the mental health consultation process and nurse role development within a variety of community mental health facilities.

In 1970, I developed the Neuman Systems Model to provide unity, or a focal point, for student learning. Graduate students requested an initial entry class that would provide an overview of the four variables of man (physiological, psychological, sociocultural, and developmental), which they would subsequently study in depth in their newly developed clinical specialty programs. I was chosen by the curriculum committee to develop and coordinate the course, in which guest faculty most knowledgeable in these four areas would lecture. Since my major concern was how to provide structure to best integrate student learning in a wholistic manner, I personally developed the model design as it still exists today and received course-teaching faculty approval of its use for student integration of their lecture material. Because of heavy time commitments with the developing community mental health program, I asked for a co-coordinator and chose a young psychiatric faculty member, Rae Jeanne Young (now Neuman Systems Model trustee Rae Jeanne Memmott), who agreed that we should evaluate the effectiveness of the model design as a teaching tool. It is important to state that was neither I knowledgeable about nursing models nor had a clear trend yet begun in nursing for developing models. The Neuman Systems Model was developed strictly as a teaching aid. However, use of the model proved positive for student learning following a two-year evaluation period; the model was first published in 1972 in the May–June issue of *Nursing Research.* The article, "A Model for Teaching Total Person Approach to Patient Problems," was the basis for the 1974 chapter, "The Betty Neuman Health-Care Systems Model: A Total Approach to Patient Problems," published in the first book on nursing conceptual models, Riehl and Roy's *Conceptual Models for Nursing Practice.*

The community mental health program continued to expand, with students from throughout the United States and other countries. Two additional faculty were added; one was Kristine Gebbie, a particularly competent program graduate, who contributed significantly to further development of the program. Several articles were coauthored by the program faculty, including a research project on "Measurement of Change in Problem Solving Ability Among Nurses Receiving Mental Health Consultation."

Concurrent with the six-and-one-half-year faculty position, beginning in the winter of 1967 I taught many on- and off-campus credit workshops (some extending through the winter of 1978), conferences, and seminars for the UCLA Extension Division Continuing Education Department and for the Western Interstate Council for Higher Education, Colorado, in states west of the Mississippi River. Teaching areas included group leadership, interviewing, family counseling, crisis intervention, mental health consultation, psychiatric community mental health issues, and curriculum development.

During this same time period, my professional activities also included community-based noncredit course teaching, workshops and conferences, interdisciplinary health care consultation, guest lectures, paper presentations, and various facilitative and leadership functions within nursing and interdisciplinary groups in several states. Mental health consultation activities both fulfilled student learning needs through role-modeling and provided community service to satisfy university requirements. I provided consultation for nursing and interdisciplinary caregiver groups in state mental hospitals, home health agencies, public health agencies, mental health centers, convalescent care centers, penal institutions, hospitals, Watts teen centers, schools, and industries. Facilitating factors for my personal and professional development during these years were both the professional need for creativity and the freedom to be creative. The challenges of continual ambiguity and risk taking, caused by rapid change and lack of mentors, also became motivational in themselves. A tribute must be paid to the UCLA School of Nursing Dean, Lulu Wolfe Hassenplug, and Nurse Continuing Education Director, Marjorie Squaires, for providing many opportunities combined with a lack of constraints related to my functioning.

During 1972, increased graduate student interest in the mental health consultation process and the Neuman Systems Model resulted in guest lectures in other UCLA clinical nurse specialist classes. Joan Riehl, a faculty friend and colleague, invited me to coauthor the first book on nursing models, *Conceptual Models for Nursing Practice*. Because of an impending move east, I directed her to Sister Callista Roy, a former UCLA classmate of mine, to coauthor the book. The Neuman Model chapter in this book was there first classified as a "systems" model.

The development of the wholistic systemic perspective of the Neuman Systems Model was facilitated by my own basic philosophy of *helping each other live,* many diverse observations and clinical experiences in teaching and encouraging positive aspects of human variables in a wide variety of community settings, and theoretical perspectives of stress related to the interactive, interrelated, interdependent, and wholistic nature of systems theory. The significance of perception and behavioral consequences cannot be overestimated. The preventions adapted from Caplan's work provided an intervention typology for nursing consistent with the systemic perspective of the model.

During the summer of 1973, I made a permanent move east to maintain my mother within her home during her aging years of declining health. Sustaining factors that kept our family viable through many challenges, both personal and professional, were my beautiful daughter Nancy's presence, creativity, spontaneity, joy of life, and many personal talents and achievements, as well as my husband Kree's consistent support, understanding, and love.

From the fall of 1973 through the summer of 1977, a part-time position as the state mental health nurse consultant for the state of West Virginia provided many challenges and professional growth activities in the statewide mental hospital system, such as consultation to and for hospital administrators, interdisciplinary groups, and program development and evaluation. Organizational development activities included conflict resolution, third-party consultation, educational conferences, workshops, seminars, and program planning.

Having been one of the first nurses licensed as a marriage, family, and child counselor in the State of California (in 1970) and also as a clinical member of the American Association of Marriage and Family Therapists and Ohio Social Work Counselors, I have continually maintained a limited private counseling practice since licensure. In 1974, I taught clergy counseling for a local Ohio mental health center. During the same year I helped initiate, develop, and support continuance of a program called "Hope" in a West Virginia state facility for the retarded. The goal was to teach, through a short-term residential program, self-help skills to retarded children so they could be maintained within the home, rather than be institutionalized; to redirect parents in their parenting efforts; and skill development to stabilize the home environment. This program evolved into a 14-year model program within the state system. I have also had limited involvement in Ohio as a licensed real estate agent, having secured original California licensure in 1971 and Ohio licensure in 1973. Continued love for the land has also led to involvement in securing selected Ohio-based land parcels for private brokerage to oil- and gas-drilling companies. Perhaps because of early work influence at Wright Field, Dayton, Ohio, I acquired a private pilot license while living in California. Another personal interest that has continued through the past few years has been in personal investments and rental housing.

In the fall of 1978, following my mother's death, personal activities focused on rental property management and other investments. These interests coincided with professional activities at nearby Ohio University, Athens, Ohio, including curriculum consultant to the School of Nursing, project planning director for development of a master's-level nursing program, and director of nursing and allied health within the University Extension Division to facilitate nursing continuing education workshops.

Following the development of several nursing models during the early 1970s, it was not until the mid-1970s that planning for their implementation began within university settings. From 1976 to the present, my major professional roles have been consultant for Neuman Systems Model implementation, lecturer at conferences, and author. Within the role of consultant for the model, a major function has been that of networking among those using the model or considering its use; clarifying the model's intent, purpose, and components; and supporting implementation plans or existing programs incorporating it. Through international travel, I have enjoyed very much the courtesies, sharing, and comparative views of other nurse professionals, along with important feedback that the model is easily used in diverse cross-cultural settings. Within the lecturer role, I have presented the model to several larger international nurse audiences in the United States and many other countries, including England, Denmark, Canada, Puerto Rico, Australia, New Zealand, Kuwait, and the Far East.

Within the author role, my publications since 1980 include a revised chapter in the second edition of *Conceptual Models for Nursing* (1980), with "tools" developed to further facilitate Neuman Systems Model implementation and for use in nursing practice; the first edition (1982) of *The Neuman Systems Model: Application to Nursing Education and*

Practice; a chapter on family use of the model in *Family Health: A Theoretical Approach to Nursing Care,* edited by Clements and Roberts (1983); an article in *Senior Nurse* (London) (fall 1985); and an invitational chapter on the model in Sweden's annual *Nursing Care Book* (winter 1986). A second book edition entitled *The Neuman Systems Model* was published in 1989, a very comprehensive third edition book was published 1995, and now this fourth edition of the book has been published. The 1986 First Biennial International Neuman Systems Model Symposium was held at Neumann College, Aston, Pennsylvania; seven others, well attended, have since been sponsored by Neuman trustee members. The trustee group was incorporated in 1988. Each symposium has shown increased international participation with increasing levels of scholarship. The trustees have introduced and facilitated model implementation throughout the world through paper presentations, publications, and consultation. The third book edition (1995) contains sections of newer areas of nursing concern for research, international model use recognition, and nurse administrative and research protocol, and this fourth edition contains integrative and scientific data.

Following several years of accumulating credit hours toward a doctoral degree at Ohio University, Athens, Ohio, in 1985 I completed a doctoral degree in clinical psychology on transfer to Pacific Western University in Los Angeles.

Several years ago, my husband Kree retired and began to pursue oil painting. We particularly enjoyed walking, reading, music, and gardening. Unfortunately, in the fall of 1992 a major stroke left him aphasic and physically debilitated. He died in 1995. Our daughter Nancy, following success in community theater during high school years, was motivated to complete an acting degree at UCLA. Now she is a licensed California PhD psychologist in a Monterey private counseling practice. She has frequently been engaged in little theater stage productions and television commercials. She has taught acting and had roles in both feature and television films. Nancy owns a beautiful ocean-view home in Pebble Beach, California, and presented me with a first grandchild, Alissa, born in the fall of 1994. Our visits are, indeed, very special occasions.

Since 1980, several important changes have been made that have enhanced the model. A Nursing Process Format was designed, using the model terminology to facilitate its implementation. A major theory for the model has been identified, in cooperation with a colleague and former Neuman trustee member, Audrey Koertvelyessy, from Ohio; it has been named *The Theory of Client System Stability.* In the 1989 book edition, a new perspective to expand the concept of environment—the created environment—was presented, and the spiritual variable was explicitly added to the model diagram as one of the client variables; further explication of the spiritual variable is presented in Chapter 1 of this fourth edition. A clearer model explanation has been offered by segmenting the model components into the four concepts of the metaparadigm of nursing—client, environment, health, and nursing. The relationship of primary prevention and health promotion has been further clarified, as well as the defense and resistance lines utilization.

The initial term *patient* was changed in the 1980 publication to *client* to fulfill the need for a qualifying term that would indicate respect and imply a collaborative lateral relationship between caregivers and the clients they serve. The model title has changed over the years, as the following chronology of publications shows:

- 1972: *A Model for Teaching Total Person Approach to Patient Problems*
- 1980: *The Betty Neuman Health Care Systems Model: A Total Approach to Patient Problems*

- 1982: *The Neuman Health Care Systems Model*
- 1989: *The Neuman Systems Model*
- 1995: *The Neuman Systems Model*
- 2002: *The Neuman Systems Model*

Until and unless research proves the need for change, the original diagram for the Neuman Systems Model will remain the same as when it was developed in 1970, since its structure and concepts are easily understood and implemented around the world.

My hope for the future remains the same as for the past—that through continued nurturance, the Neuman Systems Model will live well into the twenty-first century to benefit nursing, and other health disciplines, at all levels, and across all cultural boundaries.

USING THE NEUMAN SYSTEMS MODEL

The Neuman Systems Model has remained relevant and relatively unchanged since its inception in 1970. Although it is difficult to maintain an accurate count of the use of the Neuman Systems Model, publications, presentations, and anecdotal reports indicate that the model is used worldwide, in as many as 350 different nursing education and practice settings. A chronology of the continuing interest in and use of the Neuman Systems Model is presented below.

The implementation of nursing conceptual models began within collegiate nursing education programs in the United States during the 1970s. Planning for use of the Neuman Systems Model for nursing education first began in the early 1970s at Neumann College in Aston, Pennsylvania. Rosalie Mirenda, Neuman Systems Model trustee and current Neumann College president, guided the development of the Neuman Systems Model–based baccalaureate nursing curriculum development; the new program was implemented in 1980. During the late 1970s and early 1980s, the Neuman Systems Model also was implemented in the baccalaureate nursing education programs at Bob Jones University, Greenville, South Carolina; Delta State University, Cleveland, Mississippi; University of Pittsburgh, Pittsburgh, Pennsylvania; St. Xavier College, Chicago, Illinois; and Union College, Lincoln, Nebraska.

The faculty at the Texas Woman's University campuses at Dallas, Houston, and Denton, Texas, as well as at Northwestern State University of Louisiana in Shreveport, Louisiana, implemented the first Neuman Systems Model master's-level nursing education programs in the late 1970s. In addition, Neuman Systems Model trustee Lois Lowry guided the implementation of the Neuman Systems Model in an associate degree in nursing program at Cecil Community College in North East, Maryland.

Interest in conceptual models for theory-based nursing education increased rapidly during the late 1970s. During the early and mid-1980s, as mandated by the National League for Nursing, nursing tended toward both accelerated use of conceptual models for education and early utilization within nursing practice areas and as guides for research. Education goal clarification became a priority in relation to new nursing practice role development and expansion. Nursing models became a logical base for validation of the new nurse roles and functions and for communicating who nurses are and what they do, as being different from the past. For example, utilization of the Neuman Systems Model has either led or been concurrent with the emerging trends in nursing toward a broad systemic perspective for wholistic client care to include primary prevention and health maintenance. Its relevance should continue well into the twenty-first century in relation to evolving worldwide health care reform mandates.

To upgrade their diploma nurse education programs, the Methodist Central (four-state) Hospitals in Memphis, Tennessee, and the Altoona Hospital in Altoona, Pennsylvania, implemented the Neuman Systems Model as a theoretical base. Additional Neuman Systems Model–based associate degree in nursing programs began at Indiana University–Purdue University at Fort Wayne, Indiana (Elaine Cowan); Santa Fe Community College in Gainesville, Florida (former Neuman Systems Model trustee Gerry Green); and the University of Nevada, Las Vegas, Nevada (Rosemary Witt).

Cynthia Capers, Neuman Systems Model trustee, coordinated the first hospital-based four-year plan for nursing service implementation of the model at the Mercy Catholic Medical Center, Fitzgerald Mercy Division in Darby, Pennsylvania. Other early nursing practice areas using the Neuman Systems Model included the Hospital of the University of Pennsylvania in Philadelphia, Neonatal Clinical Care Unit; the University of Maryland, Baltimore, Institute for Emergency Medical Services–Critical Care Unit (Virginia Cardona); and the Boston City Health Department. The earliest known university outside the United States to utilize the Neuman Systems Model concepts was the University of Puerto Rico in San Juan.

The faculty at the University of Ottawa in Ontario, Canada, also found the Neuman Systems Model useful for the public health nursing courses. They also developed a joint university and community Regional Perinatal Program for Eastern Ontario, Canada (Sandra Dunn). Eugenia Story, a former public health nursing faculty member at the University of Ottawa, became an independent consultant for model implementation, contributing to both education and practice settings within the province of Ontario, Canada. Her functions included presentation of workshops for those wanting to learn more about the Neuman Systems Model and how to apply it. In the early 1980s, the model was implemented for provision of theory-based community health nursing services within the Canadian provinces of Ontario and Manitoba. At Winnipeg, Linda Drew facilitated Neuman Systems Model–based community health program development for Manitoba, and Dorothy Craig, now a former faculty member at the University of Toronto and retired Neuman Systems Model trustee, influenced development of standards for community health nurse practice, incorporating criteria from the Neuman System Model as a base for nursing care in the province of Ontario. Craig presented her work in London, England, at the Second International Primary Care Conference. Her presentation focused on a possible new direction and structure for home visiting nurse services and practice in the British Isles.

In the mid-1980s, interest in nursing conceptual models accelerated around the world. International nursing model conferences drew large audiences from many countries. The Neuman Systems Model is successfully being used in both education and practice settings in many countries. Hanne Johansen found the model concepts useful in community health nursing courses at Aarhus University, as well as in community health practice areas in Aarhus, Denmark. Furthermore, Aarhus Community Health Services sponsored publication of a handbook that Johansen wrote about the use of the Neuman Systems Model in the community for primary prevention for the aged. Ingegerd Harder, also of Aarhus University, and Hanne Seyer-Hansen published Neuman Model–based articles and a book interpreting the model for the country of Denmark. In Sweden, the Neuman Systems Model has been used for some time in clinical nursing practice and as a guide for research. Nurses in both England and Wales have found the Neuman Systems Model particularly useful in home visiting nursing. The model also is used in a variety of teaching institutions and clinical practice areas throughout the British Isles. In addition, one Australian hospital incorporated the model concepts, and several schools of nursing in Australia and New Zealand based their nursing curricula on the model. Moreover, faculty at a university in Lisbon, Portugal, utilized the model concepts in public health and critical care nursing courses and in community health nursing practice.

During the 1980s, requests for international consultation, workshops, and conference presentations of the model increased markedly. Several religious-based nurse education programs found the Neuman Systems Model particularly suitable and relevant to their curricular needs.

From the mid- to late 1980s, nursing literature reflected the trend toward increasing acceptance of wholistic and systemic concepts as a logical perspective for nursing, in its quest to become a scientific discipline. In addition, a slide presentation explaining the model has been published and marketed by the University of Michigan. At the University of Western Ontario in London, Ontario, Canada, a self-directed learning package for staff education was developed by Laurie Bernick and Diane Thompson. Bernick and Thompson also published a video presentation of the model, which includes a comprehensive health assessment and intervention tool. As a result of model implementation for their nursing service, Laura Caramanica and Lorrie Powell published programmed learning materials available to the public from the Mount Sinai Hospital in Hartford, Connecticut.

Nurses at Jefferson Davis Memorial Hospital in Natchez, Mississippi, where the Neuman Systems Model has been used since 1984, developed and implemented a nursing classification system with significant emphasis on primary prevention. Furthermore, the model is fully implemented for psychiatric nursing service at Friends Hospital (Betty Scicchitani and Patricia Maglicco) in Philadelphia, Pennsylvania; Whitby Psychiatric Hospital (Corinne Coulter) in Whitby, Ontario, Canada; and Peterborough Civic Hospital (Wendy Fucile) in Peterborough, Ontario, Canada.

The Neuman Systems Model has become a viable framework for health prevention–promotion activities in a variety of clinical nursing and research areas. For example, nurses at Lander University in Greenwood, South Carolina, Indiana University–Purdue University at Fort Wayne, Indiana, and the University of Rochester in Rochester, New York, have developed nurse-managed clinics.

The Neuman Systems Model has been widely used throughout Canada, particularly for community health nursing and education, as well as for hospital-based nursing practice. Indeed, several Canadian hospitals are known to use the model in general and/or specialized clinical areas, including Chedoke–McMaster Hospital, Ottawa Civic Hospital, and Victoria Hospital, all in Ontario, Canada; Juan de Fuca Hospitals, Victoria, British Columbia; and University Hospital of Saskatchewan, Saskatoon, Saskatchewan, Canada.

Charlene Beynon, former Neuman Systems Model trustee and supervisor of the Middlesex Health Unit in London, Ontario, Canada, and her highly motivated staff successfully implemented the model for community nursing, with workshops offered to other health district nursing units to facilitate use of the model. Manitoba nurses have implemented their province-wide plan since 1982. Queen's University, Kingston, Ontario, and the University of Saskatchewan, Saskatoon, Saskatchewan, have based their nurse education programs on the Neuman Systems Model. Neuman Systems Model concepts also are used by faculty in nursing education programs at both the University of Ottawa and the University of British Columbia.

Since the early 1980s, the model has formed the base for unilevel, multilevel, and consortium-type nurse education programs within university settings throughout the United States. At California State University in Fresno, California, Eleanor Stittich worked with faculty to develop a multilevel program for baccalaureate and master's students, including the nurse practitioner program students. Carol Frazier worked with her colleagues at Simmons College in Boston, Massachusetts, to develop a bilevel nursing program for baccalaureate and master's students. Rosemary Witt worked with faculty at the University of Nevada, Las Vegas, to develop a trilevel associate degree, baccalaureate, and master's program. Arlene Airhart worked with her colleagues at Northwestern State University in Shreveport, Louisiana, to develop a trilevel nursing education program.

The faculty of the Minnesota Intercollegiate Nursing Consortium, St. Paul, Minnesota, which included the College of St. Catherine, St. Olaf College, and Gustavus Adolphus College, jointly contributed to development of a baccalaureate nursing curriculum based on the Neuman Systems Model, with beginning computerization of courses. Lois Nelson and her colleagues at the Tri-County College Nursing Consortium Program also use the Neuman Systems Model. That program serves baccalaureate students from the State University of North Dakota in Wells Fargo, North Dakota, and Concordia College in Moorhead, Minnesota. The consortium arrangement is a unique and cost-effective method for curricular development and implementation.

Furthermore, Lander University in Greenville, South Carolina, progressed from an associate degree in nursing to a baccalaureate degree program. Faculty report a trend toward use of the Neuman Systems Model by the clinical agencies with which the Lander University students affiliate. This trend may be associated with the special education and practice information exchanges sponsored by the Lander University School of Nursing faculty, including Neuman Systems Model trustees Janet Sipple and Barbara Freese.

Moreover, international exchange programs developed as a new trend in nursing education to reduce cross-cultural differences and incorporate Neuman Systems Model concepts into community agencies where students affiliate. Seattle Pacific University in Seattle, Washington, where the baccalaureate nurse program is based on the Neuman Systems Model (formerly, Margaret Stevenson; now, Annalee Oakes), exchanges both students and faculty with the Veterans General Hospital Nursing Program (Bette Wei Wang) in Taipei, Taiwan. As a result of direct faculty exchange and ongoing consultation activities, faculty have adapted the model for Chinese culture and then developed a new baccalaureate nurse degree program at the Yang Ming Medical College in Taiwan. Seattle Pacific University also has implemented the Neuman Systems Model in Costa Rica.

Sharing information among nurses from various countries facilitates use of the Neuman Systems Model. A Lander University nurse faculty member, Nahn Joo Son Chang, who is Korean, presented a workshop on the Neuman Systems Model at Kyung Hee University in Seoul, Korea. The workshop, which was sponsored by the Korean Nurses Academic Society in Seoul, was attended by 200 nurse faculty; many indicated they were motivated to use the model in their country.

Further advances in use of the Neuman Systems Model took place as a large percentage of international nursing students from the summer master's program at the University of Portland in Portland, Oregon (Neuman Systems Model trustee, Patricia Chadwick), used the model as a guide for their master's thesis research. In addition, the results of an international survey to identify the nature and quality of Neuman Systems Model–based research, conducted with the assistance of former Neuman Systems Model trustee Audrey Koertvelyessy, was presented by University of Nevada, Las Vegas, faculty member Margaret Louis (a Neuman Systems Model trustee) at an international nursing research conference in Scotland.

Books, journal publications, paper presentations, and personal visits to other countries by myself and others over the years have greatly increased the visibility and utility of the Neuman Systems Model. Model utilization has followed a general pattern of beginning implementation within university settings followed by clinical practice areas and research (see Chapters 3, 8, 13, and 18). Educational programs and clinical agencies that have reported use of the Neuman Systems Model between 1989 and 2000 are listed in Table B-1.

Since the mid-1990s, many innovative uses of the Neuman Systems Model have been reported and are listed below. These innovations reflect, at least in part, such nursing trends as cooperative work with other disciplines. Names of contact persons are included both for recognition and networking.

Neuman Systems Model–Based Research

Nancy Cotton of Colorado developed an interdisciplinary high-risk assessment tool, based on the Neuman Systems Model, designed to predict high risk of falling for elderly rehabilitation clients. Her work is presented in a 1993 publication entitled *An Interdisciplinary High Risk Assessment Tool for Rehabilitation Inpatient Falls,* which is available from University Microfilms International, Ann Arbor, Michigan. *(Contact: Nancy C. Cotton, 700E Drake-K-11, Fort Collins, Colorado 80525)*

Jullette C. Mitre, through graduate study using the model, identified the purposeful use of "Humor as Primary and Secondary Prevention as Intervention." She describes humor as a "potent" intervention and will be pursuing her research on humor at the doctorate level. *(Contact: Jullette C. Mitre, RA, MSN, MA, 535 North Michigan Avenue, Apt. 1703, Chicago, Illinois 60611)*

Lois Lowry, a Neuman Systems Model trustee, reported that an interdisciplinary research team consisting of nurses, chaplains, and physicians designed a two-phase study to investigate client reactions, perceptions, and coping mechanisms that affect healing when clients are faced with life-threatening illness. The Neuman Systems Model provided the framework for the study because of its systems approach, breadth, understandable language, and appeal to other disciplines. This study was an outgrowth of the pilot conducted by Clark, Cross, Deane, and Lowry *(Holistic Nursing Practice,* 1991). Data were gathered through personal interviews and analyzed by qualitative methods to determine categories of commonly used, and often unconventional, therapies. Based on these findings (phase 1), clinical trials (phase 2) will be designed to test the efficacy and cost effectiveness of incorporating these modalities into the regimen of care. This proposal was enthusiastically supported by the hospital administrators and medical staff of a large institution in the Tampa Bay area where the study was to be conducted. *(Contact: Dr. Lois Lowry, RN, DNSc, Professor, East Tennessee State University, Johnson City, Tennessee; Tel: (423) 439-7168)*

TABLE B-1. Use of the Neuman Systems Model in Nursing Education and Nursing Practice, 1989–2000

Nursing Education	Nursing Practice
The University of Tennessee at Martin, Department of Nursing, Baccalaureate Nurse Program, Martin, Tennessee	The Whitby Psychiatric Hospital Nursing Service, Whitby, Ontario, Canada
Linn-Benton College, Associate Degree in Nursing, Albany, Oregon	The Collington Care Retirement Community Nursing Service and Clinic, Hyattsville, Maryland
The Los Angeles County USC Medical Center School of Nursing, Associate Degree in Nursing, Los Angeles, California	Centre de Santé, Elizabeth Bruyere Health Center (tertiary care), Ottawa, Ontario, Canada
Louisiana College, Baccalaureate Nurse Program, Pineville, Louisiana	Kuakini Health Care System Nursing Service, Honolulu, Hawaii
Auburn University, Baccalaureate Nurse Program, Auburn, Alabama	Riverside Acute Care Hospital Nursing Service, Ottawa, Ontario, Canada
William Rainey Harper College, Associate Degree Nurse Program, Palatine, Illinois	Tripler General Army Medical Center, selected nursing service areas, Honolulu, Hawaii
Mansfield University, Baccalaureate Nurse Program, Mansfield, Pennsylvania	Oregon State Psychiatric Hospital Nursing Service, Salem, Oregon
Akureye University, Baccalaureate Nurse Program, Akureye, Iceland	Anderson Hospital, Nursing Service, Marysville, Illinois
Maribor University, Baccalaureate Nurse Program, Maribor, Yugoslavia (Slovenia)	St. Luke Hospital, Nursing Service, Fargo, North Dakota
University of Guam, Baccalaureate Nurse Program, Mangilao, Guam	Mountain View Hospital, Nursing Service, Madras, Oregon
McNeese State University, trilevel nurse program and a four-school intercollegiate consortium program for a master of science in nursing, Lake Charles, Louisiana	Oklahoma State Department of Public Health, Public Health Nursing Service, Oklahoma City, Oklahoma
Bowie State University, RN–BSN Completion and Master Program, Bowie, Maryland	St. Joseph's Hospital Nursing Service, Reykjavik, Iceland
South West Medical Center Nursing Service, Oklahoma City, Oklahoma	WHO Collaborative Center for Primary Health Care Nursing, Maribor, Yugoslavia (Slovenia)
Daemen College, RN–BSN Completion Program, Amherst, New York	Lake Charles Memorial Hospital Nursing Service, Lake Charles, Louisiana
Indiana Wesleyan College, Marion, Indiana Baccalaureate and Master's Program level Community Health	West Calcasieu–Cameron Hospital Nursing Service, Sulphur, Louisiana
Milligan College, Milligan College, Tennessee, Baccalaureate Program	St. Patrick's Hospital, Nursing Service, Lake Charles, Louisiana
Loma Linda University, Loma Linda, California, Baccalaureate and Masters Programs.	Lake Area Medical Center, Lake Charles, Louisiana
Advanced Psychiatric Nursing Diploma Program at Douglas College, Vancouver, British Columbia, Canada.	Country of Holland Psychiatric Centers for Interdisciplinary Care Continuity

TABLE B-1. Use of the Neuman Systems Model in Nursing Education and Nursing Practice, 1989–2000 *(continued)*

Nursing Education	Nursing Practice
Dutch Reformed University, Zwolle, Netherlands, Baccalaureate Programs	Emergis Institute for Mental Health Care, Zealand, The Netherlands, Psychiatric Care Service
Gulf Coast University, Panama City, Florida, Associate Degree Program	
Fitchburg State College, Fitchburg, Massachusetts, Baccalaureate and Master's Programs	

The Neuman Systems Model was the conceptual model chosen by Karen Perrin, RN, MPH, as the framework for a study to investigate the perception of sexuality in relation to the five client system variables in pregnant adolescents. The purpose of the study was to determine the prevalence of physical and sexual abuse among the pregnant teen population. The relationship of the perpetrator to the victim, the pattern of assault, and demographic characteristics associated with abuse were considered. This study was conducted in the Tampa Bay area. *(Contact: Karen Perrin, RN, MPH, Adjunct Professor, College of Public Health, University of Southern Florida, Tampa, Florida)*

The Neuman Systems Model was used as a conceptual base for a study that identified self-perceived needs of Vancouver-area families with children with cancer. A dearth of information exists in the literature. An excellent interview tool is now available for gathering intra-, inter-, and extrafamily self-perceived needs data that could also be generalized for use in other family illness categories. *(Contact: Heidi Enright, BscN, RN, MSN, Instructor, General Nursing Health Sciences Department, Douglas College, 700 Royal Avenue, New Westminster, B.C. V3L5B2 Canada)*

A research project is underway at the University Hospital in Tromso, Norway, using the Neuman Systems Model to identify stressors that affect the appetites of hospitalized clients. The model was chosen because it is both understandable and practical in the work setting. Food has been identified as an important human need in providing wholistic client care. An important nursing responsibility is to create optimal nutritional conditions for hospitalized clients, which is accomplished through use of the nursing process as follows: Obtaining information about the client's eating behavior, assessing the adequacy of their nutritional status, determining the unique goals to be accomplished with regard to individual client nutrition needs, and planning and implementing nursing interventions designed to accomplish these goals. Finally, to complete the nursing process, results of the nursing interventions are evaluated to see if the desired goals have been achieved.

Helping clients respond positively to stressors to maintain system balance is viewed as an important aspect of the Neuman Systems Model's role and function in client health preservation. The current project is based on a 1991 project by the Nordic Council of Ministers on hospital food and its relationship to client well-being in five Nordic countries. *(Contact: Henny M. Olsson, PhD, RNM, Bsc in Public Health Nursing, VD in Nursing Education, Associate Professor, Center for Caring Sciences, Uppsala University, Uppsala, Sweden; Tove Forsdahl, RN, Director of Nursing, University Hospital, Tromso, Norway)*

Neuman Systems Model–Based Clinical Practice

Marilyn Schlentz developed "The Minimum Data Set and Levels of Prevention in the Long Term Care Facility," which was published in the March/April 1993 issue of *Geriatric Nursing*. In her work she demonstrated the compatibility of the Neuman Systems Model with the minimum data set, a federal data collection system mandated for long-term care. She was negotiating for use of the Neuman Systems Model with board members of the New Jersey chapter of the National Association of Directors of Nursing Administration in Long Term Care. She was also involved with the development of academic management courses specific to long-term care needs. *(Contact: Marilyn Schlentz, EdD, RN, 32 Cannon Road, Freehold, New Jersey 07728)*

A project was developed for utilizing the Neuman Systems Model, for nurse-managed health care centers in the U.S. Immigration and Naturalization Service (INS) Health Care Program. The INS maintains nine service processing centers nationwide that operate a medical facility. These medical facilities, which utilize the medical model to provide health care services, currently are under the direction of a medical officer. It is thought that the development of nurse-managed centers will provide for nurse control of practice, direct access by the patient, and wholistic, client-centered service. A goal-directed approach will be utilized to focus on primary, secondary, and tertiary prevention methods to provide health care to this diverse and poorly serviced population. Consistent with the Neuman Systems Model, evaluation of nursing care is based on stated outcomes. Long-term evaluation depends on reassessment of goals and outcomes. According to Roy C. Lopez, RNC, MSNC, CCHP, initiator of the "centers" program, the development of nurse-managed centers within the INS Health Care Program will provide nursing the opportunity to practice independently in the field of correctional health care, utilizing the Neuman Systems Model to provide client-centered, wholistic health care. Lopez, a commander in the United States Public Health Service, is assigned to the Immigration and Naturalization Service Health Care Program and currently serves as the Western Regional Supervisory Program Management Officer. Commander Lopez is also a graduate student at California State University, Dominguez Hills, Carson, California. *(Contact: Roy Lopez, MSNC, RNC, 12861 Olive Street, Garden Grove, California 92645; Tel: (714) 897-5914)*

During the past few years the Neuman Systems Model has been used for structuring the World Health Organization Collaborative Center for Primary Health Care Nursing in Maribor, Yugoslavia (Slovenia). The director has recently developed a baccalaureate nursing education program at the University of Maribor based on the Neuman Systems Model, as well as a "Hospital at Home" project in three adjoining countries. *(Contact: Majda Slajmer Japelj, International Manager, World Health Organization Collaborative Center for Primary Care Nursing, Slovenia, 62000 Maribor, UL, Talcev 9)*

Glenn Curran developed a sexual health HIV/AIDS program in the rural northwest region of Tasmania, Australia, within the 1993 criteria of the Australian Community Health Accreditation and Standards Program (CHASP), which incorporates primary health care. The Neuman Systems Model formed the base for the sexual health program as it "accommodates the complexities and dynamics of identified systems (person, group, community, or issue)." Systems thinking is considered particularly relevant to a wholistic, multidisciplinary approach to health care consistent with the principles of CHASP. *(Contact: Glenn Curran, RN RMN, B. Nurs. (Hons.), Clinical Nurse Manager, Sexual Health, HIV/AIDS Program, North West Health Region, 11 Jones Street, Burnie, 7320, Tasmania. Australia: Tel: (004) 346315)*

Janice Turner, a clinical nurse specialist, uses the Neuman Systems Model as a base for the new rural health program, a free outreach service of the Lake Charles Memorial Hospital, Lake Charles, Louisiana. From the traveling van she services rural clients, including screening for early risk factors of heart disease and stroke, fetal heart monitoring, and on-site laboratory testing. Major intervention focus at the three Neuman prevention levels is on nutrition, exercise, stress reduction, and medication monitoring. Her self-developed assessment tool is based on the five client system variables and is used in conjunction with an abbreviated checklist. She states, "The most important thing I am doing is looking at the whole person." Following initial screening, contributing stressor effects often become evident, allowing for more in-depth exploration and understanding of the entire client health condition. Once actual and potential stressors are identified, she focuses on the three preventions interventions, resource referral, and categorizing and correlating types of identified stressors with preventive intervention strategies used across the life span for the rural multiproblem community she serves. Early data suggest that clients prefer mobile health services to physician office visits. Her goal is to prove that high-quality wholistic client care is both possible and cost effective when delivered by an advanced practice nurse. *(Contact: Janice Turner, RN, MSN, Clinical Nurse Specialist, Lake Charles Memorial Hospital, Lake Charles, Louisiana 70601; Tel: (318) 494-3214)*

Through use of the Neuman Systems Model to conceptualize retirement as loss, a linkage is made between unresolved grief and illness and client loss of work and perceived health status. Since the literature reflects a dearth of health care emotional support for retirees, a Neuman Systems Model–based brief-loss counseling tool has been developed with specific guidelines to assist geriatric nurse practitioners in client rehabilitation for cost-effective wholistic care. *(Contact: Mary P. Skowronek, RN, GNP, CRNP, 918 Hawthorne Avenue, Mechanicsburg, Pennsylvania 17055)*

The Neuman Systems Model, currently used for professional nursing practice within a Canadian chronic tertiary care hospital, is facilitating policy change in the method of nursing care delivery. Thus, a major restructuring of care delivery is taking place on the assumption that through model usage, functional status of chronically ill clients will increase with the efficiency of nursing care delivery. Newer approaches to problem solving and decision making will, ideally, support nursing's adaptation to rapidly changing social/environmental forces.

A major goal is to demonstrate the efficacy of the Neuman Model for providing high-quality client care, effectively containing cost, and optimizing nursing autonomy. The proposed health delivery policy changes, it is anticipated, will foster unification of nursing theory, practice, and research, thus promoting scientific nursing interventions. The Neuman Systems Model is viewed as an alternative policy for developing a more effective and efficient health delivery system. The outcome effect should give important future direction for nursing administration and professional nursing practice within health care agencies. *(Contact: Margot Felix, RN, Bsc, (SocSc), MPA, Nurse Educator/Research and Development, Elisabeth Bruyere Health Centre, Ottawa, Ontario K1N 5G8 Canada; Tel: (613) 562-6367)*

The Neuman Systems Model is an excellent wholistic organizing structure for multi-service agencies (MSAs). It is being considered for multiservice agency development in one county of Ontario, Canada. Long-term care reform was recently introduced into Ontario's health care system in response to economic constraints, an aging population, and consumer demands for a larger role in the planning and delivery of long-term care services. Recent public consultation found existing services to be fragmented and duplicated, with inequitable access and service gaps. The reform promotes greater consumer participation in planning and controlling services they receive. This will be achieved, in part, by restructuring existing services and creating multiservice agencies with a single point of access in each county or local planning area of the province. The Neuman Systems Model was proposed to the MSA Steering Committee of one county as a fitting model for designing the MSA. The model was easily adapted to mirror the following provincial guidelines and principles:

- *Core:* seniors, adults with disabilities, and caregivers
- *Lines of resistance:* emergency response teams, short-stay beds in long-term facilities, and crisis beds
- *Normal lines of defense:* ongoing long-term care services such as in-home services, palliative care, placement coordination, meals, adult day programs, and transportation; provided by case managers, health professionals, personal support workers, and volunteers
- *Flexible line of defense:* MSA board of directors (representing local communities), executive director, education/training, volunteer coordinator, total quality management

The Neuman Model provides a framework for the structure and function of the MSA and facilitates the planning process, which is essential to the implementation of a new system. It offers a framework for future evaluation and monitoring of the MSA services within communities to ensure that the new system is meeting consumer needs. *(Contact: Nancy Smith, Case Manager, Geriatric Day Hospital, Parkwood Hospital, London, Ontario, N6C5J1 Canada; Tel: (519) 685-4019)*

The Neuman Systems Model and Nursing Information Systems

The Neuman Systems Model is relevant for nursing information systems for practice, research, education, and business. With continuing health care reform, there is a critical need for the development of nursing information systems for care of clients in community settings. The shift in the paradigm from illness care to health promotion and prevention services requires the nursing profession to respond with information systems that will track client care, their responses to preventive services, and the costs of these services for managed care.

The Neuman Systems Model, with its delineation of primary prevention, secondary prevention, and tertiary prevention interventions, is well organized for grouping services and tracking cost-effectiveness in the managed care environment. Managed care will require nursing interventions that prevent hospitalizations and/or reduce length of stay, on both the front end (primary prevention) and the back end (tertiary prevention) of health care. However, the need for organizing wholistic assessment, intervention, and outcome data for clinical and health services research is necessary for advancement of the nursing profession. Nursing informatics leaders have identified that the next generation of information systems must be flexible enough to accommodate nursing models of care and can well build on the minimum data set established by Harriet Werley. A number of classification systems for organization of client data have been suggested and discussed in the informatics literature. However, many of these are not comprehensive enough to include primary care, community care, community health, and case management.

The Community Nursing Center at the University of Rochester School of Nursing is further developing the Neuman Systems Model as a framework for nursing care and for health services research. In order to evaluate the impact of this innovative community nursing clinic model and the delivery of health care, work is beginning on a clinical information system using the Neuman Systems Model. The Omaha System, Saba's Home Health Classification System, and evolving nurse practitioner taxonomies are used with the Neuman Systems Model. Wholistic assessment and nursing interventions are viewed as critical additions to development of information systems, which have in the past reflected only medical diagnosis and treatment. In order to address social history, functional status assessment, and identification of factors that contribute to barriers and access to care, nursing must work with medicine and other disciplines toward an interdisciplinary computerized patient record that will track clients over time and across practice settings. However, consistent with the interdisciplinary focus of the Neuman Model, the Neuman client variables are used as an overall organizing framework for this new, developing information system.

Categorization of nursing interventions and outcomes across the care continuum also are critical for the future and will position this information system as an important contribution to the need for integrated information systems across care settings. Outcomes measurement, particularly in the areas of cost and quality, include specific clinical outcomes, changes in health status and health risk behaviors, changes in circumstances of living, empowerment of individuals/families, and overall quality of life. Consideration of the data elements and structure needed for interdisciplinary practice, financial analysis, and research interests of the Health Care Financing Administration, the Agency for Health Care Research and Quality, and the National Institute for Nursing Research are important for practice, education, research, and business purposes. Relevant coding and data collection by nurses about nursing assessment, interventions, and outcomes are necessary for the advancement of the profession during this evolution of health care delivery, where prevention and care outside institutions must be identified and measured.

This information system was developed for use on a microcomputer (including the laptop), which would eventually allow clinicians to enter data and review client information from remote sites. The design is being carefully considered to facilitate both clinical and health services research with attention to documenting accessible, cost-effective, and quality care outcomes. Additionally, it must be possible to export data into selected formats for further manipulation and statistical analysis for qualitative and quantitative research. Funding is being sought to facilitate practice-based research using this Neuman-focused clinical information system in a number of community nursing center sites across the United States.

(Contact: Patricia Hinton Walker, PhD, RN, FAAN, Dean, School of Nursing University of Colorado, Denver, Colorado; Tel: (303) 315-7754)

Neuman Systems Model–Based Nursing Education

At Brigham Young University in Utah, an interdisciplinary faculty group from the College of Nursing and the Departments of Religion, Business Administration, and Counseling elected to study the concept of spirituality. As they applied spiritual principles to their daily functioning, they determined the effects of spirituality on their own professional lives. It was requested by the Department of Religion that the Neuman Systems Model be interpreted by nursing. *(Contact: Rae Jeanne Memmott, Neuman trustee and Professor, Brigham Young University, 500 SWKT; Provo, Utah 84602)*

The Neuman Systems Model has been used for interdisciplinary education at East Tennessee State University in the Department of Professional Roles/Mental Health Nursing. The model became an educational cooperative base for nursing, medicine, family therapy, and social work. Clinical education settings used included private practice, mental health centers, therapeutic nursery, inpatient consultation, and public school consultation. *(Contact: Beth Brown, RN, MS, Assistant Professor, College of Nursing, East Tennessee State University, Johnson City, Tennessee 37614; Tel: (423) 929-4476)*

Janet Sipple is a pioneer in the use of nursing theory to develop and guide rural health practice as a nurse practitioner. Her use of the Neuman Systems Model both complements and facilitates the course work of her nurse practitioner accelerated seminar learning track series. The learning modules reflect the examination criteria for American Nurses Association Nurse Practitioner Certification. Dr. Sipple views the Neuman Systems Model as forming a comprehensive, flexible base with concepts relevant for establishing important health system collaborative partnerships with clients for increasing the quality of life. The three preventive interventions are used: primary prevention for health retention and promotion, secondary prevention for acute care support, and tertiary prevention for maintaining optimal client system wellness in chronic care. The model concepts define and give direction for consideration of needs and interventions for one or more clients within a particular community. This implies the identification and consideration of subsystems to benefit the larger rural community as a system and ensures delivery of appropriate health services that are responsive to the needs of all health consumers and clients. Use of the model supports both program development and evaluation. *(Contact: Janet Sipple, RN, EdD, Professor and Academic Dean, St. Luke's Hospital School of Nursing at Moravian College, Bethlehem, Pennsylvania; Tel: (610) 861-1607)*

The following shared insights are compiled from teaching experiences in using the Neuman Systems Model at the Texas Woman's University, Houston campus.

"Helping students catch the vision of theory-based nursing practice is an invigorating experience. Especially exciting is introducing the Neuman Systems Model with its inherent characteristics. The model forces the planner of health care to move within the client perspective and view both the internal and external environments from the uniqueness of the client position." The concepts within the model require a comprehensive examination of person as an open system and define preventive, therapeutic, and rehabilitative activities in a unique manner. The definitions allow the caregiver to be creative since the operationalization of the concepts does not restrict site or chronological order of use. The model encourages wholism, beginning with a comprehensive assessment and an insider view. The characteristics of the model and its application in the clinical arena provide invaluable methodologies for futuristic twenty-first-century client care.

Faculty use of the following eclectic collection of teaching–learning principles has yielded much success in guiding students into Neuman Systems Model-based practice:

- *Simple to complex:* Introducing the model with concepts and their definitions; moving from simple relationships to complex relationships, first in an abstract manner and then in applied situations

- *Familiar to unknown:* Introducing those concepts that will be most comfortable for the learner because of past associations
- *Ausubel's advance organizers:* Preparing the learner for both content and process aspects in the learning experience before beginning
- *Group process:* Progressing from the use of small groups to larger groups for assigned tasks that increase in complexity; building on the diversity (differing clinical perspectives, developmental levels, career trajectories, ethnicities, cultural variations, personal biases, etc.) of the learners within the group; capturing the affective components of responses in student interaction and helping the group deal with their behaviors
- *Use of case study:* Applying the Neuman Systems Model in analysis of clinical cases for theory-based caregiving
- *Adult learner:* Accepting students as learners with much experience on which knowledge can be built and recognizing that these students learn for future experiences

The uniqueness of utilizing the case study approach in tandem with group process facilitates learning how to use the Neuman Systems Model. *(Contact: Judith Stocks, RN, PhD, Associate Professor, Texas Women's University, College of Nursing, Houston Center, 1130 M. D. Anderson Boulevard, Houston, Texas 77030)*

For consistently effective articulation among educational programs, the constructs of the Neuman Systems Model serve well as an organizational base for presenting nursing knowledge, nursing process, and nursing roles within the Santa Fe Community College 36-week and 42-week practical nursing (PN) programs, and the associate of science in nursing (ASN) bridge and associate of science in nursing programs (36 weeks and 66 weeks in length, respectively). To facilitate articulation to the ASN bridge program, the PN faculty implemented a Neuman-based curriculum in 1993, using structure similar to the ASN program's Neuman-based curriculum implemented in 1985. Use of the model at the PN level provides structure for assessment and facilitates organization of nursing knowledge to deliver wholistic nursing care. PN graduates who articulate to the ASN bridge program continue to use the constructs of the Neuman Systems Model as they build on nursing knowledge, nursing process, and nursing roles, easily moving from PN roles as caregiver and member of the discipline of nursing to the registered nurse roles as provider of care, manager of care, and member within the discipline of nursing. General education and elective courses (including English composition, college algebra, statistics, general psychology, and humanities) are included in the curriculum, enabling graduates ' to articulate well to the university setting. *(Contact: Pat Aylward, MSN, RN, CNS, Assistant Professor, Santa Fe Community College, 3000 NW 83 Street W 201, Gainesville, Florida 32606; Tel: (W) (352) 395-5747; Fax: (904) 454-5288)*

With great interest and unique experience in international nursing, both Dean Sandra Rogers, DNSc, and Rae Jeanne Memmott, RN, MS, faculty at Brigham University College of Nursing, have explored various strategies for using the Neuman Systems Model to facilitate reaching the World Health Organization's goal of "Health for All by 2000." Many have recognized nursing as the health care profession that could most dramatically influence the achievement of that goal. However, processes by which nurses might most effectively proceed in that direction have remained obscure. It is believed that the Neuman Systems Model can provide the framework for facilitating the processes required to accomplish present and future World Health Organization goals. These nurse professionals are focusing their exploration on use of the model in schools of nursing, mother–child assessment, community assessment, and health education in underdeveloped countries. *(Contact: Dean Sandra Rogers, DNSc, and Professor Rae Jeanne Memmott, RN, MS, College of Nursing, Brigham Young University, Provo, Utah 84602-5544; Tel: (801) 378-7210; Fax (801) 378-3198)*

For the past several years, the Neuman Systems Model has been used as a curricular base for mental health psychiatric nursing education at the Escola Superior De Enfermagem Maria Fernanda Resende in Lisbon, Portugal. The model was chosen because of "the match in philosophy of approach to client centered care." The faculty have successfully used Neuman-reformulated health assessment questions for schoolchildren and also have developed a format to help students identify and relate specific stressors affecting client behavior to corresponding client system variables. *(Contact: Marta Lima Basto or Lila Mela Anjos, Escola Superior De Enfermagem De Maria Fernanda Resende, AV, DO Brasil, 53-13 1700 Lisbon, Portugal)*

Nursing faculty at Neumann College in Aston, Pennsylvania, believe that a nursing program must prepare nurses to be both accountable and responsible for providing high-quality health care within a dynamic and pluralistic society. This implies teaching nurses to assume current, dynamic roles and functions that can be adapted to rapidly changing health needs and future mandates in a reformed health care system. Based on this philosophy, faculty have developed and implemented a creative baccalaureate nurse curriculum incorporating the following concepts:

- A systems perspective of individuals, health, and nursing
- A view of individuals as complex systems, composed of interdependent variables
- Nursing as dynamic and preventive, therapeutic, and rehabilitative
- Nursing as being at the threshold of professional practice
- Nursing as requiring collaboration in multiple and interdisciplinary systems

To provide a theoretical foundation for a wholistic curriculum, the Neuman Systems Model was selected in 1976 for curricular change and will continue its relevancy for twenty-first-century learning needs. A graduate program has been developed at Neumann College to prepare advanced nurse practitioners with a managed care focus. The Neuman Systems Model again guides the curricular design for a wholistic systematic approach to nursing education.

Cooperation in interdisciplinary education, practice, and research activity is viewed as both an opportunity and a contribution to ongoing development and use of the Neuman Systems Model well into the twenty-first century. *(Contact: Rosalie Mirenda, President, Neumann College, Aston, Pennsylvania 19014; Tel: (610) 558-5570; Fax: (610) 558-5643)*

Neuman Systems Model–Based In-Service Education

Following publication of a successful study using the Neuman Systems Model for total care of the hospitalized preschool child with major focus on emotional care, Joan Orr is developing a wholistic Neuman Systems Model-based in-service training program for child health care for both community and hospital-based interdisciplinary caregivers.

(Contact: Joan P. Orr, Lecturer, Child Health, Department of Didactics, The University of South Africa, 392 Pretoria 0001 RSA)

A Proposal for Use of the Neuman Systems Model in Nursing Homes

The Neuman Systems Model has been proposed for use by directors of nursing in nursing homes to give direction for upgrading long-term client care. As one of the major components in alternative health care delivery systems, nursing homes will experience increasing demands for services well into the twenty-first century. Greater numbers of elderly and disabled persons requiring complex care will seek access to nursing home care. The health care reform movement of the 1990s does not exclude nursing homes from being held accountable for delivery of high-quality and cost-effective long-term client care. The director of nursing is in the key leadership position for change. An integrated management–Neuman Systems approach is available as an important tool for assessing, diagnosing, strategizing, monitoring, and evaluating the outcomes of care within nursing homes, thus meeting the needs and demands of the client, nursing, and organizational systems.

Nursing homes abound with a variety of stressors. One example is an increasing Foley catheter infection rate. Infections contribute to decreased quality of life for the client and increased cost for care. The stressor of an increased infection rate could affect all of the personal, nursing, and organizational systems within the facility.

The use of the Neuman Systems Management Tool in a nursing home to resolve the stressor effect of an increasing Foley catheter infection rate evolved from the following scenario: The director of nursing observed a large turnover in nursing assistants during the previous six months. The new staff were relatively inexperienced in infection control within the health care environment. The director associated the stressor of increased Foley catheter infection as originating from within the nursing system, primarily from a developmental deficit in the agency intrapersonal environment (i.e., hiring new staff). The stressor caused a reaction within the nursing system requiring secondary prevention as intervention from mobilization of internal resources to motivate, educate, and involve nursing assistants in infection control procedures. Following problem definition, a goal was set of reducing the infection rate by 10 percent within three months. This would be achieved through a mandatory in-service and continuous monitoring of Foley catheter–related infections. The predicted outcomes were expected reduction in infection rate, cost savings to consumers, and improvement in the reputation of the nursing home. If the actual outcome showed a continued increase in the infection rate, the director would reassess the nature of the stressor to develop additional strategic choices, such as obtaining the services of an infection control nurse consultant; consumer (client and family) education; and assessment of other organizational components (housekeeping, laundry, and the practices of other health care providers).

The example used here is a single, isolated stressor affecting a relatively limited segment within an agency. However, the Neuman Systems Management Tool can be equally well used more broadly to assess the interrelationships among personal, nursing, and organizational systems within an ever-changing health care environment. The state of health or instability of each interacting system affects and changes relationships among the involved systems. Thus, the tool provides a wholistic systems approach to identifying an array of stressors affecting client care that need to be analyzed as a means of determining strategic nursing actions that would retain, achieve, or maintain a desired level of quality of nursing and health care. The Neuman Systems Management Tool has great potential for use in a variety of nursing practice and education settings. As community-based nursing centers or academic nursing centers hold the promise of being the nursing practice model for the twenty-first century, managers must find ways to identify, document, and publish health care outcomes associated with care in these centers. Data gathered from use of the tool are viewed as a powerful means for demonstrating cost savings, justifying expenditures, and negotiating reimbursement for client care. The Neuman Systems Management Tool will prove to be an invaluable resource to health care providers and managers in nursing homes and other health care settings for ensuring high-quality client care outcomes.

(Contact: Authors and Consultants, Connie J. Rowles, DSN, RN, Assistant Professor, School of Nursing, Ball State University, Muncie, Indiana 47306; and Jean A. Kelley, RN, PhD, FAAN, Professor Emeritus, University of Alabama at Birmingham, 4766 Overwood Circle, Birmingham, Alabama 35222)

Appendix C:
Assessment and Intervention Based on the Neuman Systems Model

Betty Neuman

The Neuman Systems Model Nursing Process Format delineates the steps of the nursing process—nursing diagnosis, nursing goals, and nursing outcomes (Table C-1). The Neuman Systems Model Assessment and Intervention Tool is a methodology for implementation of the Nursing Process Format. The tool was first published in 1974 (Neuman, 1974). Throughout the intervening years, others have modified the original assessment and intervention tool for particular clinical situations and clinical populations (see Chapter 4). Anyone wishing to modify the original tool for other clinical situations and populations should consider the following:

- Proper assessment includes knowledge of all factors influencing the client's perceptual field.
- The meaning of a stressor should be validated by both the client and caregiver, highlighting discrepancies for resolution, and leading to relevant nursing actions.

NEUMAN SYSTEMS MODEL ASSESSMENT AND INTERVENTION TOOL

The Assessment and Intervention Tool includes the major components of the Neuman Systems Model, as well as client system–specific needs, such as age, situational differences, and special requirements. The Assessment and Intervention Tool is a generic guide for assessment and intervention within the context of the Neuman Systems Model. It is, therefore, appropriate for use with any designated client system—an individual, a family, a community, or a social issue. A unique feature of the tool is that the data obtained from client system perceptions influence the overall goals for nursing action. It is suggested that the caregiver use the tool as an interview guide rather than submitting it to the client for completion.

An overview of the Assessment and Intervention Tool is displayed in Table C-2. As can be seen, the type of stressors that are relevant, the reaction that occurs, the focus of

347

TABLE C-1. Neuman Systems Model Nursing Process Format

		Nursing Diagnosis

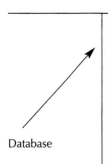

Database

Variances from
wellness are
determined by
correlations and
constraints

Hypothetical
interventions are
determined for
prescriptive
change

I. Nursing diagnosis
   A. Database—determined by:
      1. Identification and evaluation of potential or actual stressors that pose a threat to the stability of the client/client systems.
      2. Assessment of condition and strength of basic structure factors and energy resources.
      3 Assessment of characteristics of the flexible and normal lines of defense, lines of resistance, degree of potential reaction, reaction, and/or potential for reconstitution following a reaction.
      4. Identification, classification, and evaluation of potential and/or actual intra-, inter-, and extrapersonal interactions between the client and environment, considering all five variables.
      5. Evaluation of influence of past, present, and possible future life process and coping patterns on client system stability.
      6. Identification and calculation of actual and potential internal and external resources for optimal state of wellness.
      7. Identification and resolution of perceptual differences between caregivers and client/client system.
      Note: In all of the above areas of consideration the caregiver simultaneously considers five variables (dynamic interactions in the client/client system)—physiological, psychological, sociocultural, developmental, and spiritual.
   B. Variances from wellness—determined by:
      1. Synthesis of theory with client data to identify the condition from which a comprehensive diagnostic statement can be made. Goal prioritization is determinded by client/client system wellness level, system stability needs, and total available resources to accomplish desired goal outcomes.
      2. Hypothetical goals and interventions postulated to reach the desired client stability or wellness level, that is, to maintain the normal line of defense and retain the flexible line of defense, thus protecting the basic structure.

TABLE C-1. Neuman Systems Model Nursing Process Format *(continued)*

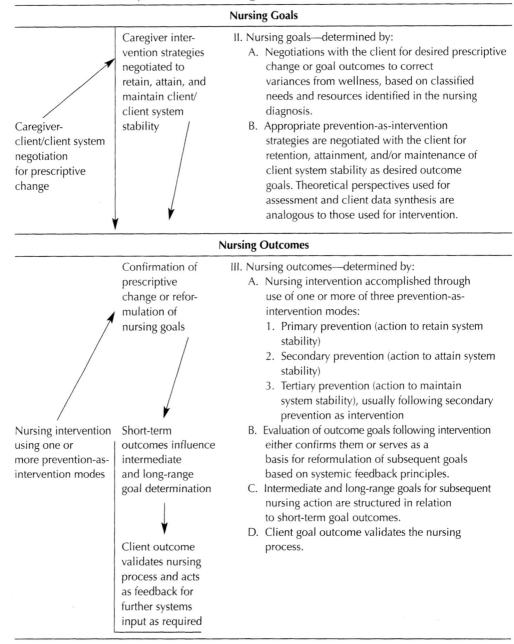

Nursing Goals

Caregiver inter-
vention strategies
negotiated to
retain, attain, and
maintain client/
client system
stability

Caregiver-
client/client system
negotiation
for prescriptive
change

II. Nursing goals—determined by:
  A. Negotiations with the client for desired prescriptive
     change or goal outcomes to correct
     variances from wellness, based on classified
     needs and resources identified in the nursing
     diagnosis.
  B. Appropriate prevention-as-intervention
     strategies are negotiated with the client for
     retention, attainment, and/or maintenance of
     client system stability as desired outcome
     goals. Theoretical perspectives used for
     assessment and client data synthesis are
     analogous to those used for intervention.

Nursing Outcomes

Confirmation of
prescriptive
change or refor-
mulation of
nursing goals

Nursing intervention
using one or
more prevention-as-
intervention modes

Short-term
outcomes influence
intermediate
and long-range
goal determination

Client outcome
validates nursing
process and acts
as feedback for
further systems
input as required

III. Nursing outcomes—determined by:
  A. Nursing intervention accomplished through
     use of one or more of three prevention-as-
     intervention modes:
     1. Primary prevention (action to retain system
        stability)
     2. Secondary prevention (action to attain system
        stability)
     3. Tertiary prevention (action to maintain
        system stability), usually following secondary
        prevention as intervention
  B. Evaluation of outcome goals following intervention
     either confirms them or serves as a
     basis for reformulation of subsequent goals
     based on systemic feedback principles.
  C. Intermediate and long-range goals for subsequent
     nursing action are structured in relation
     to short-term goal outcomes.
  D. Client goal outcome validates the nursing
     process.

Copyright © 1980 by Betty Neuman. Revised 1987 by Betty Neuman.

assessment, and the intervention goals for each prevention-as-intervention modality are listed. The Assessment and Intervention Tool Overview can be used as a checklist in conjunction with the Assessment and Intervention Tool. The Assessment and Intervention Tool is displayed in Tables C-3, C-4, C-5, and C-6.

TABLE C-2. Assessment and Intervention Tool Overview

Primary Prevention	secondary Prevention	tertiary Prevention
Stressors[a] Convert or potential	Stressors[a] Overt, actual, or known	Stressors[a] Overt, or residual—Possible convert
Reaction Hypothetical or possible, based on available knowledge	Reaction Identified symptoms or known stress factors	Reaction Hypothetical or known residual symptoms of known stress factors
Assessment Based on client assessment, experience, and theory Risk or possible hazard based on client and caregiver perceptions Meaning of experience to client Lifestyle factors Coping patterns (past, present, possible) Individual differences identified	Assessment Determined by nature and degree of reaction Determine internal and external available resources to resist the reaction Rationale for goals-collaborative goal setting with client	Assessment Determined by degree of stability following treatment and futher potential reconstitution for possible regression factors
Intervention as prevention Strengthen client flexible line of defense Client education and desensitization to stressors Stressor avoidance Strengthen individual resistance factors	Intervention as treatment Wellness variance—overt symptoms—nursing diagnosis Need priority and related goals Client strengths and weaknesses related to the five client system variables Shift of need priorities as client responds to treatment (primary prevention needs and tertiary prevention may occur simultaneously with treatment of secondary prevention) Intervention in maladaptive processes Optimal use of internal and external resources, such as energy conservation, noise reduction, and financial aid	Intervention as reconstitution following treatment Motivation Education and Reeducation Behavior modification Reality orientation Progressive goal setting Optimal use of available internal and external resources Maintenance of client's optimal functional level

[a]*Assessment should include information concerning the relationship of the four variables—physiological, psychological, sociocultural, and developmental. (Since 1989, a fifth variable has been added—spiritual.)*

Reproduced, with revision (1987), from B. Neuman, "The Betty Neuman Health Care Systems Model: A Total Approach to Patient Problems," in Conceptual Models for Nursing Practice, *edited by J. P. Riehl and C. Roy (New York: Appleton-Century-Crofts, 1974).*

TABLE C-3. Neuman Systems Model Assessment and Intervention Tool: Client Assessment and Nursing Diagnosis

---

Client

A. *Intake Summary*

    1. Name_____

       Age_____

       Sex_____

       Marital status_____

    2. Referral source and related information.

B. *Stressors as Perceived by Client* (If client is incapacitated, secure data from family or other resources)

    1. What do you consider your major stress area, or areas of health concern? (Identify three areas.)

    2. How do present circumstances differ from your usual pattern of living? (Identify lifestyle patterns.)

    3. Have you ever experienced a similar problem? If so, what was that problem and how did you handle it? Were you successful? (Identify past coping patterns.)

    4. What do you anticipate for yourself in the future as a consequence of your present situation? (Identify perceptual factors, that is, reality versus distortions–expectations, present and possible future coping patterns.)

    5. What are you doing and what can you do to help yourself? (Identify perceptual factors, that is, reality versus distortions–expectations, present and possible future coping patterns.)

    6. What do you expect caregivers, family, friends, or others to do for you? (Identify perceptual factors, that is, reality versus distortions–expectations, present and possible future coping patterns.)

C. *Stressors as Perceived by Caregiver*

    1. What do you consider your major stress area, or areas of health concern? (Identify three areas.)

    2. How do present circumstances differ from your usual pattern of living? (Identify lifestyle patterns.)

    3. Have you ever experienced a similar problem? If so, what was that problem and how did you handle it? Were you successful? (Identify past coping patterns.)

    4. What do you anticipate for yourself in the future as a consequence of your present situation? (Identify perceptual factors, that is, reality versus distortions–expectations, present and possible future coping patterns.)

    5. What are you doing and what can you do to help yourself? (Identify perceptual factors, that is, reality versus distortions–expectations, present and possible future coping patterns.)

    6. What do you expect caregivers, family, friends, or others to do for you? (Identify perceptual factors, that is, reality versus distortions-expectations, present and possible future coping patterns.)

D. *Summary of Impressions:* Note any discrepancies or distortions between the client perception and that of the caregiver related to the situation.

    1. *Intrapersonal Factors*

       a. Physical (examples: degree of mobility, range of body function)

       b. Psychosociocultural (examples: attitudes, values, expectations, behavior patterns, and nature of coping patterns)

TABLE C-3. Neuman Systems Model Assessment and Intervention Tool: Client Assessment and Nursing Diagnosis *(continued)*

D. *Summary of Impressions:* Note any discrepancies or distortions between the client perception and that of the caregiver related to the situation *(continued).*

    c. Developmental (examples: age, degree of normalcy, factors related to present situation)

    d. Spiritual belief system (examples: hope and sustaining factors)

  2. Interpersonal Factors

    Examples are resources and relationship of family, friends, or caregivers that either influence or could influence Area D.

  3. Extrapersonal Factors

    Examples are resources and relationship of community facilities, finances, employment, or other areas that either influence or could influence Areas D and E.

E. *Formulation of a Comprehensive Nursing Diagnosis*

This is accomplished by identifying and ranking the priority of needs based on total data obtained from the client's perception, the caregiver's perception, or other resources, such as laboratory reports, other caregivers, or agencies. Appropriate theory is related to the above data.

Reassessment is a continuous process and is related to the effectiveness of intervention based on the prior stated goals. Effective reassessment would include the following as they relate to the total client situation:

1. Changes in nature of stressors and priority assignments
2. Changes in intrapersonal factors
3. Changes in interpersonal factors
4. Changes in extrapersonal factors

In reassessment, it is important to note the change of priority of goals in relation to the primary, secondary, and tertiary prevention-as-intervention categories. An assessment tool of this nature should offer a current, progressive, and comprehensive analysis of the client's total circumstances and relationship of the five client variables (physiological, psychological, sociocultural, developmental, and spiritual) to environmental influences.

DIRECTIONS FOR USE OF THE ASSESSMENT AND INTERVENTION TOOL

Table C-3. Neuman Systems Model Assessment and Intervention Tool: Client Assessment and Nursing Diagnosis

CATEGORY A—Biographical Data

A-1. This section includes general biographical data. However, certain agencies may require additional data in this area.

A-2. Referral source and related information are important. They provide a background history about the client and make possible any contacts with those who interviewed the client earlier. Requests from agencies for reciprocal relationships might be recorded in this area.

TABLE C-4. Neuman Systems Model Assessment and Intervention Tool: Summary of Goals with Rationale

	Primary Prevention (Prevention of treatment)	Secondary Prevention (Treatment)	Tertiary Prevention (Follow-up after treatment)
Immediate Goals: 1. 2. 3. Rationale:			
Intermediate Goals: 1. 2. 3. Rationale:			
Future Goals: 1. 2. 3. Rationale:			

CATEGORY B—Stressors as Perceived by Client

B-1. It is important to find out from clients how they perceive or experience their particular health situation or condition. By clarifying the client's perception, data are obtained for optimal care planning.

TABLE C-5. Neuman Systems Model Assessment and Intervention Tool: Intervention Plan to Support Stated Goals

Primary Prevention	Secondary Prevention	Tertiary Prevention
Date		
Goals[a]	Goals[a]	Goals[a]
1.	1.	1.
2.	2.	2.
3.	3.	3.
Intervention:	Intervention:	Intervention:
Outcome:	Outcome:	Outcome:
Comments:	Comments:	Comments:

[a]Goals are stated in order of priority.

TABLE C-6. Neuman Systems Model Assessment and Intervention Tool: Format for Prevention as Intervention

Nursing Action		
Primary Prevention	*Secondary Prevention*	*Tertiary Prevention*
1. Classify stressors that threaten stability of the client/client system. Prevent stressor invasion.	1. Following stressor invasion, protect basic structure.	1. During reconstitution, attain and maintain maximum level of wellness or stability following treatment.
2. Provide information to retain or strengthen existing client/client systems strengths.	2. Mobilize and optimize internal/external resources to attain stability and energy conservation.	2. Educate, reeducate, and/or reorient as needed.
3. Support positive coping and functioning.	3. Facilitate purposeful manipulation of stressors and reactions to stressors.	3. Support client/client system toward appropriate goals.
4. Desensitize existing or possible noxious stressors.	4. Motivate, educate, and involve client/client system in health care goals.	4. Coordinate and integrate health service resources.
5. Motivate toward wellness.	5. Facilitate appropriate treatment and intervention measures.	5. Provide primary and/or secondary preventive intervention required.
6. Coordinate and intergrate interdisciplinary theories and epidemiological input.	6. Support positive factors toward wellness.	
7. Educate or reeducate.	7. Promote advocacy by coordination and integration.	
8. Use stress as a positive intervention strategy.	8. Provide primary preventive intervention as required.	

Note: *A first priority for nursing action in each of the areas of prevention as intervention is to determine the nature of stressors and their threat to the client/client system. Some general categorical functions for nursing action are initiation, planning, organization, monitoring, coordinating, implementing, integrating, advocating, supporting, and evaluating. An example of a limited classification system for stressors is illustrated by the following four categories: (1) deprivation, (2) excess, (3) change, and (4) intolerance.*

Copyright © 1980 by Betty Neuman. Revised 1987 by Betty Neuman.

B-2. The client should be encouraged to discuss how present lifestyle is related to past or usual lifestyle patterns. A marked change may be significantly related to the course of an illness or possible illness.

B-3. This area relates to coping patterns. It is important to learn what similar conditions may have existed in the past and how the client has coped with them. Such data provide insight about the type of resources available that were mobilized to deal with the situation. Past coping patterns may be significantly related to the present situation, making possible certain predictions as to what a client may or may not be able to accomplish based on system strengths and weaknesses. For example, symptoms of present loss might be exaggerated following unresolved past losses.

B-4.   The area of client expectations is important in planning health care interventions. Goals for care could be inappropriate if not based on clarification of how the client perceives his or her situation or condition. For example, a client might erroneously think the situation is terminal while the caregiver attempts to prepare the client for living.

B-5.   If the extent of client motivation to help him- or herself can be known, available internal and external resources can be more wisely used on the client's behalf.

B-6.   The health care cost factor can often be a source of stress for the client. Sufficient data should be obtained from the client about the health care services the client thinks are needed. However, the caregiver should bear in mind that the client frequently requires help in determining what services are realistic and how they can best facilitate wellness.

CATEGORY C—Stressors as Perceived by Caregiver. The fact that caregivers have a perspective different from that of the client is considered a positive factor. Education, past experiences, values, personal biases, and unresolved personal conflicts can, however, distort the caregiver's clear conception of the client's actual condition. Category C was included to reduce this possibility. Questions 1 through 6 are essentially the same as those in Category B so that the client's perception can be compared with the caregiver's perception of the client. The interviewer should know the basis for his or her own perceptions, as well as the client's, so that the reality of the client's situation or condition can be fairly accurately described in a summary of impressions.

CATEGORY D—As Perceived by Both Client and Caregiver. These categories deal with the intra-, inter-, and extrapersonal factors illustrated on the model diagram. In order to assess an individual's total situation or condition at any point, it is necessary to know the relationships among internal environmental factors, factors occurring between the individual and the environment, and as external environmental factors that affect or could affect the individual. This set of questions attempts to clarify these relationships so that goal priorities can be established.

CATEGORY E—Nursing Diagnosis. A clear, comprehensive statement of the client condition requires the reconciliation of perceptual differences between client and caregiver. All pertinent aspects of client data must be ordered according to need priority before appropriate client goals can be determined.

Table C-4. Neuman Systems Model Assessment and Intervention Tool: Summary of Goals with Rationale

Once the major problem has been defined in relation to all factors affecting the client situation or condition, further classification is needed. A decision must be made as to what form of intervention should take priority. For example, if a reaction has not yet occurred and the client has been assessed as being in a high-risk category, intervention should begin at the primary prevention-as-intervention level. Moreover, one should be able to state the logic or rationale for the intervention. If a reaction is noted on assessment (i.e., symptoms are obvious), intervention should begin at the secondary prevention level (treatment). When assessment is made following treatment, intervention should begin at the tertiary prevention level (this is known as maintenance following treatment).

By relating all factors affecting the client, it is possible to determine fairly accurately what type of intervention is needed (primary, secondary, or tertiary), as well as the rationale to support the stated goals. At whatever point interventions are begun, it is important to attempt to project possible future health care requirements. These data may not be readily available on initial assessment but should be noted when possible to provide a comprehensive and progressive view of the client's total condition. It is important to relate this section of the assessment and intervention tool to the intervention plan.

Table C-5. Neuman Systems Model Assessment and Intervention Tool: Intervention Plan to Support Stated Goals

This portion of the Assessment and Intervention Tool is in the form of a worksheet that provides progressive data about the type of intervention given, by goal, as listed and ranked by priority. The type of interventions, and their outcomes are noted. The comment section might include data useful for future planning, such as new goal priorities based on changes in the client's condition or responses and success or failure of past or present intervention, or both. This format classifies each intervention in a consistent, progressive, and comprehensive manner to which any caregiver can meaningfully relate. This process of classifying data allows one to see the relationship of parts to the whole system thereby reducing care fragmentation and costs.

Because there are conflicting views about how to arrive at and state the nursing diagnosis, it is important to provide such information for use of the Neuman Systems Model. To date, no definitive or satisfactory answer has been offered to the question, "How do you use theory in making a nursing diagnosis based on the Neuman Systems Model?"

In addition to the general problem of conflicting views on how the nursing diagnosis is arrived at and best stated, there are some specific factors that contribute to a confusing and faulty nursing diagnosis: (1) existing North American Nursing Diagnosis Association (NANDA) diagnostic nomenclature does not "fit" the entirety of nursing models; (2) interpretation of client data may be faulty or information may be insufficient; (3) theory may not be explicitly used or it may be improperly related to client data. It is more common for theory to be explicitly related to intervention than to assessment and the nursing diagnosis.

Table C-6. Neuman Systems Model Assessment and Intervention Tool: Format for Prevention as Intervention

This portion of the Assessment and Intervention Tool lists the actions that can be taken as part of each prevention-as-intervention modality.

USING THE ASSESSMENT AND INTERVENTION TOOL: A FAMILY CASE STUDY

To best resolve the nursing diagnosis dilemma in using the Neuman Systems Model and the Neuman Systems Model Nursing Process Format (Table C-1), a brief family case study is presented here. The case study is followed by an illustration of the way client data and theory are synthesized into what is known as "variance from wellness," that is, the difference from the normal or usual wellness condition. The areas of wellness variance, or those of major concern that provide the basis for a wholistic and comprehensive nursing diagnostic statement, include the entire client–family condition as a system. Since theory is related to client data, defensible and logical client goals are readily determined from the diagnostic statement for subsequent appropriate intervention, in order to retain, attain, and maintain system stability or wellness. Theory appropriate to the nursing diagnostic statement also will be found to be relevant for nursing intervention.

The B Family

The B family moved from a metropolitan area, with Mr. B assuming the superintendency of a rural school district. Mrs. B had worked very hard at various jobs to help her husband acquire his doctoral degree and to advance his career goals. She had not wanted to make this move because of her mother's terminal condition with bone cancer, which would necessitate long trips every other weekend for family visits. Mr. and Mrs. B were both in their late thirties and had two teenage daughters aged 14 and 16.

Mrs. B devoted all her time to family needs, keeping the home and environment immaculate. The family profile was one of happiness, togetherness, and religious centeredness, though there was little socialization in the home. Both daughters were obese and shy, with social contacts only while at school. The younger daughter was in competition with the older daughter, who was favored by the parents. There were frequent purchases of the newest styles in clothing for all family members. A public image of the ideal proper family prevailed.

Then, to supplement the family income, Mrs. B assumed a position in a nearby dairy, rising early in the morning and riding to work with a close neighbor, Mrs. P, who also worked there. During their one-and-one-half-year stay, the family had won the respect of all residents of the small village in which they lived. Mr. B had excelled in the school system. All family members kept a low social profile.

During the winter preceding the elder daughter's high school graduation and soon following her eighteenth birthday, she suddenly told the family that she was "in love" with the neighbor's wife with whom the mother rode to work. Following attempted violence toward Mrs. P, the mother collapsed and was hospitalized for hypoglycemic shock; the elder daughter promptly moved into Mrs. P's home, with her husband present.

Two days following hospital discharge, Mrs. B attempted suicide with an overdose of sleeping medication. Mrs. B improved to some degree because of counseling while hospitalized. Neither the younger daughter nor Mr. B became involved, but rather continued with usual school activities. The older daughter completed high school while continuing to live across the street with Mrs. P, whose husband finally moved out of their residence. She remained estranged from her family. Though the school system invited

Mr. B to continue, he relinquished his position at the end of the school year, assuming a position near Mrs. B's mother, who died one week prior to their move. Mr. B's major concern was that he might lose his new position if the family crisis should become known. The younger daughter became more withdrawn, and the crisis remained essentially unresolved for all family members. Since the family chose not to share their dilemma with distant family members, there was no support from relatives, neighbors were immobilized, and there was no appropriate follow-up therapeutic family intervention from the community agencies. The family moved away and failed to keep contact with the villagers.

Major Stressors for Each Family Member

- Mr. B—loss of status
- Mrs. B—questionable mothering role and loss
- Younger daughter—unmet developmental needs
- Older daughter—unmet developmental needs

Family Perception of Their Condition

Mrs. P had unjustly invaded the B family system, creating the major crises that occurred.

Caregiver Perception of Their Condition

The parents had failed to relate effectively to their daughters' developmental needs and to those of the family as a system.

Rigid family interaction patterns were considered a major causal factor in the crisis situation. Mr. B also failed to recognize and support the needs of his wife before and after the crisis. Community resources failed to provide appropriate family intervention, and unresolved family crises remained.

Determination of the Nursing Diagnosis

Variance from wellness is first determined by the following synthesis or integration of the database, with various appropriate theories (placed in parentheses in relation to analyses of the database) as follows:

- The family's past accumulated energy drain weakened the flexible line of defense, allowing stressors to penetrate the solid or normal defense line of the family, causing a series of near-fatal crises. A serious threat to the basic structure of the family existed for which there had been no previous coping mechanisms developed as internal lines of resistance (crisis, systems, communication, and nursing process theories).
- Social role and function as well as educational differences can influence family behavior. Integrating differing expectations, which can become internal and external stressors, into the intrafamily system is often difficult to accomplish while maintaining family stability (role and systems theories). Unless individual needs are identified and met, family integrity may be jeopardized, especially when new

coping strategies are required (personality, developmental, change, and family theories).

- Excessive energy was required to maintain the public image of Mr. B, while the growth and development needs of the two daughters and their mother were grossly compromised over the years (growth and development theory). The autocratic, rigid family interaction patterns failed to allow for free expression of emotions, differences, ideas, and individuation. The needs of one family part or member, Mr. B, superseded the needs of the other three, creating a dysfunction of the family system (systems and family theories).

Variance from Wellness

1. Mother's suicide attempt
2. Father's public image
3. Younger daughter's immobilization
4. Older daughter's abandonment

From the specific areas of variance from wellness (theory and database synthesis), the following wholistic and comprehensive nursing diagnostic statement was made:

Erosion of the family system because of the continuous, unresolved stressor of rigid family rules to maintain Mr. B's public image resulted in bankruptcy of family emotions and energy, negating sustaining family communications during the crises.

Once a meaningful and comprehensive diagnostic statement of the overall situation can be made, major areas for goal setting and subsequent intervention can logically be determined and defended as required. The use of theory, then, is circular; that is, the same theories used in determining major wellness variance also can be used for purposeful outcome goals and intervention. Nurse professionalism is related to skill in synthesis of established scientific theory with client data to frame an accurate client diagnostic statement and present a logical, defensible justification for the decisions made.

REFERENCE

Neuman, B. (1974). The Betty Neuman health-care systems model: A total person approach to patient problems. In J. P. Riehl & C. Roy (Eds.), *Conceptual models for nursing practice* (pp. 99–114). Norwalk, CT: Appleton-Century-Crofts.

Appendix D:
The Neuman Systems Model Trustees Group, Inc.

Betty Neuman

When the Neuman Systems Model was first published, it was intended for nursing; I thought that if it proved valuable, the profession would recognize the fact and further develop, refine, and nurture it. Until such time as it either proved or disproved its utility, I considered myself a servant of the model, shepherding it during the struggles of its early years. My goal was to provide visibility through attempts to clarify its concepts, develop tools for its use, and motivate and network with those who were using or planned to use it, until it reached maturity. My hope is that the nursing profession, in its continuing efforts to be creative with the Neuman Systems Model, will preserve the integrity and identity of the model in future development and utilization of its concepts. The model is now used worldwide, providing new parameters, concepts, and terminology for nursing and other health disciplines appropriate for the twenty-first century.

I am most appreciative of the work of many fine people who in various ways have facilitated the visibility and mature state of the model. Much time, talent, faith, pioneering spirit, effort, and nurturance was required for it to withstand the test of time in proving its value for organizing health care activities and giving direction for high-quality care.

The model is now officially placed with personally chosen Neuman Systems Model Trustee Group members, whose internalization of the model components, competency, and dedication offer assurance that the model will live on. The Neuman Systems Model Trustees Agreement follows.

THE NEUMAN SYSTEMS MODEL TRUSTEES AGREEMENT
Purpose

The purpose of this Neuman Systems Model Trustees Agreement, established in the fall of 1988 by the Trustor, Betty M. Neuman, RN, PhD, is to preserve, protect, and perpetuate the integrity of the model for the future of nursing.

Membership

The membership will be called The Neuman Systems Model Trustees Group, Inc., and will initially include professional nurses from the United States and other countries who for the past two years have been committed to and engaged in the development or use of the Neuman Systems Model. Upon resignation, the current member may appoint a successor with the above qualifications for majority-vote acceptance by the current membership group. A two-thirds vote is required for decision making.

Functions

1. Present or facilitate presentation of the model and its usage at conferences and meetings.
2. Achieve unanimous agreement on any future permanent changes in the original Neuman Systems Model diagram.
3. Consult or provide consultation activities for nursing education and practice implementation.
4. Provide information, networking, and support to those requiring or requesting it.
5. Trustee member sharing and updating of information and activities related to the model on a continuing basis with a commitment to its further development.
6. Plan, promote, and conduct national and international conferences on the Neuman Systems Model.
7. Establish by-laws or protocol for Trustee Group membership involvement as required for continued functional relevancy.

Active Membership

The active members of the Neuman Systems Model Trustees Group, as of fall 2000, are listed in Table D-1.

TABLE D-1. The Neuman Systems Model Trustees Group, Fall 2000

Patricia Aylward, RN, MSN,CNS 5364 SW 89 Street Ocala, Florida 34476 Tel: (H) (352) 237-5223 (Fax) (352) 237-5223 *Pataylward@aol.com*	**Diane Breckenridge, RN, PhD** University of Pennsylvania School of Nursing 420 Guardian Drive Philadelphia, Pennsylvania 19104-6096 Tel: (W) (215) 898-0088 (Fax) (215) 836-2194 (H) (215) 836-2193 *breckenr@nursing.upenn.edu*
Barbara Cammuso, PhD, EdD, RNCS Fitchburg State College Fitchburg, Massachusetts Tel: (W) (508) 665-3365 (Fax) (508) 845-9402 (H) (508) 842-3579 *BCammuso@fsc.edu*	**Cynthia Flynn Capers, PhD, RN** College of Nursing University of Akron 209 Carroll Street Akron, Ohio 44325 Tel: (W) (303) 972-7552 (Fax) (303) 972-5737 (H) (303) 882-4327 *capers@uakron.edu*

TABLE D-1. The Neuman Systems Model trustees Group, Fall 2000 *(continued)*

TABLE D-1. The Neuman Systems Model trustees Group, Fall 2000 *(continued)*

Appendix E: Neuman Systems Model Bibliography

Citations compiled by Jacqueline Fawcett,
September 2000.

PRIMARY SOURCES

Hinton-Walker, P., & Neuman, B. (Eds.). (1996). *Blueprint for use of nursing models.* New York: NLN Press.

Huch, M. H. (1991). Perspectives on health. *Nursing Science Quarterly, 4,* 33–40.

Neuman, B. (1974). The Betty Neuman Health-Care Systems Model: A total person approach to patient problems. In J. P. Riehl & C. Roy (Eds.), *Conceptual models for nursing practice* (pp. 99–114). New York: Appleton-Century-Crofts.

Neuman, B. (1980). The Betty Neuman Health-Care Systems Model: A total person approach to patient problems. In J. P. Riehl & C. Roy (Eds.), *Conceptual models for nursing practice* (2nd ed., pp. 119–34). New York: Appleton-Century-Crofts.

Neuman, B. (1982). The Neuman Health-Care Systems Model: A total approach to client care. In B. Neuman (Ed.), *The Neuman Systems Model: Application to nursing education and practice* (pp. 8–29). Norwalk, CT: Appleton-Century-Crofts.

Neuman, B. (1982). *The Neuman Systems Model: Application to nursing education and practice.* Norwalk, CT: Appleton-Century-Crofts.

Neuman, B. (1982). The systems concept and nursing. In B. Neuman (Ed.), *The Neuman Systems Model: Application to nursing education and practice* (pp. 3–7). Norwalk, CT: Appleton-Century-Crofts.

Neuman B. (1983). Family intervention using the Betty Neuman health care systems model. In I. W. Clements & F. B. Roberts (Eds.), *Family health: A theoretical approach to nursing care* (pp. 239–54). New York: Wiley.

Neuman B. (1985). The Neuman Systems Model. *Senior Nurse, 5*(3), 20–23.

Neuman, B. (1989). The Neuman nursing process format: Family. In J. P. Riehl-Sisca (Ed.), *Conceptual models for nursing practice* (3rd ed., pp. 49–62). Norwalk, CT: Appleton & Lange.

Neuman, B. (1989). In conclusion—in transition. In B. Neuman (Ed.), *The Neuman Systems Model* (2nd ed., pp. 453–70). Norwalk, CT: Appleton & Lange.

Neuman, B. (1989). *The Neuman Systems Model* (2nd ed.). Norwalk, CT: Appleton & Lange.

Neuman, B. (1989). The Neuman Systems Model. In B. Neuman (Ed.), *The Neuman Systems Model* (2nd ed., pp. 3–63). Norwalk, CT: Appleton & Lange.

Neuman, B. (1990). The Neuman Systems Model: A theory for practice. In M. E. Parker (Ed.), *Nursing theories in practice* (pp. 241–61). New York: National League for Nursing.

Neuman, B. M. (1990). Health as a continuum based on the Neuman Systems Model. *Nursing Science Quarterly, 3,* 129–35.

Neuman, B., & Young, R. J. (1972). A model for teaching total person approach to patient problems. *Nursing Research, 21,* 264–69.

Neuman, B. (1995). *The Neuman Systems Model* (3rd ed.). Norwalk, CT: Appleton & Lange.

Neuman, B. (1995). In conclusion—toward new beginnings. In B. Neuman (Ed.), *The Neuman Systems Model* (3rd ed., pp. 671–703). Norwalk, CT: Appleton & Lange.

Neuman, B. (1995). The Neuman Systems Model. In B. Neuman (Ed.), *The Neuman Systems Model* (3rd ed., pp. 3–61). Norwalk, CT: Appleton & Lange.

Neuman, B. (1996). The Neuman Systems Model in research and practice. *Nursing Science Quarterly, 9,* 67–70.

Neuman, B., Chadwick, P. L., Beynon, C. E., et al. (1997). The Neuman Systems Model: Reflections and projections. *Nursing Science Quarterly, 10,* 18–21.

COMMENTARY: GENERAL

Aggleton, P., & Chalmers, H. (1989). Neuman's Systems Model. *Nursing Times, 85*(51), 27–29.

Beckman, S. J., Boxley-Harges, S., Bruick-Sorge, C., et al. (1994). Betty Neuman: Systems Model. In A. Marriner-Tomey (Ed.), *Nursing theorists and their work* (3rd ed., pp. 269–304). St. Louis: Mosby.

Biley, F. (1990). The Neuman model: An analysis. *Nursing (London), 4*(4), 25–28.

Brouse, S. H. (1992). Analysis of nurse theorists' definition of health for congruence with holism. *Journal of Holistic Nursing, 10,* 324–36.

Burney, M. A. (1992). King and Newman: In search of the nursing paradigm. *Journal of Advanced Nursing, 17,* 601–603.

Campbell, V. (1989). The Betty Neuman health care systems model. An analysis. In J. P. Riehl-Sisca (Ed.), *Conceptual models for nursing practice* (3rd ed., pp. 63–72). Norwalk, CT: Appleton & Lange.

Capers, C. F. (1996). The Neuman Systems Model: A culturally relevant perspective. *Association of Black Nursing Faculty Journal, 7,* 113–17.

Christensen, P. J., & Kenney, J. W. (Eds.) (1995). Nursing process: Application of conceptual models (4th ed.). St. Louis: Mosby.

Cross, J. R. (1985). Betty Neuman. In J. B. George (Ed.), *Nursing theories: The base for professional nursing practice* (2nd ed., pp. 258–86). Englewood Cliffs, NJ: Prentice Hall.

Cross, J. R. (1990). Betty Neuman. In J. B. George (Ed.), *Nursing theories: The base for professional nursing practice* (3rd ed., pp. 259–78). Norwalk, CT: Appleton & Lange.

Curran, G. (1995). The Neuman Systems Model revisited. In B. Neuman (Ed.), *The Neuman Systems Model* (3rd ed., pp. 93–99). Norwalk, CT: Appleton & Lange.

Curran, G. (1995). The spiritual variable: A world view. In B. Neuman (Ed.), *The Neuman Systems Model* (3rd ed., pp. 581–89). Norwalk, CT: Appleton & Lange.

Fawcett, J. (1989). Analysis and evaluation of the Neuman Systems Model. In B. Neuman (Ed.), *The Neuman Systems Model* (2nd ed., pp. 65–92). Norwalk, CT: Appleton & Lange.

Fawcett, J., Carpenito, J. J., Efinger, J., et al. (1982). A framework for analysis and evaluation of conceptual models of nursing with an analysis and evaluation of the Neuman Systems Model: In B. Neuman (Ed.), *The Neuman Systems Model: Application to nursing education and practice* (pp. 30–43). Norwalk, CT: Appleton-Century-Crofts.

Forchuk, C. (1991). Reconceptualizing the environment of the individual with a chronic mental illness. *Issues in Mental Health Nursing, 12,* 159–70.

Freese, B., Beckman, S. J., Boxley-Harges, S., et al. (1998). Betty Neuman: Systems Model. In A. Marriner-Tomey & M. R. Alligood (Eds.), *Nursing theorists and their work* (4th ed., pp. 267–99). St. Louis: Mosby.

Fulton, R. A. B., & Carson, V. (1995). The spiritual variable: Essential to the client system. In B. Neuman (Ed.), *The Neuman Systems Model* (3rd ed., pp. 77–91). Norwalk, CT: Appleton & Lange.

George, J. B. (1995). Betty Neuman. In J. B. George (Ed.), *Nursing theories: The base for professional nursing practice* (4th ed., pp. 251–79). Norwalk, CT: Appleton & Lange.

Harris, S. M., Hermiz, M. E., Meininger, M., & Steinkeler, S. E. (1989). Betty Neuman: Systems Model. In A. Marriner-Tomey (Ed.), *Nursing theorists and their work* (2nd ed., pp. 361–88). St. Louis: Mosby.

Hermiz, M. E., & Meininger, M. (1986). Betty Neuman: Systems Model. In A. Marriner (Ed.), *Nursing theorists and their work* (pp. 313–31). St. Louis: Mosby.

Lancaster, D. R. (1996). Neuman's Systems Model. In J. J. Fitzpatrick & A. L. Whall (Eds.), *Conceptual models of nursing: Analysis and application* (3rd ed., pp. 199–223). Stamford, CT: Appleton & Lange.

Lancaster, D. R., & Whall, A. L. (1989). The Neuman Systems Model. In J. J. Fitzpatrick & A. L. Whall (Eds.), *Conceptual models of nursing: Analysis and application* (2nd ed., pp. 255–70). Bowie, MD: Brady.

Lowry, L. W., Hinton Walker, P., & Mirenda, R. (1995). Through the looking glass back to the future. In B. Neuman (Ed.), *The Neuman Systems Model* (3rd ed., pp. 63–76). Norwalk, CT: Appleton & Lange.

Martsolf, D. S., & Mickley, J. R. (1998). The concept of spirituality in nursing theories: Differing world views and extent of focus. *Journal of Advanced Nursing, 27,* 294–303.

Meleis, A. I. (1997). *Theoretical nursing: Development and progress* (3rd ed.). Philadelphia: Lippincott.

Mirenda, R. M., & Wright, C. (1987). Using nursing model to affirm Catholic identity. *Health Progress, 68*(2), 63–67, 94.

Neuman, B., Newman, D. M. L., & Holder, P. (2000). Leadership–scholarship integration: Using the Neuman Systems Model. *Nursing Science Quarterly, 13,* 60–63.

Reed, K. S. (1993). *Betty Neuman: The Neuman Systems Model.* Newbury Park, CA: Sage.

Stevens, B. J. (1982). Foreword. In B. Neuman (Ed.), *The Neuman Systems Model: Application to nursing education and practice* (pp. xiii–xiv). Norwalk, CT: Appleton-Century-Crofts.

Thibodeau, J. A. (1983). *Nursing models: Analysis and evaluation.* Monterey, CA: Wadsworth.

Torres, G. (1986). *Theoretical foundations of nursing.* Norwalk, CT: Appleton-Century-Crofts.

Venable, J. F. (1974). The Neuman Health-Care Systems Model: An analysis. In J. P. Riehl & C. Roy (Eds.), *Conceptual models for nursing practice* (pp. 115–22). New York: Appleton-Century-Crofts. Reprinted in J. P. Riehl & C. Roy (1980), *Conceptual models for nursing practice* (2nd ed., pp. 135–41). New York: Appleton-Century-Crofts.

Walker, L. O., & Avant, K. C. (1983). *Strategies for theory construction in nursing.* Norwalk, CT: Appleton-Century-Crofts.

Whall, A. L. (1983). The Betty Neuman Health Care System Model. In J. J. Fitzpatrick & A. L. Whall (Eds.), *Conceptual models of nursing: Analysis and application* (pp. 203–19). Bowie, MD: Brady.

Wheeler, K. (1989). Self-psychology's contributions to understanding stress and implications for nursing. *Journal of Advanced Medical-Surgical Nursing, 1*(4), 1–10.

COMMENTARY: RESEARCH

Barrett, M. (1991). A thesis is born. *Image: Journal of Nursing Scholarship, 23,* 261–62.

Breckenridge, D. M. (1995). Nephrology practice and directions for research. In B. Neuman (Ed.), *The Neuman Systems Model* (3rd ed., pp. 499–507). Norwalk, CT: Appleton & Lange.

Fawcett, J. (1995). Constructing conceptual–theoretical–empirical structures for research: Future implications for use of the Neuman Systems Model. In B. Neuman (Ed.), *The Neuman Systems Model* (3rd ed., pp. 459–71). Norwalk, CT: Appleton & Lange.

Gigliotti, E. (1997). Use of Neuman's lines of defense and resistance in nursing research: Conceptual and empirical considerations. *Nursing Science Quarterly, 10,* 136–43.

Grant, J. S., Kinney, M. R., & Davis, L. L. (1993). Using conceptual frameworks or models to guide nursing research. *Journal of Neuroscience Nursing, 25,* 52–56.

Hoffman, M. K. (1982). From model to theory construction: An analysis of the Neuman Health-Care Systems Model: In B. Neuman (Ed.), *The Neuman Systems Model: Ap-*

plication to nursing education and practice (pp. 44–54). Norwalk, CT: Appleton-Century-Crofts.

Louis, M. (1995). The Neuman model in nursing research: An update. In B. Neuman (Ed.), *The Neuman Systems Model* (3rd ed., pp. 473–95). Norwalk, CT: Appleton & Lange. [See also Capers, C. F. (1995). Editorial comments. In B. Neuman (Ed.), *The Neuman Systems Model* (3rd ed., pp. 496–97). Norwalk, CT: Appleton & Lange.]

Louis, M., & Koertvelyessy, A. (1989). The Neuman model in research. In B. Neuman (Ed.), *The Neuman Systems Model* (2nd ed., pp. 93–114). Norwalk, CT: Appleton & Lange.

Meleis, A. I. (1995). Theory testing and theory support: Principles, challenges, and sojourn into the future. In B. Neuman (Ed.), *The Neuman Systems Model* (3rd ed., pp. 447–57). Norwalk, CT: Appleton & Lange.

Smith, M. C., & Edgil, A. E. (1995). Future directions for research with the Neuman Systems Model. In B. Neuman (Ed.), *The Neuman Systems Model* (3rd ed., pp. 509–17). Norwalk, CT: Appleton & Lange.

COMMENTARY: EDUCATION

Arndt, C. (1982). Systems theory and educational programs for nursing service administration. In B. Neuman (Ed.), *The Neuman Systems Model: Application to nursing education and practice* (pp. 182–87). Norwalk, CT: Appleton-Century-Crofts.

Bower, F. L. (1982). Curriculum development and the Neuman Model. In B. Neuman (Ed.), *The Neuman Systems Model: Application to nursing education and practice* (pp. 94–99). Norwalk, CT: Appleton-Century-Crofts.

Damant, M. (1995). Community nursing in the United Kingdom: A case for reconciliation using the Neuman Systems Model. In B. Neuman (Ed.), *The Neuman Systems Model* (3rd ed., pp. 607–20). Norwalk, CT: Appleton & Lange.

Freiburger, O. A. (1998). Overview of strategies that integrate the Neuman Systems Model, critical thinking, and cooperative learning. In L. Lowry (Ed.), *The Neuman Systems Model and nursing education: Teaching strategies and outcomes* (pp. 31–36). Indianapolis: Sigma Theta Tau International Center Nursing Press.

Gunter, L. M. (1982). Application of the Neuman Systems Model to gerontic nursing. In B. Neuman (Ed.), *The Neuman Systems Model: Application to nursing education and practice* (pp. 196–210). Norwalk, CT: Appleton-Century-Crofts.

Karmels, P. (1993). Conundrum game for nursing theorists: Neuman, King, and Johnson. *Nurse Educator, 18*(6), 8–9.

Lowry, L. (1998). Creative teaching and effective evaluation. In L. Lowry (Ed.), *The Neuman Systems Model and nursing education: Teaching strategies and outcomes* (pp. 17–29). Indianapolis: Sigma Theta Tau International Center Nursing Press.

Lowry, L. (1998). Vision, values, and verities. In L. Lowry (Ed.), *The Neuman Systems Model and nursing education: Teaching strategies and outcomes* (pp. 167–74). Indianapolis: Sigma Theta Tau International Center Nursing Press.

Lowry, L. W., Burns, C. M., Smith, A. A., & Jacobson, H. (2000). Compete or complement? An interdisciplinary approach to training health professionals. *Nursing and Health Care Perspectives, 21*, 76–80.

Major, S. (1989). Neuman's systems model and experiential taxonomy. *Senior Nurse, 9*(6), 25–27.

Meiner, S. (1998). General systems theory. In A. S. Luggen, S. S. Travis, S. Meiner, & National Gerontological Nursing Association Staff (Eds.), *NGNA core curriculum for gerontological advance practice nurses* (pp. 20–22). Thousand Oaks, CA: Sage.

Neuman, B. (1998). NDs should be future coordinators of health care (letter to the Editor). *Image: Journal of Nursing Scholarship, 30,* 106.

Newsome, G. G., & Lowry, L. (1998). Evaluation in nursing: History, models, and Neuman's framework. In L. Lowry (Ed.), *The Neuman Systems Model and nursing education: Teaching strategies and outcomes* (pp. 37–51). Indianapolis: Sigma Theta Tau International Center Nursing Press.

Toot, J. L., & Schmoll, B. J. (1995). The Neuman Systems Model and physical therapy educational curricula. In B. Neuman (Ed.), *The Neuman Systems Model* (3rd ed., pp. 231–46). Norwalk, CT: Appleton & Lange.

COMMENTARY: ADMINISTRATION

Arndt, C. (1982). Systems concepts for management of stress in complex health-care organizations. In B. Neuman (Ed.), *The Neuman Systems Model: Application to nursing education and practice* (pp. 97–114). Norwalk, CT: Appleton-Century-Crofts.

Bennett, S., Hulkes, C., Jones, J., et al. (1998). Models of care: Developing a trust-wide philosophy. *Community Practitioner, 71,* 334, 336.

Bowles, L., Oliver, N., & Stanley, S. (1995). A fresh approach. *Nursing Times, 91*(1), 40–41.

Fawcett, J., Botter, M. L., Burritt, J., Crossley, J. D., & Fink, B. B. (1989). Conceptual models of nursing and organization theories. In B. Henry, M. DiVincenti, C. Arndt, & A. Marriner (Eds.), *Dimensions of nursing administration: Theory, research, education, and practice* (pp. 143–54). Boston: Blackwell Scientific Publications.

Hinton-Walker, P. (1995). TQM and the Neuman Systems Model: Education for health care administration. In B. Neuman (Ed.), *The Neuman Systems Model* (3rd ed., pp. 365–76). Norwalk, CT: Appleton & Lange.

Kelley, J. A., & Sanders, N. F. (1995). A systems approach to the health of nursing and health care organizations. In B. Neuman (Ed.), *The Neuman Systems Model* (3rd ed., pp. 347–64). Norwalk, CT: Appleton & Lange.

Kelley, J. A., Sanders, N. F., & Pierce, J. D. (1989). A systems approach to the role of the nurse administrator in education and practice. In B. Neuman (Ed.), *The Neuman Systems Model* (2nd ed., pp. 115–38). Norwalk, CT: Appleton & Lange.

Latimer, J., & Spuhler-Gaughan, M. J. (1991). Quality assurance and risk management. In C. Birdsall (Ed.), *Management issues in critical care* (pp. 113–30). St. Louis: Mosby-Year Book.

Neuman, B., & Martin, K. S. (1998). Neuman Systems Model and the Omaha system (letter to the editor). *Image: Journal of Nursing Scholarship, 30,* 8.

Russell, J., & Hezel, L. (1994). Role analysis of the advanced practice nurse using the Neuman health care systems model as a framework. *Clinical Nurse Specialist, 8,* 215–20.

Simmons, L., & Borgdon, C. (1991). The clinical nurse specialist in HIV care. *The Kansas Nurse, 66*(1), 6–7.

Vokaty, D. A. (1982). The Neuman Systems Model applied to the clinical nurse specialist role. In B. Neuman (Ed.), *The Neuman Systems Model: Application to nursing education and practice* (pp. 165–67). Norwalk, CT: Appleton-Century-Crofts.

COMMENTARY: PRACTICE

Balch, C. (1974). Breaking the lines of resistance. In J. P. Riehl & C. Roy (Eds.), *Conceptual models for nursing practice* (pp. 130–34). New York: Appleton-Century-Crofts.

Bennett, S., Hulkes, C., Jones, J., et al. (1998). Models of care: Developing a trust-wide philosophy. *Community Practitioner, 71,* 334, 336.

Bigbee, J. (1984). The changing role of rural women: Nursing and health implications. *Health Care of Women International, 5,* 307–22.

Black, P., Deeny, P., & McKenna, H. (1997). Sensoristrain: An exploration of nursing interventions in the context of the Neuman Systems Model. *Intensive and Critical Care Nursing, 13,* 249–58.

Brown, M. W. (1988). Neuman's Systems Model in risk factor reduction. *Cardiovascular Nursing, 24*(6), 43.

Buchanan, B. F. (1987). Human–environment interaction: A modification of the Neuman Systems Model for aggregates, families, and the community. *Public Health Nursing, 4,* 52–64.

Coutu-Wakulczyk, G., & Beckingham, A. C. (1993). Selected nursing models applicable to gerontological practice. In A. C. Beckingham & B. DuGas (Eds.), *Promoting healthy aging: A nursing and community perspective* (pp. 80–110). St. Louis: Mosby-Year Book.

Craddock, R. B., & Stanhope, M. K. (1980). The Neuman Health-Care Systems Model: Recommended adaptation. In J. P. Riehl & C. Roy (Eds.), *Conceptual models for nursing practice* (2nd ed., pp. 159–69). New York: Appleton-Century-Crofts.

Cross, J. R. (1995). Nursing process of the family client: Application of Neuman's Systems Model. In P. J. Christensen & J. W. Kenney (Eds.), *Nursing process: Application of conceptual models* (4th ed., pp. 246–69). St. Louis: Mosby-Year Book.

Davis, L. H. (1982). Aging: A social and preventive perspective. In B. Neuman (Ed.), *The Neuman Systems Model: Application to nursing education and practice* (pp. 211–14). Norwalk, CT: Appleton-Century-Crofts.

Engberg, I. B. (1995). Brief abstracts: Use of the Neuman Systems Model in Sweden. In B. Neuman (Ed.), *The Neuman Systems Model* (3rd ed., pp. 653–56). Norwalk, CT: Appleton & Lange.

Fawcett, J. (1998). Conceptual models and therapeutic modalities in advanced psychiatric nursing practice. In A. W. Burgess (Ed.), *Advanced practice psychiatric nursing* (pp. 41–48). Stamford, CT: Appleton & Lange.

Fawcett, J., Tulman, L., & Samarel, N. (1995). Enhancing function in life transitions and serious illness. *Advanced Practice Nursing Quarterly, 1*(3), 50–57.

Goodman, H. (1995). Patients' views count as well. *Nursing Standard, 9*(40), 55.

Haggart, M. (1993). A critical analysis of Neuman's Systems Model in relation to public health nursing. *Journal of Advanced Nursing, 18,* 1917–22.

Helland, W. Y. (1995). Nursing diagnosis: Diagnostic process. In P. J. Christensen & J. W. Kenney (Eds.), *Nursing process: Application of conceptual models* (4th ed., pp. 120–38). St. Louis: Mosby-Year Book.

Hinton-Walker, P. (1993). Care of the chronically ill: Paradigm shifts and directions for the future. *Holistic Nursing Practice, 8*(1), 56–66.

Kinservik, M. A., & Friedhoff, M. M. (2000). Control issues in toilet training. *Pediatric Nursing, 26,* 267–74.

Molassiotis, A. (1997). A conceptual model of adaptation to illness and quality of life for cancer patients treated with bone marrow transplants. *Journal of Advanced Nursing, 26,* 572–79.

Pierce, A. G., & Fulmer, T. T. (1995). Application of the Neuman Systems Model to gerontological nursing. In B. Neuman (Ed.), *The Neuman Systems Model* (3rd ed., pp. 293–308). Norwalk, CT: Appleton & Lange.

Procter, N. G., & Cheek, J. (1995). Nurses' role in world catastrophic events: War dislocation effects on Serbian Australians. In B. Neuman (Ed.), *The Neuman Systems Model* (3rd ed., pp. 119–31). Norwalk, CT: Appleton & Lange.

Quayhagen, M. P., & Roth, P. A. (1989). From models to measures in assessment of mature families. *Journal of Professional Nursing, 5,* 144–51.

Reed, K. S. (1989). Family theory related to the Neuman Systems Model. In B. Neuman (Ed.), *The Neuman Systems Model* (2nd ed., pp. 385–96). Norwalk, CT: Appleton & Lange.

Reed, K. S. (1993). Adapting the Neuman Systems Model for family nursing. *Nursing Science Quarterly, 6,* 93–97.

Salvage, J., & Turner, C. (1989). Brief abstracts: The Neuman model use in England. In B. Neuman (Ed.), *The Neuman Systems Model* (2nd ed., pp. 445–50). Norwalk, CT: Appleton & Lange.

Sohier, R. (1989). Nursing care for the people of a small planet: Culture and the Neuman Systems Model. In B. Neuman (Ed.), *The Neuman Systems Model* (2nd ed., pp. 139–54). Norwalk, CT: Appleton & Lange.

Sohier, R. (1995). Nursing care for the people of a small planet: Culture and the Neuman Systems Model. In B. Neuman (Ed.), *The Neuman Systems Model* (3rd ed., pp. 101–17). Norwalk, CT: Appleton & Lange.

Spradley, B. W. (1990). Community health nursing: Concepts and practice. Glenview, IL: Scott, Foresman/Little, Brown Higher Education.

Stuart, G. W., & Wright, L. K. (1995). Applying the Neuman Systems Model to psychiatric nursing practice. In B. Neuman (Ed.), *The Neuman Systems Model* (3rd ed., pp. 263–73). Norwalk, CT: Appleton & Lange.

Tomlinson, P. S., & Anderson, K. H. (1995). Family health and the Neuman Systems Model. In B. Neuman (Ed.), *The Neuman Systems Model* (3rd ed., pp. 133–44). Norwalk, CT: Appleton & Lange.

Vaughan, B., & Gough, P. (1995). Use of the Neuman Systems Model in England: Abstracts. In B. Neuman (Ed.), *The Neuman Systems Model* (3rd ed., pp. 599–605). Norwalk, CT: Appleton & Lange.

Wright, K. B. (1998). Professional, ethical, and legal implications for spiritual care in nursing. *Image: Journal of Nursing Scholarship, 30,* 81–83.

RESEARCH

Ali, N. S., & Khalil, H. Z. (1989). Effect of psychoeducational intervention on anxiety among Egyptian bladder cancer patients. *Cancer Nursing, 12,* 236–42.

Andersen, J. E., & Briggs, L. L. (1988). Nursing diagnosis: A study of quality and supportive evidence. *Image: Journal of Nursing Scholarship, 20,* 141–44.

Barker, E., Robinson, D., & Brautigan, R. (1999). The effect of psychiatric home nurse follow-up on readmission rates of patients with depression. *Journal of the American Psychiatric Nurses Association, 5,* 111–16.

Bass, L. S. (1991). What do parents need when their infant is a patient in the NICU? *Neonatal Network, 10*(4), 25–33.

Beynon, C., & Laschinger, H. K. (1993). Theory-based practice: Attitudes of nursing managers before and after educational sessions. *Public Health Nursing, 10,* 183–88.

Blank, J. J., Clark, L., Longman, A. J., & Atwood, J. R. (1989). Perceived home care needs of cancer patients and their caregivers. *Cancer Nursing, 12,* 78–84.

Bowdler, J. E., & Barrell, L. M. (1987). Health needs of homeless persons. *Public Health Nursing, 4,* 135–40.

Bowman, A. M. (1997). Sleep satisfaction, perceived pain and acute confusion in elderly clients undergoing orthopaedic procedures. *Journal of Advanced Nursing, 26,* 550–64.

Breckenridge, D. M. (1997a). Decisions regarding dialysis treatment modality: A holistic perspective. *Holistic Nursing Practice, 12*(1), 54–61.

Breckenridge, D. M. (1997b). Patients' perception of why, how, and by whom dialysis treatment modality was chosen. *Association of Nephrology Nurses Journal, 24,* 313–21.

Brown, K. C., Sirles, A. T., Hilyer, J. C., & Thomas, M. J. (1992). Cost-effectiveness of a back school intervention for municipal employees. *Spine, 17,* 1224–28.

Bueno, M. N., Redeker, N., & Norman, E. M. (1992). Analysis of motor vehicle crash data in an urban trauma center: Implications for nursing practice and research. *Heart and Lung, 21,* 558–67.

Cantin, B., & Mitchell, M. (1989). Nurses' smoking behavior. *The Canadian Nurse, 85*(1), 20–21.

Capers, C. F. (1991). Nurses' and lay African Americans' views about behavior. *Western Journal of Nursing Research, 13,* 123–35.

Carroll, T. L. (1989). Role deprivation in baccalaureate nursing students pre and post curriculum revision. *Journal of Nursing Education, 28,* 134–39.

Cava, M. A. (1992). An examination of coping strategies used by long-term cancer survivors. *Canadian Oncology Nursing Journal, 2,* 99–102.

Chiverton, P., Tortoretti, D., LaForest, M., & Walker, P. H. (1999). Bridging the gap between psychiatric hospitalization and community care: Cost and quality outcomes. *Journal of the American Psychiatric Association, 5,* 46–53.

Clark, C. C., Cross, J. R., Deane, D. M., & Lowry, L. W. (1991). Spirituality: Integral to quality care. *Holistic Nursing Practice, 5,* 67–76.

Collins, M. A. (1996). The relation of work stress, hardiness, and burnout among full-time hospital staff nurses. *Journal of Nursing Staff Development, 12,* 81–85.

Courchene, V. S., Patalski, E., & Martin, J. (1991). A study of the health of pediatric nurses administering cyclosporine A. *Pediatric Nursing, 17,* 497–500.

Decker, S. D., & Young, E. (1991). Self-perceived needs of primary caregivers of home-hospice clients. *Journal of Community Health Nursing, 8,* 147–54.

Fields, W. L., & Loveridge, C. (1988). Critical thinking and fatigue: How do nurses on 8-& 12-hour shifts compare? *Nursing Economic$, 6,* 189–91.

Flanders-Stepans, M. B., & Fuller, S. G. (1999). Physiological effects of infant exposure to environmental tobacco smoke: A passive observation study. *Journal of Perinatal Nursing, 8,* 10–21.

Flannery, J. (1995). Cognitive assessment in the acute care setting: Reliability and validity of the Levels of Cognitive Functioning Assessment Scale (LOCFAS). *Journal of Nursing Measurement, 3,* 43–58.

Fowler, B. A., & Risner, P. B. (1994). A health promotion program evaluation in a minority industry. *Association of Black Nursing Faculty Journal, 5*(3), 72–76.

Freiberger, D., Bryant, J., & Marino, B. (1992). The effects of different central venous line dressing changes on bacterial growth in a pediatric oncology population. *Journal of Pediatric Oncology Nursing, 9,* 3–7.

Gavigan, M., Kline-O'Sullivan, C., & Klumpp-Lybrand, B. (1990). The effect of regular turning on CABG patients. *Critical Care Nursing Quarterly, 12*(4), 69–76.

Gellner, P., Landers, S., O'Rourke, D., & Schlegel, M. (1994). Community health nursing in the 1990s: Risky business? *Holistic Nursing Practice, 8*(2), 15–21.

George, J. (1997). Nurses' perceived autonomy in a shared governance setting. *Journal of Shared Governance, 3*(2), 17–21.

Gifford, D. K. (1996). Monthly incidence of stroke in rural Kansas. *Kansas Nurse, 71*(5), 3–4.

Gigliotti, E. (1999). Women's multiple role stress: Testing Neuman's flexible line of defense. *Nursing Science Quarterly, 12,* 36–44.

Grant, J. S., & Bean, C. A. (1992). Self-identified needs of informal caregivers of head-injured adults. *Family and Community Health, 15*(2), 49–58.

Gries, M., & Fernsler, J. (1988). Patient perceptions of the mechanical ventilation experience. *Focus on Critical Care, 15,* 52–59.

Hainsworth, D. S. (1996). The effect of death education on attitudes of hospital nurses toward care of the dying. *Oncology Nursing Forum, 23,* 963–67.

Hanson, M. J. S. (1999). Cross-cultural study of beliefs about smoking among teenaged females. *Western Journal of Nursing Research, 21,* 635–51.

Heffline, M. S. (1991). A comparative study of pharmacological versus nursing interventions in the treatment of postanesthesia shivering. *Journal of Post Anesthesia Nursing, 6,* 311–20.

Hinds, C. (1990). Personal and contextual factors predicting patients' reported quality of life: Exploring congruency with Betty Neuman's assumptions. *Journal of Advanced Nursing, 15,* 456–62.

Hoch, C. C. (1987). Assessing delivery of nursing care. *Journal of Gerontological Nursing, 13,* 1–17.

Johnson, P. (1983). Black hypertension: A transcultural case study using the Betty Neuman model of nursing care. *Issues in Health Care of Women, 4,* 191–210.

Jones, W. R. (1996). Stressors in the primary caregivers of traumatic head injured persons. *AXON, 18,* 9–11.

Kahn, E. C. (1992). A comparison of family needs based on the presence or absence of DNR orders. *Dimensions of Critical Care Nursing, 11,* 286–92. [See also Schare, B. L. (1993). Commentary on "A comparison of family needs based on the presence or absence of DNR orders." *Nursing Scan in Research, 6*(2), 16.]

Koku, R. V. (1992). Severity of low back pain: A comparison between participants who did and did not receive counseling. *American Association of Occupational Health Nurses Journal, 40,* 84–89.

Leja, A. M. (1989). Using guided imagery to combat postsurgical depression. *Journal of Gerontological Nursing, 15*(4), 6–11.

Lin, M, Ku, N., Leu, J., Chen, J., & Lin, L. (1996). An exploration of the stress aspects, coping behaviors, health status and related aspects in family caregivers of hepatoma patients. *Nursing Research (China), 4,* 171–85. [Chinese, English abstract]

Loescher, L. J. , Clark, L., Atwood, J. R., Leigh, S., & Lamb, G. (1990). The impact of the cancer experience on long-term survivors. *Oncology Nursing Forum, 17,* 223–29.

Louis, M. (1989). An intervention to reduce anxiety levels for nurses working with long-term care clients using Neuman's model. In J. P. Riehl-Sisca (Ed.), *Conceptual models for nursing practice* (3rd ed., pp. 95–103). Norwalk, CT: Appleton & Lange.

Lowry, L. W., & Anderson, B. (1993). Neuman's framework and ventilator dependency: A pilot study. *Nursing Science Quarterly, 6,* 195–200.

Lowry, L. W., Saeger, J., & Barnett, S. (1997). Client satisfaction with prenatal care and pregnancy outcomes. *Outcomes Management for Nursing Practice, 1*(1), 29–35.

Mackenzie, S. J., & Laschinger, H. K. S. (1995). Correlates of nursing diagnosis quality in public health nursing. *Journal of Advanced Nursing, 21,* 800–808.

Maligalig, R. M. L. (1994). Parents' perceptions of the stressors of pediatric ambulatory surgery. *Journal of Post Anesthesia Nursing, 9,* 278–82.

Mannina, J. (1997). Finding an effective hearing testing protocol to identify hearing loss and middle ear disease in school-aged children. *Journal of School Nursing, 13*(5), 23–28.

Marsh, V., Beard, M. T., & Adams, B. N. (1999). Job stress and burnout: The mediational effect of spiritual well-being and hardiness among nurses. *Journal of Theory Construction and Testing, 3,* 13–19.

Montgomery, P., & Craig, D. (1990). Levels of stress and health practices of wives of alcoholics. *Canadian Journal of Nursing Research, 22,* 60–70.

Moody, N. B. (1996). Nurse faculty job satisfaction: A national survey. *Journal of Professional Nursing, 12*, 277–88.

Nortridge, J. A., Mayeux, V., Anderson, S. J., & Bell, M. L. (1992). The use of cognitive style mapping as a predictor for academic success of first semester diploma nursing students. *Journal of Nursing Education, 31*, 352–56.

Nuttall, P., & Flores, F. C. (1997). Hmong healing practices used for common childhood illnesses. *Pediatric Nursing, 23*, 247–51.

Picot, S. J. F., Zauszniewski, J. A., Debanne, S. M., & Holston, E. C. (1999). Mood and blood pressure responses in Black female caregivers and noncaregivers. *Nursing Research, 48*, 150–61.

Purushotham, D., & Walker, G. (1994). The Neuman Systems Model: A conceptual framework for clinical teaching/learning process. In R. M. Carroll-Johnson & M. Paquette (Eds.), *Classification of nursing diagnoses: Proceedings of the tenth conference* (pp. 271–73). Philadelphia: Lippincott.

Radwanski, M. (1992). Self-medicating practices for managing chronic pain after spinal cord injury. *Rehabilitation Nursing, 17*, 312–18.

Rodrigues-Fisher, L., Bourguignon, C., & Good, B. V. (1993). Dietary fiber nursing intervention: Prevention of constipation in older adults. *Clinical Nursing Research, 2*, 464–77.

Roggensack, J. (1994). The influence of perioperative theory and clinical in a baccalaureate nursing program on the decision to practice perioperative nursing. *Prairie Rose, 63*(2), 6–7.

Semple, O. D. (1995). The experiences of family members of persons with Huntington's Disease. *Perspectives, 19*(4), 4–10.

Sirles, A. T., Brown, K., & Hilyer, J. C. (1991). Effects of back school education and exercise in back injured municipal workers. *American Association of Occupational Health Nursing Journal, 39*, 7–12.

Skipwith, D. H. (1994). Telephone counseling interventions with caregivers of elders. *Journal of Psychosocial Nursing and Mental Health Services, 32*(3), 7–12, 34–35.

Speck, B. J. (1990). The effect of guided imagery upon first semester nursing students performing their first injections. *Journal of Nursing Education, 29*, 346–50.

Vaughn, M., Cheatwood, S., Sirles, A. T., & Brown, K. C. (1989). The effect of progressive muscle relaxation on stress among clerical workers. *American Association of Occupational Health Nurses Journal, 37*, 302–306.

Waddell, K. L., & Demi, A. S. (1993). Effectiveness of an intensive partial hospitalization program for treatment of anxiety disorders. *Archives of Psychiatric Nursing, 7*, 2–10.

Williamson, J. W. (1992). The effects of ocean sounds on sleep after coronary artery bypass graft surgery. *American Journal of Critical Care, 1*, 91–97.

Wilson, L. C. (2000). Implementation and evaluation of church–based health fairs. *Journal of Community Health Nursing, 17*, 39–48.

Wilson, V. S. (1987). Identification of stressors related to patients' psychological responses to the surgical intensive care unit. *Heart and Lung, 16*, 267–73.

Ziemer, M. M. (1983). Effects of information on postsurgical coping. *Nursing Research, 32*, 282–87.

DOCTORAL DISSERTATIONS

Al-Nagshabandi, E. A. H. (1994). An exploration of the physical and psychological responses of surgically-induced menopausal Saudi women using the Neuman Systems Model. *Dissertation Abstracts International, 55,* 1374B.

Ark, P. D. (1997). Health risk behaviors and coping strategies of African American sixth graders. *Dissertation Abstracts International, 58,* 1205B.

Barnes-McDowell, B. M. (1997). Home apnea monitoring: Family functioning, concerns, and coping. *Dissertation Abstracts International, 58,* 1205B.

Bemker, M. A. (1997). Adolescent female substance abuse: Risk and resiliency factors. *Dissertation Abstracts International, 57,* 75446B.

Bittinger, J. P. (1996). Case management and satisfaction with nursing care of patients hospitalized with congestive heart failure. *Dissertation Abstracts International, 56,* 3866B.

Burritt, J. E. (1988). The effects of perceived social support on the relationship between job stress and job satisfaction and job performance among registered nurses employed in acute care facilities. *Dissertation Abstracts International, 49,* 2123B.

Butts, M. J. (1998). Outcomes of comfort touch in institutionalized elderly female residents. *Dissertation Abstracts International, 59,* 3344B.

Cagle, R. (1997). The relationship between health care provider advice and the initiation of breast-feeding. *Dissertation Abstracts International, 57,* 4974B.

Cammuso, B. S. (1994). Caring and accountability in nursing practice in Ireland and the United States: Helping Irish nurses bridge the gap when they choose to practice in the United States. *Dissertation Abstracts International, 55,* 76B.

Capers, C. F. (1987). Perceptions of problematic behavior as held by lay black adults and registered nurses. *Dissertation Abstracts International, 47,* 4467B.

Chilton, L. L. A. (1997). The influence of behavioral cues on immunization practices of elders. *Dissertation Abstracts International, 57,* 5572B.

Collins, A. S. (1992). Effects of positional changes on selected physiological and psychological measurements in clients with atrial fibrillation. *Dissertation Abstracts International, 53,* 200B.

Collins, C. R. (1999). The older widow-adult child relationship as an influence upon health promoting behaviors. *Dissertation Abstracts International, 60,* 1527B.

Cox, D. D. (1996). The impact of stress, coping, constructive thinking and hardiness on health and academic performance of female registered nurse students pursuing a baccalaureate degree in nursing. *Dissertation Abstracts International, 57,* 237B.

Doherty, D. C. Spousal abuse: An African-American female perspective. *Dissertation Abstracts International, 58,* 1798B.

Downing, B. H. (1995). Evaluation of a computer assisted intervention for musculoskeletal discomfort, strength, and flexibility and job satisfaction of video display operators. *Dissertation Abstracts International, 55,* 3237B.

Dunbar, S. B. (1982). The effect of formal patient education on selected psychological and physiological variables of adaptation after acute myocardial infarction. *Dissertation Abstracts International, 43,* 1794B.

Flannery, J. C. (1988). Validity and reliability of Levels of Cognitive Functioning Assessment Scale for adults with closed head injuries. *Dissertation Abstracts International, 48*, 3248B.

Fulton, B. J. (1993). Evaluation of the effectiveness of the Neuman Systems Model as a theoretical framework for baccalaureate nursing programs. *Dissertation Abstracts International, 53*, 5641B.

Gibson, D. E. (1989). A Q-analysis of interpersonal trust in the nurse–client relationship. *Dissertation Abstracts International, 50*, 493B.

Gibson, M. H. (1996). The quality of life of adult hemodialysis patients. *Dissertation Abstracts International, 56*, 5416B.

Gigliotti, E. (1997). The relations among maternal and student role involvement, perceived social support and perceived multiple role stress in mothers attending college: A study based on Betty Neuman's Systems Model. *Dissertation Abstracts International, 58*, 135B.

Glazer, G. L. (1985). The relationship between pregnant women's anxiety levels and stressors and their partners' anxiety levels and stressors. *Dissertation Abstracts International, 46*, 1869B.

Goble, D. S. (1991). A curriculum framework for the prevention of child sexual abuse. *Dissertation Abstracts International, 52*, 2004A.

Hanson, M. J. S. (1996). Beliefs, attitudes, subjective norms, perceived behavioral control, and cigarette smoking in White, African-American, and Puerto Rican-American teenage women. *Dissertation Abstracts International, 56*, 4240B.

Hanson, P. A. (1998). An application of Bowen family systems theory: Triangulation, differentiation of self and nurse manager job stress responses. *Dissertation Abstracts International, 58*, 5889B.

Harbin, P. D. O. (1990). A Q-analysis of the stressors of adult female nursing students enrolled in baccalaureate schools of nursing. *Dissertation Abstracts International, 50*, 3919B.

Hayes, K. V. D. (1995). Diagnostic content validation and operational definitions of risk factors for the nursing diagnosis high risk for disuse syndrome. *Dissertation Abstracts International, 55*, 5284B.

Heaman, D. J. (1992). Perceived stressors and coping strategies of parents with developmentally disabled children. *Dissertation Abstracts International, 52*, 6316B.

Henze, R. L. (1994). The relationship among selected stress variables and white blood count in severely head injured patients. *Dissertation Abstracts International, 55*, 365B.

Herald, P. A. (1994). Relationship between hydration status and renal function in patients receiving aminoglycoside antibiotics. *Dissertation Abstracts International, 55*, 365B.

Hood, L. J. (1998). The effects of nurse faculty hardiness and sense of coherence on perceived stress, scholarly productivity, and job satisfaction. *Dissertation Abstracts International, 58*, 4720B.

Jennings, K. (1998). Predicting intention to obtain a Pap smear among African American and Latina women. *Dissertation Abstracts International, 58*, 3557B.

Lamb, K. A. (1999). Baccalaureate nursing students' perception of empathy and stress in their interactions with clinical instructors: Testing a theory of optimal student system stability according to the Neuman Systems Model. *Dissertation Abstracts International, 60,* 1028B.

Lancaster, D. R. N. (1992). Coping with appraised threat of breast cancer: Primary prevention coping behaviors utilized by women at increased risk. *Dissertation Abstracts International, 53,* 202B.

Lapvongwatana, P. (2000). Perinatal risk assessment for low birthweight in Thai mothers: Using the Neuman Systems Model. *Dissertation Abstracts International, 61,* 1325B.

Lee, P. L. (1996). Caregiver stress as experienced by wives of institutionalized and in-home dementia husbands. *Dissertation Abstracts International, 56,* 4241B.

Marsh, V. (1998). Job stress and burnout among nurses: The mediational effect of spiritual well-being and hardiness. *Dissertation Abstracts International, 58,* 4142B.

McDaniel, G. M. S. (1990). The effects of two methods of dangling on heart rate and blood pressure in postoperative abdominal hysterectomy patients. *Dissertation Abstracts International, 50,* 3923B.

Mirenda, R. M. (1996). A conceptual–theoretical strategy for curriculum development in baccalaureate nursing programs. *Dissertation Abstracts International, 56,* 5421B.

Monahan, G. L. (1997). A profile of pregnant drug-using female arrestees in California: The relationships among sociodemographic characteristics, reproductive and drug additional histories, HIV/STD risk behaviors, and utilization of prenatal care services and substance abuse treatment programs. *Dissertation Abstracts International, 57,* 5576B.

Moody, N. B. (1991). Selected demographic variables, organizational characteristics, role orientation, and job satisfaction among nurse faculty. *Dissertation Abstracts International, 52,* 1356B.

Norman, S. E. (1991). The relationship between hardiness and sleep disturbances in HIV-infected men. *Dissertation Abstracts International, 51,* 4780B.

Norris, E. W. (1990). Physiologic response to exercise in clients with mitral valve prolapse syndrome. *Dissertation Abstracts International, 50,* 5549B.

Parodi, V. A. (1998). Neuman based analysis of women's health needs aboard a deployed Navy ship: Can nursing make a difference? *Dissertation Abstracts International, 58,* 6491B.

Payne, P. L. (1994). A study of the teaching of primary prevention competencies as recommended by the report of the PEW Health Professions Commission in bachelor of science in nursing programs and associate in nursing programs. *Dissertation Abstracts International, 54,* 3553B.

Peoples, L. T. (1991). The relationship between selected client, provider, and agency variables and the utilization of home care services. *Dissertation Abstracts International, 51,* 3782B.

Peterson, G. A. (1998). Nursing perceptions of the spiritual dimension of patient care: The Neuman Systems Model in curricular formations. *Dissertation Abstracts International, 59,* 605B.

Poole, V. L. (1992). Pregnancy wantedness, attitude toward pregnancy, and use of alcohol, tobacco, and street drugs during pregnancy. *Dissertation Abstracts International, 52,* 5193B.

Pothiban, L. (1993). Risk factor prevalence, risk status, and perceived risk for coronary heart disease among Thai elderly. *Dissertation Abstracts International, 54,* 1337B.

Quinn, A. T. (1992). A hospice death education course: Evaluating effectiveness in meeting goals. *Dissertation Abstracts International, 53,* 728A.

Riley-Lawless, K. (2000). The relationship among characteristics of the family environment and behavioral and physiologic cardiovascular risk factors in parents and their adolescent twins. *Dissertation Abstracts International, 61,* 1328B.

Rowe, M. L. (1990). The relationship of commitment and social support to the life satisfaction of caregivers to patients with Alzheimer's disease. *Dissertation Abstracts International, 51,* 1747B.

Rowles, C. J. (1993). The relationship of selected personal and organizational variables and the tenure of directors of nursing in nursing homes. *Dissertation Abstracts International, 53,* 4593B.

Schlosser, S. P. (1985). The effect of anticipatory guidance on mood state in primiparas experiencing unplanned cesarean delivery (metropolitan area, Southeast). *Dissertation Abstracts International, 46,* 2627B.

Schmidt, C. S. (1983). A comparison of the effectiveness of two nursing models in decreasing depression and increasing life satisfaction of retired individuals. *Dissertation Abstracts International, 43,* 2856B.

Sipple, J. E. A. (1989). A model for curriculum change based on retrospective analysis. *Dissertation Abstracts International, 50,* 1927A.

South, L. D. (1995). The relationship of self-concept and social support in school age children with leukemia. *Dissertation Abstracts International, 56,* 1939B.

Tarmina, M. S. (1992). Self-selected diet of adult women with families. *Dissertation Abstracts International, 53,* 777B.

Tennyson, M. G. (1992). Becoming pregnant: Perceptions of black adolescents. *Dissertation Abstracts International, 52,* 5196B.

Terhaar, M. F. (1989). The influence of physiologic stability, behavioral stability and family stability on the preterm infant's length of stay in the neonatal intensive care unit. *Dissertation Abstracts International, 50,* 1328B.

Thornhill, B. E. (1986). A Q-analysis of stressors in the primipara during the immediate postpartal period. *Dissertation Abstracts International, 47,* 135B.

Underwood, P. W. (1986). Psychosocial variables: Their prediction of birth complications and relation to perception of childbirth. *Dissertation Abstracts International, 47,* 997B.

Vincent, J. L. M. (1988). A Q analysis of the stressors of fathers with an infant in an intensive care unit. *Dissertation Abstracts International, 49,* 3111B.

Watson, L. A. (1991). Comparison of the effects of usual, support, and informational nursing interventions on the extent to which families of critically ill patients perceived their needs were met. *Dissertation Abstracts International, 52,* 2999B.

Webb, C. A. (1988). A cross-sectional study of hope, physical status, cognitions and meaning and purpose of pre- and post-retirement adults. *Dissertation Abstracts International, 49,* 1922A.

Whatley, J. H. (1989). Effects of health locus of control and social network on risk-taking in adolescents. *Dissertation Abstracts International, 50,* 129B.

Williamson, J. W. (1990). The influence of self-selected monotonous sounds on the night sleep pattern of postoperative open heart surgery patients. *Dissertation Abstracts International, 51,* 1750B.

Yoder, R. E. (1995). Primary prevention emphasis and self-reported health behaviors of nursing students. *Dissertation Abstracts International, 56,* 747B.

Ziemer, M. M. (1982). Providing patients with information prior to surgery and the reported frequency of coping behaviors and development of symptoms following surgery. *Dissertation Abstracts International, 43,* 2165B.

MASTER'S THESES

Alford, D. L. (1994). Differences in levels of anxiety of spouses of critical care surgical patients when the spouse participates in preoperative care. *Master's Abstracts International, 32,* 222.

Allen, K. S. (1997). The effect of cancer diagnosis information on the anxiety of patients with an initial diagnosis of first cancer. *Master's Abstracts International, 35,* 996.

Anderson, R. R. (1992). Indicators of nutritional status as a predictor of pressure ulcer development in the critically ill adult. *Master's Abstracts International, 30,* 92.

Averill, J. B. (1989). The impact of primary prevention as an intervention strategy. *Master's Abstracts International, 27,* 89.

Baloush, N. A. (1991). Social support and maternal reaction in Saudi Arabian women with premature births from a Neuman framework. *Master's Abstracts International, 29,* 432.

Barnes, M. E. (1994). Knowledge, experiences, attitudes, and assessment practices of nurse practitioners with regard to stressors related to childhood sexual abuse. *Master's Abstracts International, 32,* 223.

Barron, L. A. (1999). Diabetes self-management and psychosocial adjustment. *Master's Abstracts International, 37,* 587.

Baskin-Nedzelski, J. (1992). Job stressors among visiting nurses. *Master's Abstracts International, 30,* 79.

Baumle, W. M. (1993). A comparison study of the psychological pain response of persons on long-term intermittent intravenous antibiotic therapy. *Master's Abstracts International, 31,* 1199.

Besseghini, C. (1990). Stressful life events and angina in individuals undergoing exercise stress testing. *Master's Abstracts International, 28,* 569.

Bischoff, S. M. (1988). Job stress in nurses working in correctional settings. *Master's Abstracts International, 26,* 323.

Blount, K. R. (1989). The relationship between the parent's and five to six-year-old child's perception of life events as stressors within the Neuman health care systems framework. *Master's Abstracts International, 27,* 487.

Boyes, L. M. (1994). The effects of permanent night shift versus night shift rotation on job performance in the critical care area. *Master's Abstracts International, 32,* 1366.

Briggs, L. L. (1985). Nursing diagnoses generated from assessment data in a medical or nursing data base. *Master's Abstracts International, 23,* 470.

Brown, F. A. (1995). The effects of an eight-hour affective education program on fear of AIDS and homophobia in student nurses. *Master's Abstracts International, 33,* 1487.

Burnett, H. M. (2000). An exploratory study on the perceived health status changes in criminally victimized older adults. *Master's Abstracts International, 38,* 418.

Cava, M. A. (1991). A descriptive study of the use of coping strategies to promote wellness by individuals who have survived cancer. *Master's Abstracts International, 29,* 89.

Clevenger, M. D. (1995). Nursing activities and patient control. *Master's Abstracts International, 33,* 1835.

Cole, B. A. (1995). Patient compliance with tuberculosis preventive treatmen. *Master's Abstracts International, 33,* 1835.

Columbus, L. A. (1991). Effectiveness of a health promotion program in improving older women's ability to cope. *Master's Abstracts International, 29,* 274.

Cotten, N. C. (1993). An interdisciplinary high risk assessment tool for rehabilitation inpatient falls. *Master's Abstracts International, 31,* 1732.

Cullen, L. M. (1994). Nurses' perceptions of humor as a preventive intervention to promote the health of clients in a health care setting. *Master's Abstracts International, 32,* 592.

Donner, P. L. (1994). Maternal anxiety related to the care of an infant requiring pharmacological management for apnea of prematurity. *Master's Abstracts International, 32,* 937.

Elgar, S. J. (1992). The influence of companion animals on perceived social support and perceived stress among family caregivers. *Master's Abstracts International, 30,* 732.

Ferguson, M. J. (1995). Relationship between quiz game participation and final exam performance for nursing models. *Master's Abstracts International, 33,* 173.

Fields, W. L. (1988). The effects of the 12-hour shift on fatigue and critical thinking performance in critical care nurses. *Master's Abstracts International, 26,* 237.

Fillmore, J. A. (1993). The effects of preoperative teaching on anxiety levels of hysterectomy patients. *Master's Abstracts International, 31,* 761.

Finney, G. A. H. (1990). Spiritual needs of patients. *Master's Abstracts International, 28,* 272.

Freund, C. H. (1993). The use of nursing and related theory in school nursing practice. *Master's Abstracts International, 31,* 271.

Fukuzawa, M. (1996). Nursing care behaviors which predict patient satisfaction. *Master's Abstracts International, 34,* 1547.

Gaeta, T. V. (1990). A study to determine client satisfaction with home care services. *Master's Abstracts International, 28,* 408.

Geiger, P. A. (1996). Participation in a phase II cardiac rehabilitation program and perceived quality of life. *Master's Abstracts International, 34,* 1548.

Goldstein, L. A. (1988). Needs of spouses of hospitalized cancer patients. *Master's Abstracts International, 26,* 105.

Good, B. A. V. (1993). Efficacy of nursing intervention as secondary prevention of chronic nonorganic constipation in older adult nursing home residents: A replication study. *Master's Abstracts International, 31*, 1736.

Gray, R. (1998). The lived experience of children, ages 8-12 years, who witness family violence in the home. *Master's Abstracts International, 36*, 1327.

Greve, D. L. (1993). An examination of the efficacy of increased fiber and fluids on the establishment of voluntary bowel movements in terminally ill older adults receiving antibiotics. *Master's Abstracts International, 31*, 1203.

Gulliver, K. M. (1997). Hopelessness and spiritual well-being in persons with HIV infection. *Master's Abstracts International, 35*, 1374.

Harper, B. (1993). Nurses' beliefs about social support and the effect of nursing care on cardiac clients' attitudes in reducing cardiac risk status. *Master's Abstracts International, 31*, 273.

Haskill, K. M. (1988). Sources of occupational stress of the community health nurse. *Master's Abstracts International, 26*, 106.

Higgs, K. T. (1995). Preterm labor risk factors identified in an ambulatory perinatal setting with home uterine activity monitoring support. *Master's Abstracts International, 33*, 1490.

Holloway, C. (1995). Stress perceived among nurse managers in community health settings. *Master's Abstracts International, 33*, 1490.

Ivey, B. M. (1994). Social support and the woman with breast cancer: Issues of measurement. *Master's Abstracts International, 32*, 1628.

Johnson, K. M. (1996). Stressors of local Ontario Nurses' Association presidents. *Master's Abstracts International, 34*, 1149.

Kazakoff, K. J. (1991). The evaluation of return to work and retention of employment of cardiac patients following cardiac rehabilitation programs. *Master's Abstracts International, 29*, 450.

Kelleher, J. J. (1991). Health behaviors of HIV positive people. *Master's Abstracts International, 29*, 645.

Klimek, S. C. (1995). Identification and comparison of factors affecting breast self-examination between professional nurses and non-nursing professional women. *Master's Abstracts International, 33*, 516.

LaReau, R. M. (2000). The effect of an initial clinical nursing experience in a nursing hme on associate degree nursing student attitudes toward the elderly. *Master's Abstracts International, 38*, 420.

Larino, E. A. (1997). Determining the level of care provided by the family nurse practitioner during a deployment. *Master's Abstracts International, 35*, 1376.

Lenhart, E. M. (1994). The effect of preoperative intensive care orientation on postoperative anxiety levels in spouses of coronary artery bypass clients. *Master's Abstracts International, 32*, 1372.

Lesmond, J. S. G. (1993). Clients' perceptions of the effects of social support in their adjustment to breast cancer in a visiting nursing environment in central Ontario, Canada. *Master's Abstracts International, 31*, 276.

Lijauco, C. C. (1998). Factors related to length of stay in coronary artery bypass graft patients. *Master's Abstracts International, 36*, 512.

Maligalig, R. M. L. (1994). Parents' perceptions of the stressors of pediatric ambulatory surgery. *Master's Abstracts International, 32,* 597.

Mann, N. J. (1996). Risk behavior of adolescents who have liver disease. *Master's Abstracts International, 34,* 1150.

Mannina, J. M. (1995). The use of puretone audiometry and tympanometry to identify hearing loss and middle ear disease in school age children. *Master's Abstracts International, 33,* 1823.

Marini, S. L. (1991). A comparison of predictive validity of the Norton scale, the Daly scale, and the Braden scale. *Master's Abstracts International, 29,* 648.

Marlett, L. A. (1999). The breast feeding practices of women with a history of breast cancer. *Master's Abstracts International, 37,* 1180.

McCue, M. M. (1991). The caregiving experience of the elderly female caregiver of a spouse impaired by stroke. *Master's Abstracts International, 29* 218.

McMillan, D. E. (1997). Impact of therapeutic support of inherent coping strategies on chronic low back pain: A nursing intervention study. *Master's Abstracts International, 35,* 520.

Micevski, V. (1997). Gender differences in the presentation of physiological symptoms of myocardial infarction. *Master's Abstracts International, 35,* 520.

Miller, C. A. (1988). Effects of support on the level of anxiety for family members and/or significant others of emergency room patients. *Master's Abstracts International, 26,* 177.

Morris, D. C. (1991). Occupational stress among home care first line managers. *Master's Abstracts International, 29,* 443.

Morrison, L. A. (1993). Palliative care volunteers' descriptions of the stressors experienced in their relationship with clients coping with terminal illness at home. *Master's Abstracts International, 31,* 301.

Moynihan, B. A. (1995). A descriptive study of three male adolescent sex offenders. *Master's Abstracts International, 33,* 873.

Murphy, N. G. (1990). Factors associated with breastfeeding success and failure: A systematic integrative review (Infant nutrition). *Master's Abstracts International, 28,* 275.

Murray, M. M. (1994). Relationships among the frequency of pressure ulcer risk assessment, nursing, interventions, and the occurrence and severity of pressure ulcers. *Master's Abstracts International, 32,* 1630.

Neabel, B. (1999). A comparison of family needs perceived by nurses and family members of acutely ill brain-injured patients. *Master's Abstracts International, 37,* 592.

Newman, S. K. (1995). Perceived stressors between partnered and unpartnered women. *Master's Abstracts International, 33,* 178.

Nicholson, C. H. (1995). Client's perceptions of preparedness for discharge home following total hip or knee replacement surgery. *Master's Abstracts International, 33,* 873.

Occhi, A. M. (1993). Donation: The family's perspective. *Master's Abstracts International, 31,* 1208.

O'Neal, C. A. S. (1993). Effects of BSE on depression/anxiety in women diagnosed with breast cancer. *Master's Abstracts International, 31,* 1747.

Parker, V. J. (1995). Stress of discharge in men and women following cardiac surgery. *Master's Abstracts International, 33,* 518.

Peper, K. R. (1992). Concerns/problems experienced after discharge from an acute care setting: The patient's perspective. *Master's Abstracts International, 30,* 714.

Peters, M. R. (1998). An exploratory study of job stress and stressors in hospice administration. *Master's Abstracts International, 36,* 502.

Petock, A. M. (1991). Decubitus ulcers and physiological stressors. *Master's Abstracts International, 29,* 267.

Porritt See, J. A. S. (1994). The effects of a prenatal education program on the identification and reporting of the stressors of postpartum depression. *Master's Abstracts International, 32,* 1632.

Ramsey, B. A. (1999). Can a multidisciplinary team decrease hospital length of stay for elderly trauma patients? *Master's Abstracts International, 37,* 1182.

Robinson, C. A. (1999). The difference in perception of quality of life in patients one year after an infrainguinal bypass for critical limb ischemia. *Master's Abstracts International, 37,* 914.

Sabati, N. (1995). Relationship between Neuman's systems model's buffering property of the flexible line of defense and active participation in support groups for women. *Master's Abstracts International, 33,* 179.

St. John-Spadafore, M. J. (1994). The impact of a primary prevention program on women's perceived ability to manage stressors. *Master's Abstracts International, 32,* 943.

Sammarco, C. C. A. (1990). The study of stressors of the operating room nurse versus those of the intensive care unit nurse. *Master's Abstracts International, 28,* 276.

Scalzo Tarrant, T. (1993). Improving the frequency and proficiency of breast self examination. *Master's Abstracts International, 31,* 1211.

Scarpino, L. L. (1988). Family caregivers' perception associated with the chemotherapy treatment setting for the oncology client. *Master's Abstracts International, 26,* 424.

Semple, O. D. (1995). The experiences of family members of patients with Huntington's disease. *Master's Abstracts International, 33,* 1847.

Smith, J. A. (1995). Caregiver wellness following interventions based on interdisciplinary geriatric assessment. *Master's Abstracts International, 33,* 1707.

Story, M. (1993). Stressful life events of women. *Master's Abstracts International, 31,* 1212.

Sullivan, M. M. (1991). Comparisons of job satisfaction scores of school nurses with job satisfaction normative scores of hospital nurses. *Master's Abstracts International, 29,* 652.

Tomson, D. C. (1994). The impact of previous experience in nursing, educational background, and marital status on self-esteem among community health care workers. *Master's Abstracts International, 32,* 1172.

Triggs, D. R. (1992). The influence of a stress management class on job satisfaction and related occupational tensions in registered nurses. *Master's Abstracts International, 30,* 718.

Tudini, J. B. (1992). A survey of the psychological variables of burnout and depression among nurses. *Master's Abstracts International, 30,* 1302.

Tweed, S. A. (2000). Affective and biological responses to the inhalation of the essential oil lavender. *Master's Abstracts International, 38,* 986.

Vitthuhn, K. M. (1999). Delivery of analgesics for the postoperative thoracotomy patient. *Master's Abstracts International, 37,* 1185.

Vujakovich. M. A. (1996). Family stress and coping behaviors in families of head-injured individuals. *Master's Abstracts International, 34,* 286.

Wilkey, S. F. (1990). The effects of an eight-hour continuing education course on the death anxiety levels of registered nurses. *Master's Abstracts International, 28,* 480.

Wright, J. G. (1997). The impact of preoperative education on health locus of control, self-efficacy, and anxiety for patients undergoing total joint replacement surgery. *Master's Abstracts International, 35,* 216.

Wullschleger, L. A. (2000). Fetal infant mortality in Kalamazoo. *Master's Abstracts International, 38,* 422.

Zeliznak, C. M. (1991). Sources of occupational stress of the community health nurse. *Master's Abstracts International, 29,* 654.

CLINICAL TOOLS/EDUCATIONAL TOOLS

Baker, N. A. (1982). Use of the Neuman model in planning for the psychological needs of the respiratory disease patient. In B. Neuman (Ed.), *The Neuman Systems Model: Application to nursing education and practice* (pp. 241–51). Norwalk, CT: Appleton-Century-Crofts.

Beckman, S. J., Boxley-Harges, S., Bruick-Sorge, C., & Eichenauer, J. (1998). Evaluation modalities for assessing student and program outcomes. In L. Lowry (Ed.), *The Neuman Systems Model and nursing education: Teaching strategies and outcomes* (pp. 149–60). Indianapolis: Sigma Theta Tau International Center Nursing Press.

Beddome, G. (1989). Application of the Neuman Systems Model to the assessment of community-as-client. In B. Neuman (Ed.), *The Neuman Systems Model* (2nd ed., pp. 363–74). Norwalk, CT: Appleton & Lange.

Beddome, G. (1995). Community-as-client assessment: A Neuman-based guide for education and practice. In B. Neuman (Ed.), *The Neuman Systems Model* (3rd ed., pp. 567–79). Norwalk, CT: Appleton & Lange.

Beitler, B., Tkachuck, B., & Aamodt, D. (1980). The Neuman model applied to mental health, community health, and medical-surgical nursing. In J. P. Riehl & C. Roy (Eds.), *Conceptual models for nursing practice* (2nd ed., pp. 170–78). New York: Appleton-Century-Crofts.

Benedict, M. B., & Sproles, J. B. (1982). Application of the Neuman model to public health nursing practice. In B. Neuman (Ed.), *The Neuman Systems Model: Application to nursing education and practice* (pp. 223–40). Norwalk, CT: Appleton-Century-Crofts.

Bowman, G. E. (1982). The Neuman assessment tool adapted for child day-care centers. In B. Neuman (Ed.), *The Neuman Systems Model: Application to nursing education and practice* (pp. 324–34). Norwalk, CT: Appleton-Century-Crofts.

Breckenridge, D. M. (1982). Adaptation of the Neuman Systems Model for the renal client. In B. Neuman (Ed.), *The Neuman Systems Model: Application to nursing education and practice* (pp. 267–77). Norwalk, CT: Appleton-Century-Crofts.

Breckenridge, D. M., Cupit, M. C., & Raimondo, J. M. (1982). Systematic nursing assessment tool for the CAPD client. *Nephrology Nurse* (January/February), 24, 26–27, 30–31.

Burke, M. E. Sr., Capers, C. F., O'Connell, R. K., Quinn, R. M., & Sinnott, M. (1989). Neuman-based nursing practice in a hospital setting. In B. Neuman (Ed.), *The Neuman Systems Model* (2nd ed., pp. 423–44). Norwalk, CT: Appleton & Lange.

Cardona, V. D. (1982). Client rehabilitation and the Neuman model. In B. Neuman (Ed.), *The Neuman Systems Model: Application to nursing education and practice* (pp. 278–90). Norwalk, CT: Appleton-Century-Crofts.

Carrigg, K. C., & Weber, R. (1997). Development of the Spiritual Care Scale. Image: *Journal of Nursing Scholarship, 29*, 293.

Clark, F. (1982). The Neuman Systems Model: A clinical application for psychiatric nurse practitioners. In B. Neuman (Ed.), *The Neuman Systems Model: Application to nursing education and practice* (pp. 335–53). Norwalk, CT: Appleton-Century-Crofts.

Cotten, N. C. (1993). An interdisciplinary high risk assessment tool for rehabilitation inpatient falls. *Master's Abstracts International, 31*, 1732.

Cunningham, S. G. (1982). The Neuman model applied to an acute care setting: Pain. In B. Neuman (Ed.), *The Neuman Systems Model: Application to nursing education and practice* (pp. 291–96). Norwalk, CT: Appleton-Century-Crofts.

Dunbar, S. B. (1982). Critical care and the Neuman model. In B. Neuman (Ed.), *The Neuman Systems Model: Application to nursing education and practice* (pp. 297–307). Norwalk, CT: Appleton-Century-Crofts.

Dunn, S. I., & Trepaniér, M. J. (1989). Application of the Neuman model to perinatal nursing. In B. Neuman (Ed.), *The Neuman Systems Model* (2nd ed., pp. 407–22). Norwalk, CT: Appleton & Lange.

Felix, M., Hinds, C., Wolfe, S. C., & Martin, A. (1995). The Neuman Systems Model in a chronic care facility: A Canadian experience. In B. Neuman (Ed.), *The Neuman Systems Model* (3rd ed., pp. 549–65). Norwalk, CT: Appleton & Lange.

Flannery, J. (1991). FAMLI-RESCUE: A family assessment tool for use by neuroscience nurses in the acute care setting. *Journal of Neuroscience Nursing, 23*, 111–15.

Fulbrook, P. R. (1991). The application of the Neuman Systems Model to intensive care. *Intensive Care Nursing, 7*, 28–39.

Gunter, L. M. (1982). Application of the Neuman Systems Model to gerontic nursing. In B. Neuman (Ed.), *The Neuman Systems Model: Application to nursing education and practice* (pp. 196–210). Norwalk, CT: Appleton-Century-Crofts.

Hinton-Walker, P., & Raborn, M. (1989). Application of the Neuman model in nursing administration and practice. In B. Henry, C. Arndt, M. DiVincenti, & A. Marriner-Tomey (Eds.), *Dimensions of nursing administration: Theory, research, education, and practice* (pp. 711–23). Boston: Blackwell Scientific Publications.

Johnson, M. N., Vaughn-Wrobel, B., Ziegler, S., et al. (1982). Use of the Neuman Health-Care Systems Model in the master's curriculum: Texas Woman's University.

In B. Neuman (Ed.), *The Neuman Systems Model: Application to nursing education and practice* (pp. 130–52). Norwalk, CT: Appleton-Century-Crofts.

Kelley, J. A., & Sanders, N. F. (1995). A systems approach to the health of nursing and health care organizations. In B. Neuman (Ed.), *The Neuman Systems Model* (3rd ed., pp. 347–64). Norwalk, CT: Appleton & Lange.

Kelley, J. A., Sanders, N. F., & Pierce, J. D. (1989). A systems approach to the role of the nurse administrator in education and practice. In B. Neuman (Ed.), *The Neuman Systems Model* (2nd ed., pp. 115–38). Norwalk, CT: Appleton & Lange.

Lowry, L. (1998). Efficacy of the Neuman Systems Model as a curriculum framework: A longitudinal study. In L. Lowry (Ed.), *The Neuman Systems Model and nursing education: Teaching strategies and outcomes* (pp. 139–47). Indianapolis: Sigma Theta Tau International Center Nursing Press.

Lowry, L. W., & Jopp, M. C. (1989). An evaluation instrument for assessing an associate degree nursing curriculum based on the Neuman Systems Model. In J. P. Riehl-Sisca (Ed.), *Conceptual models for nursing practice* (3rd ed., pp. 73–85). Norwalk, CT: Appleton & Lange.

Lowry, L. W., & Newsome, G. G. (1995). Neuman–based associate degree programs: Past, present, and future. In B. Neuman (Ed.), *The Neuman Systems Model* (3rd ed., pp. 197–214). Norwalk, CT: Appleton & Lange.

McGee, M. (1995). Implications for use of the Neuman Systems Model in occupational health nursing. In B. Neuman (Ed.), *The Neuman Systems Model* (3rd ed., pp. 657–67). Norwalk, CT: Appleton & Lange.

McHolm, F. A., & Geib, K. M. (1998). Application of the Neuman Systems Model to teaching health assessment and nursing process. Nursing Diagnosis: *The Journal of Nursing Language and Classification, 9,* 23–33.

McInerney, K. A. (1982). The Neuman Systems Model applied to critical care nursing of cardiac surgery clients. In B. Neuman (Ed.), *The Neuman Systems Model: Application to nursing education and practice* (pp. 308–15). Norwalk, CT: Appleton-Century-Crofts.

Mirenda, R. M. (1986). The Neuman model in practice. *Senior Nurse, 5*(3), 26–27.

Mischke-Berkey, K., & Hanson, S. M. H. (1991). *Pocket guide to family assessment and intervention.* St. Louis: Mosby-Year Book.

Mischke-Berkey, K., Warner, P., & Hanson, S. (1989). Family health assessment and intervention. In P. J. Bomar (Ed.), *Nurses and family health promotion: Concepts, assessment, and interventions* (pp. 115–54). Baltimore: Williams and Wilkins.

Murphy, N. G. (1990). Factors associated with breastfeeding success and failure: A systematic integrative review (infant nutrition). *Master's Abstracts International, 28,* 275.

Neuman, B. (1989). The Neuman Systems Model. In B. Neuman (Ed.), *The Neuman Systems Model* (2nd ed., pp. 3–63). Norwalk, CT: Appleton & Lange.

Neuman, B. (1995a). In conclusion—toward new beginnings. In B. Neuman (Ed.), *The Neuman Systems Model* (3rd ed., pp. 671–703). Norwalk, CT: Appleton & Lange.

Neuman, B. (1995b). The Neuman Systems Model. In B. Neuman (Ed.), *The Neuman Systems Model* (3rd ed., pp. 3–61). Norwalk, CT: Appleton & Lange.

Reed, K. (1982). The Neuman Systems Model: A basis for family psychosocial assessment. In B. Neuman (Ed.), *The Neuman Systems Model: Application to nursing education and practice* (pp. 188–95). Norwalk, CT: Appleton-Century-Crofts.

Schlentz, M. D. (1993). The minimum data set and the levels of prevention in the long-term care facility. *Geriatric Nursing, 14,* 79–83.

Strickland-Seng, V. (1995). The Neuman Systems Model in clinical evaluation of students. In B. Neuman (Ed.), *The Neuman Systems Model* (3rd ed., pp. 215–25). Norwalk, CT: Appleton & Lange.

Strickland-Seng, V. (1998). Clinical evaluation: The heart of clinical performance. In L. Lowry (Ed.), *The Neuman Systems Model and nursing education: Teaching strategies and outcomes* (pp. 129–34). Indianapolis: Sigma Theta Tau International Center Nursing Press.

Tollett, S. M. (1982). Teaching geriatrics and gerontology: use of the Neuman Systems Model. In B. Neuman (Ed.), *The Neuman Systems Model: Application to nursing education and practice* (pp. 1159–64). Norwalk, CT: Appleton-Century-Crofts.

Trépanier, M. J., Dunn, S. I., & Sprague, A. E. (1995). Application of the Neuman Systems Model to perinatal nursing. In B. Neuman (Ed.), *The Neuman Systems Model* (3rd ed., pp. 309–20). Norwalk, CT: Appleton & Lange.

Ziegler, S. M. (1982). Taxonomy for nursing diagnosis derived from the Neuman Systems Model. In B. Neuman (Ed.), *The Neuman Systems Model: Application to nursing education and practice* (pp. 55–68). Norwalk, CT: Appleton-Century-Crofts.

EDUCATION

Baker, N. A. (1982a). The Neuman Systems Model as a conceptual framework for continuing education in the work place. In B. Neuman (Ed.), *The Neuman Systems Model: Application to nursing education and practice* (pp. 260–64). Norwalk, CT: Appleton-Century-Crofts.

Baker, N. A. (1982b). Use of the Neuman model in planning for the psychological needs of the respiratory disease patient. In B. Neuman (Ed.), *The Neuman Systems Model: Application to nursing education and practice* (pp. 241–51). Norwalk, CT: Appleton-Century-Crofts.

Beckman, S. J., Boxley-Harges, S., Bruick-Sorge, C., & Eichenauer, J. (1998a). Critical thinking, the Neuman Systems Model, and associate degree education. In L. Lowry (Ed.), *The Neuman Systems Model and nursing education: Teaching strategies and outcomes* (pp. 53–58). Indianapolis: Sigma Theta Tau International Center Nursing Press.

Beckman, S. J., Boxley-Harges, S., Bruick-Sorge, C., & Eichenauer, J. (1998b). Evaluation modalities for assessing student and program outcomes. In L. Lowry (Ed.), *The Neuman Systems Model and nursing education: Teaching strategies and outcomes* (pp. 149–60). Indianapolis: Sigma Theta Tau International Center Nursing Press.

Beitler, B., Tkachuck, B., & Aamodt, D. (1980). The Neuman model applied to mental health, community health, and medical-surgical nursing. In J. P. Riehl & C. Roy (Eds.), *Conceptual models for nursing practice* (2nd ed., pp. 170–78). New York: Appleton-Century-Crofts.

Beyea, S., & Matzo, M. (1989). Assessing elders using the functional health pattern assessment model. *Nurse Educator, 14*(5), 32–37.

Bloch, C., & Bloch, C. (1995). Teaching content and process of the Neuman Systems Model. In B. Neuman (Ed.), *The Neuman Systems Model* (3rd ed., pp. 175–82). Norwalk, CT: Appleton & Lange.

Bourbonnais, F. F., & Ross, M. M. (1985). The Neuman Systems Model in nursing education: Course development and implementation. *Journal of Advanced Nursing, 10,* 117–23.

Bruton, M. R., & Matzo, M. (1989). Curriculum revisions at Saint Anselm College: Focus on the older adult. In B. Neuman (Ed.), *The Neuman Systems Model* (2nd ed., pp. 201–10). Norwalk, CT: Appleton & Lange.

Busch, P., & Lynch, M. H. (1998). Creative teaching strategies in a Neuman-based baccalaureate curriculum. In L. Lowry (Ed.), *The Neuman Systems Model and nursing education: Teaching strategies and outcomes* (pp. 59–69). Indianapolis: Sigma Theta Tau International Center Nursing Press.

Capers, C. F. (1986). Some basic facts about models, nursing conceptualizations, and nursing theories. *Journal of Continuing Education, 16,* 149–54.

Chang, N. J., & Freese, B. T. (1998). Teaching culturally competent care: A Korean-American experience. In L. Lowry (Ed.), *The Neuman Systems Model and nursing education: Teaching strategies and outcomes* (pp. 85–90). Indianapolis: Sigma Theta Tau International Center Nursing Press.

Conners, V. L. (1982). Teaching the Neuman Systems Model: An approach to student and faculty development. In B. Neuman (Ed.), *The Neuman Systems Model: Application to nursing education and practice* (pp. 176–81). Norwalk, CT: Appleton-Century-Crofts.

Conners, V. L. (1989). An empirical evaluation of the Neuman Systems Model: The University of Missouri-Kansas City. In B. Neuman (Ed.), *The Neuman Systems Model* (2nd ed., pp. 249–58). Norwalk, CT: Appleton & Lange.

Conners, V., Harmon, V. M., & Langford, R. W. (1982). Course development and implementation using the Neuman Systems Model as a framework: Texas Woman's University (Houston Campus). In B. Neuman (Ed.), *The Neuman Systems Model: Application to nursing education and practice* (pp. 153–58). Norwalk, CT: Appleton-Century-Crofts.

Craig, D. M. (1995). The Neuman model: Examples of its use in Canadian educational programs. In B. Neuman (Ed.), *The Neuman Systems Model* (3rd ed., pp. 521–27). Norwalk, CT: Appleton & Lange.

Dale, M. L., & Savala, S.M. (1990). A new approach to the senior practicum. *Nursing-Connections, 3*(1), 45–51.

Dyck, S. M., Innes, J. E., Rae, D. I., & Sawatzky, J. E. (1989). The Neuman Systems Model in curriculum revision: A baccalaureate program, University of Saskatchewan. In B. Neuman (Ed.), *The Neuman Systems Model* (2nd ed., pp. 225–36). Norwalk, CT: Appleton & Lange.

Edwards, P. A., & Kittler, A. W. (1991). Integrating rehabilitation content in nursing curricula. *Rehabilitation Nursing, 16,* 70–73.

Engberg, I. B. (1995). Brief abstracts: Use of the Neuman Systems Model in Sweden. In

B. Neuman (Ed.), *The Neuman Systems Model* (3rd ed., pp. 653–56). Norwalk, CT: Appleton & Lange.

Engberg, I. B., Bjälming, E., & Bertilson, B. (1995). A structure for documenting primary health care in Sweden using the Neuman Systems Model. In B. Neuman (Ed.), *The Neuman Systems Model* (3rd ed., pp. 637–51). Norwalk, CT: Appleton & Lange.

Evans, B. (1998). Fourth-generation evaluation and the Neuman Systems Model. In L. Lowry (Ed.), *The Neuman Systems Model and nursing education: Teaching strategies and outcomes* (pp. 117–27). Indianapolis: Sigma Theta Tau International Center Nursing Press.

Freese, B. T., & Scales, C. J. (1998). NSM-based care as an NLN program evaluation outcome. In L. Lowry (Ed.), *The Neuman Systems Model and nursing education: Teaching strategies and outcomes* (pp. 135–38). Indianapolis: Sigma Theta Tau International Center Nursing Press.

Freiburger, O. A. (1998). The Neuman Systems Model, critical thinking, and cooperative learning in a nursing issues course. In L. Lowry (Ed.), *The Neuman Systems Model and nursing education: Teaching strategies and outcomes* (pp. 79–84). Indianapolis: Sigma Theta Tau International Center Nursing Press.

Glazebrook, R. S. (1995). The Neuman Systems Model in cooperative baccalaureate nursing education: The Minnesota Intercollegiate Nursing Consortium experience. In B. Neuman (Ed.), *The Neuman Systems Model* (3rd ed., pp. 227–30). Norwalk, CT: Appleton & Lange.

Harty, M. B. (1982). Continuing education in nursing and the Neuman model. In B. Neuman (Ed.), *The Neuman Systems Model: Application to nursing education and practice* (pp. 100–106). Norwalk, CT: Appleton-Century-Crofts.

Hassell, J. S. (1998). Critical thinking strategies for family and community client systems. In L. Lowry (Ed.), *The Neuman Systems Model and nursing education: Teaching strategies and outcomes* (pp. 71–77). Indianapolis: Sigma Theta Tau International Center Nursing Press.

Hilton, S. A., & Grafton, M. D. (1995). Curriculum transition based on the Neuman Systems Model: Los Angeles County Medical Center School of Nursing. In B. Neuman (Ed.), *The Neuman Systems Model* (3rd ed., pp. 163–74). Norwalk, CT: Appleton & Lange.

Johansen, H. (1989). Neuman model concepts in joint use—community health practice and student teaching—School of Advanced Nursing Education, Aarhus University, Aarhus, Denmark. In B. Neuman (Ed.), *The Neuman Systems Model* (2nd ed., pp. 334–62). Norwalk, CT: Appleton & Lange.

Johnson, M. N., Vaughn-Wrobel, B., Ziegler, S., Hough, L., Bush, H. A., & Kurtz, P. (1982). Use of the Neuman Health-Care systems model in the master's curriculum: Texas Woman's University. In B. Neuman (Ed.), *The Neuman Systems Model: Application to nursing education and practice* (pp. 130–52). Norwalk, CT: Appleton-Century-Crofts.

Johnson, S. E. (1989). A picture is worth a thousand words: Helping students visualize a conceptual model. *Nurse Educator, 14*(3), 21–24.

Kilchenstein, L., & Yakulis, I. (1984). The birth of a curriculum: Utilization of the Betty Neuman health care systems model in an integrated baccalaureate program. *Journal of Nursing Education, 23,* 126–27.

Klotz, L. C. (1995). Integration of the Neuman Systems Model into the BSN curriculum at the University of Texas at Tyler. In B. Neuman (Ed.), *The Neuman Systems Model* (3rd ed., pp. 183–95). Norwalk, CT: Appleton & Lange.

Knox, J. E., Kilchenstein, L., & Yakulis, I. M. (1982). Utilization of the Neuman model in an integrated baccalaureate program: University of Pittsburgh. In B. Neuman (Ed.), *The Neuman Systems Model: Application to nursing education and practice* (pp. 117–23). Norwalk, CT: Appleton-Century-Crofts.

Laschinger, S. J., Maloney, R., & Tranmer, J. E. (1989). An evaluation of student use of the Neuman Systems Model: Queen's University, Canada. In B. Neuman (Ed.), *The Neuman Systems Model* (2nd ed., pp. 211–24). Norwalk, CT: Appleton & Lange.

Lebold, M., & Davis, L. (1980). A baccalaureate nursing curriculum based on the Neuman health systems model. In. J. P. Riehl & C. Roy (Eds.), *Conceptual models for nursing practice* (2nd ed., pp 151–58). New York: Appleton-Century-Crofts.

Lebold, M. M., & Davis, L. H. (1982). A baccalaureate nursing curriculum based on the Neuman Systems Model: Saint Xavier College. In B. Neuman (Ed.), *The Neuman Systems Model: Application to nursing education and practice* (pp. 124–29). Norwalk, CT: Appleton-Century-Crofts.

Louis, M., Witt, R., & LaMancusa, M. (1989). The Neuman Systems Model in multilevel nurse education programs: University of Nevada, Las Vegas. In B. Neuman (Ed.), *The Neuman Systems Model* (2nd ed., pp. 237–48). Norwalk, CT: Appleton & Lange.

Lowry, L. (1986). Adapted by degrees. *Senior Nurse, 5*(3), 25–26.

Lowry, L. (1988). Operationalizing the Neuman Systems Model: A course in concepts and process. *Nurse Educator, 13*(3), 19–22.

Lowry, L. (1998). Efficacy of the Neuman Systems Model as a curriculum framework: A longitudinal study. In L. Lowry (Ed.), *The Neuman Systems Model and nursing education: Teaching strategies and outcomes* (pp. 139–47). Indianapolis: Sigma Theta Tau International Center Nursing Press.

Lowry, L., Bruick-Sorge, C., Freese, B. T., & Sutherland, R. (1998). Development and renewal of faculty for Neuman-based teaching. In L. Lowry (Ed.), *The Neuman Systems Model and nursing education: Teaching strategies and outcomes* (pp. 161–66). Indianapolis: Sigma Theta Tau International Center Nursing Press.

Lowry, L., & Green, G. H. (1989). Four Neuman-based associate degree programs: Brief description and evaluation. In B. Neuman (Ed.), *The Neuman Systems Model* (2nd ed., pp. 283–12). Norwalk, CT: Appleton & Lange.

Lowry, L. W., & Jopp, M. C. (1989). An evaluation instrument for assessing an associate degree nursing curriculum based on the Neuman Systems Model. In J. P. Riehl-Sisca (Ed.), *Conceptual models for nursing practice* (3rd ed., pp. 73–85). Norwalk, CT: Appleton & Lange.

Lowry, L. W., & Newsome, G. G. (1995). Neuman-based associate degree programs: Past, present, and future. In B. Neuman (Ed.), *The Neuman Systems Model* (3rd ed., pp. 197–214). Norwalk, CT: Appleton & Lange.

McCulloch, S. J. (1995). Utilization of the Neuman Systems Model: University of South Australia. In B. Neuman (Ed.), *The Neuman Systems Model* (3rd ed., pp. 591–97). Norwalk, CT: Appleton & Lange.

McHolm, F. A., & Geib, K. M. (1998). Application of the Neuman Systems Model to teaching health assessment and nursing process. Nursing Diagnosis: *The Journal of Nursing Language and Classification, 9,* 23–33.

Mirenda, R. M. (1986). The Neuman Systems Model: Description and application. In P. Winstead-Fry (Ed.), *Case studies in nursing theory* (pp. 127–66). New York: National League for Nursing.

Moxley, P. A., & Allen, L. M. H. (1982). The Neuman Systems Model approach in a master's degree program: Northwestern State University. In B. Neuman (Ed.), *The Neuman Systems Model: Application to nursing education and practice* (pp. 168–75). Norwalk, CT: Appleton-Century-Crofts.

Mrkonich, D. E., Hessian, M., & Miller, M. W. (1989). A cooperative process in curriculum development using the Neuman health-care systems model. In J. P. Riehl-Sisca (Ed.), *Conceptual models for nursing practice* (3rd ed., pp. 87–94). Norwalk, CT: Appleton & Lange.

Mrkonich, D., Miller, M., & Hessian, M. (1989). Cooperative baccalaureate education: The Minnesota intercollegiate nursing consortium. In B. Neuman (Ed.), *The Neuman Systems Model* (2nd ed., pp. 175–82). Norwalk, CT: Appleton & Lange.

Nelson, L. F., Hansen, M., & McCullagh, M. (1989). A new baccalaureate North Dakota-Minnesota nursing education consortium. In B. Neuman (Ed.), *The Neuman Systems Model* (2nd ed., pp. 183–92). Norwalk, CT: Appleton & Lange.

Neuman, B. (1995). In conclusion—toward new beginnings. In B. Neuman (Ed.), *The Neuman Systems Model* (3rd ed., pp. 671–703). Norwalk, CT: Appleton & Lange.

Neuman, B., & Wyatt, M. (1980). The Neuman Stress/Adaptation systems approach to education for nurse administrators. In J. P. Riehl & C. Roy (Eds.), *Conceptual models for nursing practice* (2nd ed., pp. 142–50). New York: Appleton-Century-Crofts.

Nichols, E. G., Dale, M. L., & Turley, J. (1989). The University of Wyoming evaluation of a Neuman–based curriculum. In B. Neuman (Ed.), *The Neuman Systems Model* (2nd ed., pp. 259–82). Norwalk, CT: Appleton & Lange.

Nuttall, P., Stittich, E. M., & Flores, F. C. (1998). The Neuman Systems Model in advanced practice nursing. In L. Lowry (Ed.), *The Neuman Systems Model and nursing education: Teaching strategies and outcomes* (pp. 109–14). Indianapolis: Sigma Theta Tau International Center Nursing Press.

Peternelj-Taylor, C. A., & Johnson, R. (1996). Custody and caring: Clinical placement of student nurses in a forensic setting. *Perspectives in Psychiatric Care, 32*(4), 23–29.

Reed-Sorrow, K., Harmon, R. L., & Kitundu, M.E. (1989). Computer-assisted learning and the Neuman Systems Model. In B. Neuman (Ed.), *The Neuman Systems Model* (2nd ed., pp. 155–60). Norwalk, CT: Appleton & Lange.

Roberts, A. G. (1994). Effective inservice education process. *Oklahoma Nurse, 39*(4), 11.

Ross, M. M., Bourbonnais, F. F., & Carroll, G. (1987). Curricular design and the Betty Neuman Systems Model: A new approach to learning. *International Nursing Review, 34,* 75–79.

Sipple, J. A., & Freese, B. T. (1989). Transition from technical to professional-level nursing education. In B. Neuman (Ed.), *The Neuman Systems Model* (2nd ed., pp. 193–200). Norwalk, CT: Appleton & Lange.

Stittich, E. M., Avent, C. L., & Patterson, K. (1989). Neuman-based baccalaureate and graduate nursing programs, California State University, Fresno. In B. Neuman (Ed.), *The Neuman Systems Model* (2nd ed., pp. 163–74). Norwalk, CT: Appleton & Lange.

Stittich, E. M., Flores, F. C., & Nuttall, P. (1995). Cultural considerations in a Neuman–based curriculum. In B. Neuman (Ed.), *The Neuman Systems Model* (3rd ed., pp. 147–62). Norwalk, CT: Appleton & Lange.

Story, E. L., & DuGas, B. W. (1988). A teaching strategy to facilitate conceptual model implementation in practice. *Journal of Continuing Education in Nursing, 19,* 244–47.

Story, E. L., & Ross, M. M. (1986). Family centered community health nursing and the Betty Neuman Systems Model. *Nursing Papers, 18*(2), 77–88.

Strickland-Seng, V. (1995). The Neuman Systems Model in clinical evaluation of students. In B. Neuman (Ed.), *The Neuman Systems Model* (3rd ed., pp. 215–25). Norwalk, CT: Appleton & Lange.

Strickland-Seng, V. (1998). Clinical evaluation: The heart of clinical performance. In L. Lowry (Ed.), *The Neuman Systems Model and nursing education: Teaching strategies and outcomes* (pp. 129–34). Indianapolis: Sigma Theta Tau International Center Nursing Press.

Strickland-Seng, V., Mirenda, R., & Lowry, L. W. (1996). The Neuman Systems Model in nursing education. In P. Hinton Walker & B. Neuman (Eds.), *Blueprint for use of nursing models* (pp. 91–140). New York: NLN Press.

Sutherland, R. & Forrest, D. L. (1998). Primary prevention in an associate of science curriculum. In L. Lowry (Ed.), *The Neuman Systems Model and nursing education: Teaching strategies and outcomes* (pp. 99–108). Indianapolis: Sigma Theta Tau International Center Nursing Press.

Tollett, S. M. (1982). Teaching geriatrics and gerontology: use of the Neuman Systems Model. In B. Neuman (Ed.), *The Neuman Systems Model: Application to nursing education and practice* (pp. 1159–64). Norwalk, CT: Appleton-Century-Crofts.

Weitzel, A., & Wood, K. (1998). Community health nursing: Keystone of baccalaureate education. In L. Lowry (Ed.), *The Neuman Systems Model and nursing education: Teaching strategies and outcomes* (pp. 91–98). Indianapolis: Sigma Theta Tau International Center Nursing Press.

ADMINISTRATION

Beynon, C. E. (1995). Neuman–based experiences of the Middlesex-London health unit. In B. Neuman (Ed.), *The Neuman Systems Model* (3rd ed., pp. 537–47). Norwalk, CT: Appleton & Lange.

Burke, M. E. Sr., Capers, C. F., O'Connell, R. K., Quinn, R. M., & Sinnott, M. (1989). Neuman–based nursing practice in a hospital setting. In B. Neuman (Ed.), *The Neuman Systems Model* (2nd ed., pp. 423–44). Norwalk, CT: Appleton & Lange.

Capers, C. F., & Kelly, R. (1987). Neuman nursing process: A model of holistic care. *Holistic Nursing Practice, 1*(3), 19–26.

Capers, C. F., O'Brien, C., Quinn, R., Kelly, R., & Fenerty, A. (1985). The Neuman Systems Model in practice. Planning phase. *Journal of Nursing Administration, 15*(5), 29–39.

Caramanica, L., & Thibodeau, J. (1987). Nursing philosophy and the selection of a model for practice. *Nursing Management, 10*(10), 71.

Caramanica, L., & Thibodeau, J. (1989). Developing a hospital nursing philosophy and selecting a model for practice. In B. Neuman (Ed.), *The Neuman Systems Model* (2nd ed., pp. 441–43). Norwalk, CT: Appleton & Lange.

Craig, D. M. (1995). Community/public health nursing in Canada: Use of the Neuman Systems Model in a new paradigm. In B. Neuman (Ed.), *The Neuman Systems Model* (3rd ed., pp. 529–35). Norwalk, CT: Appleton & Lange.

Craig, D., & Beynon, C. (1996). Nursing administration and the Neuman Systems Model. In P. Hinton Walker & B. Neuman (Eds.), *Blueprint for use of nursing models* (pp. 251–74). New York: NLN Press.

Craig, D. M., & Morris-Coulter, C. (1995). Neuman implementation in a Canadian psychiatric facility. In B. Neuman (Ed.), *The Neuman Systems Model* (3rd ed., pp. 397–406). Norwalk, CT: Appleton & Lange.

Davies, P. (1989). In Wales: Use of the Neuman Systems Model by community psychiatric nurses. In B. Neuman (Ed.), *The Neuman Systems Model* (2nd ed., pp. 375–84). Norwalk, CT: Appleton & Lange.

Davies, P., & Proctor, H. (1995). In Wales: Using the model in community mental health nursing. In B. Neuman (Ed.), *The Neuman Systems Model* (3rd ed., pp. 621–27). Norwalk, CT: Appleton & Lange.

Drew, L. L., Craig, D. M., & Beynon, C. E. (1989). The Neuman Systems Model for community health administration and practice: Provinces of Manitoba and Ontario, Canada. In B. Neuman (Ed.), *The Neuman Systems Model* (2nd ed., pp. 315–42). Norwalk, CT: Appleton & Lange.

Dunn, S. I., & Trepaniér, M. J. (1989). Application of the Neuman model to perinatal nursing. In B. Neuman (Ed.), *The Neuman Systems Model* (2nd ed., pp. 407–22). Norwalk, CT: Appleton & Lange.

Dwyer, C. M., Walker, P. H., Suchman, A., & Coggiola, P. (1995). Opportunities and obstacles: Development of a true collaborative practice with physicians. In B. Murphy (Ed.), *Nursing centers: The time is now* (pp. 135–55). New York: National League for Nursing.

Echlin, D. J. (1982). Palliative care and the Neuman model. In B. Neuman (Ed.), *The Neuman Systems Model: Application to nursing education and practice* (pp. 257–59). Norwalk, CT: Appleton-Century-Crofts.

Engberg, I. B. (1995). Brief abstracts: Use of the Neuman Systems Model in Sweden. In B. Neuman (Ed.), *The Neuman Systems Model* (3rd ed., pp. 653–56). Norwalk, CT: Appleton & Lange.

Felix, M., Hinds, C., Wolfe, S. C., & Martin, A. (1995). The Neuman Systems Model in a chronic care facility: A Canadian experience. In B. Neuman (Ed.), *The Neuman Systems Model* (3rd ed., pp. 549–65). Norwalk, CT: Appleton & Lange.

Frioux, T. D., Roberts, A. G., & Butler, S. J. (1995). Oklahoma state public health nursing: Neuman-based. In B. Neuman (Ed.), *The Neuman Systems Model* (3rd ed., pp. 407–14). Norwalk, CT: Appleton & Lange.

Fulbrook, P. R. (1991). The application of the Neuman Systems Model to intensive care. *Intensive Care Nursing, 7,* 28–39.

Hinton-Walker, P. (1994). Dollars and sense in health reform: Interdisciplinary practice and community nursing centers. *Nursing Administration Quarterly, 19*(1), 1–11.

Hinton-Walker, P. (1995). Neuman-based education, practice, and research in a community nursing center. In B. Neuman (Ed.), *The Neuman Systems Model* (3rd ed., pp. 415–30). Norwalk, CT: Appleton & Lange.

Hinton-Walker, P. (1996). Blueprint example: An integrated model for evaluation, research, and policy analysis in the context of managed care. In P. Hinton-Walker & B. Neuman (Eds.), *Blueprint for use of nursing models* (pp. 11–30). New York: NLN Press.

Hinton-Walker, P., & Raborn, M. (1989). Application of the Neuman model in nursing administration and practice. In B. Henry, C. Arndt, M. DiVincenti, & A. Marriner-Tomey (Eds.), *Dimensions of nursing administration. Theory, research, education, and practice* (pp. 711–23). Boston: Blackwell Scientific Publications.

Johns, C. (1991). The Burford Nursing Development Unit holistic model of nursing practice. *Journal of Advanced Nursing, 16,* 1090–98.

Mann, A. H., Hazel, C., Geer, C., Hurley, C. M., & Podrapovic, T. (1993). Development of an orthopaedic case manager role. *Orthopaedic Nursing, 12*(4), 23–27, 62.

Moynihan, M. M. (1990). Implementation of the Neuman Systems Model in an acute care nursing department. In M. E. Parker (Ed.), *Nursing theories in practice* (pp. 263–73). New York: National League for Nursing.

Mytka, S., & Beynon, C. (1994). A model for public health nursing in the Middlesex-London, Ontario, schools. *Journal of School Health, 64,* 85–88.

Neuman, B. (1995). In conclusion—toward new beginnings. In B. Neuman (Ed.), *The Neuman Systems Model* (3rd ed., pp. 671–703). Norwalk, CT: Appleton & Lange.

Pinkerton, A. (1974). Use of the Neuman model in a home health-care agency. In J. P. Riehl & C. Roy (Eds.), *Conceptual models for nursing practice* (pp. 122–29). New York: Appleton-Century-Crofts.

Reitano, J. K. (1997). Learning through experience—Chester Community Nursing Center: A Healthy Partnership. *Accent Magazine* [Neumann College], fall, 11.

Roberts, A. G. (1994). Effective inservice education process. *Oklahoma Nurse, 39*(4), 11.

Rodriguez, M. L. (1995). The Neuman Systems Model adapted to a continuing care retirement community. In B. Neuman (Ed.), *The Neuman Systems Model* (3rd ed., pp. 431–42). Norwalk, CT: Appleton & Lange.

Schlentz, M. D. (1993). The minimum data set and the levels of prevention in the long-term care facility. *Geriatric Nursing, 14,* 79–83.

Scicchitani, B., Cox, J. G., Heyduk, L. J., Maglicco, P. A., & Sargent, N. A. (1995). Implementing the Neuman model in a psychiatric hospital. In B. Neuman (Ed.), *The Neuman Systems Model* (3rd ed., pp. 387–95). Norwalk, CT: Appleton & Lange.

Verberk, F. (1995). In Holland: Application of the Neuman model in psychiatric nursing. In B. Neuman (Ed.), *The Neuman Systems Model* (3rd ed., pp. 629–36). Norwalk, CT: Appleton & Lange.

PRACTICE

Anderson, E., McFarlane, J., & Helton, A. (1986). Community-as-Client: A model for practice. *Nursing Outlook, 34,* 220–24.

Baerg, K. L. (1991). Using Neuman's model to analyze a clinical situation. *Rehabilitation Nursing, 16,* 38–39.

Baker, N. A. (1982). Use of the Neuman model in planning for the psychological needs of the respiratory disease patient. In B. Neuman (Ed.), *The Neuman Systems Model: Application to nursing education and practice* (pp. 241–51). Norwalk, CT: Appleton-Century-Crofts.

Beckingham, A. C., & Baumann, A. (1990). The ageing family in crisis: Assessment and decision-making models. *Journal of Advanced Nursing, 15,* 782–87.

Beddome, G. (1989). Application of the Neuman Systems Model to the assessment of community-as-client. In B. Neuman (Ed.), *The Neuman Systems Model* (2nd ed., pp. 363–74). Norwalk, CT: Appleton & Lange.

Beitler, B., Tkachuck, B., & Aamodt, D. (1980). The Neuman model applied to mental health, community health, and medical-surgical nursing. In J. P. Riehl & C. Roy (Eds.), *Conceptual models for nursing practice* (2nd ed., pp. 170–78). New York: Appleton-Century-Crofts.

Benedict, M. B., & Sproles, J. B. (1982). Application of the Neuman model to public health nursing practice. In B. Neuman (Ed.), *The Neuman Systems Model: Application to nursing education and practice* (pp. 223–40). Norwalk, CT: Appleton-Century-Crofts.

Bergstrom, D. (1992). Hypermetabolism in multisystem organ failure: A Neuman systems perspective. *Critical Care Nursing Quarterly, 15*(3), 63–70.

Beyea, S., & Matzo, M. (1989). Assessing elders using the functional health pattern assessment model. *Nurse Educator, 14*(5), 32–37.

Biley, F. C. (1989). Stress in high dependency units. *Intensive Care Nursing, 5,* 134–41.

Breckenridge, D. M. (1982). Adaptation of the Neuman Systems Model for the renal client. In B. Neuman (Ed.), *The Neuman Systems Model: Application to nursing education and practice* (pp. 267–77). Norwalk, CT: Appleton-Century-Crofts.

Breckenridge, D. M. (1989). Primary prevention as an intervention modality for the renal client. In B. Neuman (Ed.), *The Neuman Systems Model* (2nd ed., pp. 397–406). Norwalk, CT: Appleton & Lange.

Bueno, M. M., & Sengin, K. K. (1995). The Neuman Systems Model for critical care nursing: A framework for practice. In B. Neuman (Ed.), *The Neuman Systems Model* (3rd ed., pp. 275–91). Norwalk, CT: Appleton & Lange.

Bullock, L. F. C. (1993). Nursing interventions for abused women on obstetrical units. *AWHONN's Clinical Issues in Perinatal and Women's Health Nursing, 4*(3), 371–77.

Cardona, V. D. (1982). Client rehabilitation and the Neuman model. In B. Neuman (Ed.), *The Neuman Systems Model: Application to nursing education and practice* (pp. 278–90). Norwalk, CT: Appleton-Century-Crofts.

Cheung, Y. L. (1997). The application of Neuman System Model to nursing in Hong Kong? *Hong Kong Nursing Journal, 33*(4), 17–21.

Chiverton, P., & Flannery, J. C. (1995). Cognitive impairment; use of the Neuman Systems Model. In B. Neuman (Ed.), *The Neuman Systems Model* (3rd ed., pp. 249–61). Norwalk, CT: Appleton & Lange.

Clark, F. (1982). The Neuman Systems Model: A clinical application for psychiatric nurse practitioners. In B. Neuman (Ed.), *The Neuman Systems Model: Application to nursing education and practice* (pp. 335–53). Norwalk, CT: Appleton-Century-Crofts.

Clark, J. (1982). Development of models and theories on the concept of nursing. *Journal of Advanced Nursing, 7,* 129–34.

Cook, K. R. (1999). Assessment of potential inhalant use by students. *Journal of School Nursing, 15*(5), 20–23.

Cookfair, J. M. (1996). Community as client. In J. M. Cookfair (Ed.), *Nursing care in the community* (2nd ed., pp. 19–37). St. Louis: Mosby-Year Book.

Cowperthwaite, B., LaPlante, K., Mahon, B., & Markowski, T. (1997). Latex allergy in the nursing population. *Canadian Operating Room Nursing Journal, 15*(2), 23–24, 26–28, 30–32.

Cunningham, S. G. (1982). The Neuman model applied to an acute care setting: Pain. In B. Neuman (Ed.), *The Neuman Systems Model: Application to nursing education and practice* (pp. 291–96). Norwalk, CT: Appleton-Century-Crofts.

Cunningham, S. G. (1983). The Neuman Systems Model applied to a rehabilitation setting. *Rehabilitation Nursing, 8*(4), 20–22.

Delunas, L. R. (1990). Prevention of elder abuse: Betty Neuman health care systems approach. *Clinical Nurse Specialist, 4,* 54–58.

Echlin, D. J. (1982). Palliative care and the Neuman model. In B. Neuman (Ed.), *The Neuman Systems Model: Application to nursing education and practice* (pp. 257–59). Norwalk, CT: Appleton-Century-Crofts.

Fawcett, J. (1997). Conceptual models as guides for psychiatric nursing practice. In A. W. Burgess (Ed.), *Psychiatric nursing: Promoting mental health* (pp. 627–42). Stamford, CT: Appleton & Lange.

Fawcett, J., Archer, C. L., Becker, D., Brown, K. K., Gann, S., Wong, M. J., & Wurster, A. B. (1992). Guidelines for selecting a conceptual model of nursing: Focus on the individual patient. *Dimensions of Critical Care Nursing, 11,* 268–77.

Fawcett, J., Cariello, F. P., Davis, D. A., Farley, J., Zimmaro, D. M., & Watts, R. J. (1987). Conceptual models of nursing: Application to critical care nursing practice. *Dimensions of Critical Care Nursing, 6,* 202–13.

Foote, A. W., Piazza, D., & Schultz, M. (1990). The Neuman Systems Model: Application to a patient with a cervical spinal cord injury. *Journal of Neuroscience Nursing, 22,* 302–06.

Galloway, D. A. (1993). Coping with a mentally and physically impaired infant: A self-analysis. *Rehabilitation Nursing, 18,* 34–36.

Fuller, C. C., & Hartley, B. (2000). Linear scleroderma: A Neuman nursing perspective. *Journal of Pediatric Nursing, 15*, 168–74.

Gavan, C. A. S., Hastings-Tolsma, M. T., & Troyan, P. J. (1988). Explication of Neuman's model: A holistic systems approach to nutrition for health promotion in the life process. *Holistic Nursing Practice, 3*(1), 26–38.

Gibson, M. (1996). Health promotion for a group of elderly clients. *Perspectives, 20*(3), 2–5.

Gigliottti, E. (1998). You make the diagnosis. Case study: Integration of the Neuman Systems Model with the theory of nursing diagnosis in postpartum nursing. *Nursing Diagnosis: The Journal of Nursing Language and Classification, 9, 14*, 34–38.

Goldblum-Graff, D., & Graff, H. (1982). The Neuman model adapted to family therapy. In B. Neuman (Ed.), *The Neuman Systems Model: Application to nursing education and practice* (pp. 217–22). Norwalk, CT: Appleton-Century-Crofts.

Hassell, J. S. (1996). Improved management of depression through nursing model application and critical thinking. *Journal of the American Academy of Nurse Practitioners, 8*, 161–66.

Herrick, C. A., & Goodykoontz, L. (1989). Neuman's systems model for nursing practice as a conceptual framework for a family assessment. *Journal of Child and Adolescent Psychiatric and Mental Health Nursing, 2*, 61–67.

Herrick, C. A., Goodykoontz, L., & Herrick, R. H. (1992). Selection of treatment modalities. In P. West & C. L. Evans (Eds.), *Psychiatric and mental health nursing with children and adolescents* (pp. 98–115). Gaithersburg, MD: Aspen.

Herrick, C. A., Goodykoontz, L., Herrick, R. H., & Hackett, B. (1991). Planning a continuum of care in child psychiatric nursing: A collaborative effort. *Journal of Child and Adolescent Psychiatric and Mental Health Nursing, 4*, 41–48.

Hiltz, D. (1990). The Neuman Systems Model: An analysis of a clinical situation. *Rehabilitation Nursing, 15*, 330–32.

Hoeman, S. P., & Winters, D. M. (1990). Theory-based case management: High cervical spinal cord injury. *Home Healthcare Nurse, 8*, 25–33.

Kido, L. M. (1991). Sleep deprivation and intensive care unit psychosis. *Emphasis: Nursing, 4*(1), 23–33.

Knight, J. B. (1990). The Betty Neuman Systems Model applied to practice: A client with multiple sclerosis. *Journal of Advanced Nursing, 15*, 447–55.

Lile, J. L. (1990). A nursing challenge for the 90s: Reducing risk factors for coronary heart disease in women. *Health Values: Achieving High-Level Wellness, 14*(4), 17–21.

Lindell, M., & Olsson, H. (1991). Can combined oral contraceptives be made more effective by means of a nursing care model? *Journal of Advanced Nursing, 16*, 475–79.

Mayers, M. A., & Watson, A. B. (1982). Nursing care plans and the Neuman Systems Model: In B. Neuman (Ed.), *The Neuman Systems Model: Application to nursing education and practice* (pp. 69–84). Norwalk, CT: Appleton-Century-Crofts.

McInerney, K. A. (1982). The Neuman Systems Model applied to critical care nursing of cardiac surgery clients. In B. Neuman (Ed.), *The Neuman Systems Model: Application to nursing education and practice* (pp. 308–15). Norwalk, CT: Appleton-Century-Crofts.

Mill, J. E. (1997). The Neuman Systems Model: Application in a Canadian HIV setting. *British Journal of Nursing, 6,* 163–66.

Millard, J. (1992). Health visiting an elderly couple. *British Journal of Nursing, 1,* 769–73.

Miner, J. (1995). Incorporating the Betty Neuman Systems Model into HIV clinical practice. *AIDS Patient Care, 9*(1), 37–39.

Mirenda, R. M. (1986). The Neuman Systems Model: Description and application. In P. Winstead-Fry (Ed.), *Case studies in nursing theory* (pp. 127–66). New York: National League for Nursing.

Moore, S. L., & Munro, M. F. (1990). The Neuman Systems Model applied to mental health nursing of older adults. *Journal of Advanced Nursing, 15,* 293–99.

Mynatt, S. L., & O'Brien, J. (1993). A partnership to prevent chemical dependency in nursing using Neuman's Systems Model. *Journal of Psychosocial Nursing and Mental Health Services, 31*(4), 27–34.

Narsavage, G. L. (1997). Promoting function in clients with chronic lung disease by increasing their perception of control. *Holistic Nursing Practice, 12*(1), 17–26.

Neal, M. C. (1982). Nursing care plans and the Neuman Systems Model: II. In B. Neuman (Ed.), *The Neuman Systems Model: Application to nursing education and practice* (pp. 85–93). Norwalk, CT: Appleton-Century-Crofts.

Neuman, B. (1983). The family experiencing emotional crisis. Analysis and application of Neuman's health care systems model. In I. W. Clements & F. B. Roberts (Eds.), Family health: A theoretical approach to nursing care (pp. 353–67). New York: John Wiley & Sons.

Orr, J. P. (1993). An adaptation of the Neuman Systems Model to the care of the hospitalized preschool child. *Curationis, 16*(3), 37–44.

Owens, M. (1995). Care of a woman with Down's syndrome using the Neuman Systems Model. *British Journal of Nursing, 4,* 752–58.

Piazza, D., Foote, A., Wright, P., & Holcombe, J. (1992). Neuman Systems Model used as a guide for the nursing care of an 8-year-old child with leukemia. *Journal of Pediatric Oncology Nursing, 9*(1), 17–24.

Picton, C. E. (1995). An exploration of family-centered care in Neuman's model with regard to the care of the critically ill adult in an accident and emergency setting. *Accident and Emergency Nursing, 3*(1), 33–37.

Pierce, J. D., & Hutton, E. (1992). Applying the new concepts of the Neuman Systems Model. *Nursing Forum, 27,* 15–18.

Poole, V. L., & Flowers, J. S. (1995). Care management of pregnant substance abusers using the Neuman Systems Model. In B. Neuman (Ed.), *The Neuman Systems Model* (3rd ed., pp. 377–86). Norwalk, CT: Appleton & Lange.

Redheffer G. (1985). Application of Betty Neuman's Health Care Systems Model to emergency nursing practice: Case review. *Point of View, 22*(2), 4–6.

Reed, K. (1982). The Neuman Systems Model: A basis for family psychosocial assessment. In B. Neuman (Ed.), *The Neuman Systems Model: Application to nursing education and practice* (pp. 188–95). Norwalk, CT: Appleton-Century-Crofts.

Rice, M. J. (1982). The Neuman Systems Model applied in a hospital medical unit. In B.

Neuman (Ed.), *The Neuman Systems Model: Application to nursing education and practice* (pp. 316–23). Norwalk, CT: Appleton-Century-Crofts.

Robichaud-Ekstrand, S., & Delisle, L. (1989). Neuman en médecine-chirurgie [The Neuman model in medical-surgical settings]. *The Canadian Nurse, 85*(6), 32–35.

Ross, M., & Bourbonnais, F. (1985). The Betty Neuman Systems Model in nursing practice: A case study approach. *Journal of Advanced Nursing, 10,* 199–207.

Ross, M. M., & Helmer, H. (1988). A comparative analysis of Neuman's model using the individual and family as the units of care. *Public Health Nursing, 5,* 30–36.

Russell, J., Hileman, J. W., & Grant, J. S. (1995). Assessing and meeting the needs of home caregivers using the Neuman Systems Model. In B. Neuman (Ed.), *The Neuman Systems Model* (3rd ed., pp. 331–41). Norwalk, CT: Appleton & Lange.

Shaw, M. C. (1991). A theoretical base for orthopaedic nursing practice: The Neuman Systems Model. *Canadian Orthopaedic Nurses Association Journal, 13*(2), 19–21.

Smith, M. C. (1989). Neuman's model in practice. *Nursing Science Quarterly, 2,* 116–17.

Sohier, R. (1997). Neuman's systems model in nursing practice. In M. R. Alligood & A. Marriner-Tomey (Eds.), *Nursing theory: Utilization and application* (pp. 109–27). St. Louis: Mosby-Year Book.

Sullivan, J. (1986). Using Neuman's model in the acute phase of spinal cord injury. *Focus on Critical Care, 13*(5), 34–41.

Torkington, S. (1988). Nourishing the infant. *Senior Nurse, 8*(2), 24–25.

Trépanier, M. J., Dunn, S. I., & Sprague, A. E. (1995). Application of the Neuman Systems Model to perinatal nursing. In B. Neuman (Ed.), *The Neuman Systems Model* (3rd ed., pp. 309–20). Norwalk, CT: Appleton & Lange.

Utz, S. W. (1980). Applying the Neuman model to nursing practice with hypertensive clients. *Cardio-Vascular Nursing, 16,* 29–34.

Wallingford, P. (1989). The neurologically impaired and dying child: Applying the Neuman Systems Model. *Issues in Comprehensive Pediatric Nursing, 12,* 139–57.

Ware, L. A., & Shannahan, M. K. (1995). Using Neuman for a stable parent support group in neonatal intensive care. In B. Neuman (Ed.), *The Neuman Systems Model* (3rd ed., pp. 321–30). Norwalk, CT: Appleton & Lange.

Waters, T. (1993). Self-efficacy, change, and optimal client stability. *Addictions Nursing Network, 5*(2), 48–51.

Weinberger, S. L. (1991). Analysis of a clinical situation using the Neuman System Model. *Rehabilitation Nursing, 16,* 278, 280–81.

Wormald, L. (1995). Samuel—the boy with tonsillitis: A care study. *Intensive and Critical Care Nursing, 11,* 157–60.

Wright, P. S., Piazza, D., Holcombe, J., & Foote, A. (1994). A comparison of three theories of nursing used as a guide for the nursing care of an 8-year-old child with leukemia. *Journal of Pediatric Oncology Nursing, 11,* 14–19.

Index

Savala, S., 239

Scales, C. J., 224, 230

Schlentz, M., 67, 337

Schmoll, B. J., 193, 230

Scicchitani, B., 332

Scope and Standards of Forensic Nursing Practice, 248

Seattle Pacific University, 333

Sebastian, L., 80, 82, 84

Secondary prevention
    administration of health care services, 267–269, 295–297
    Assessment and Intervention Tool, Neuman Systems Model, 353
    community/aggregate clients, 54
    defining, 14
    educational tools, 239–240
    guidelines, clinical practice, 40
    literature, review of the, 47–48, 54
    pain, 47
    postpartum mood disorders, 84–86
    prevention as intervention, 26–28
    research, 114–115, 160–163
    rural health care, 341

Seely, S., 74

Self-Care Framework, Orem's, 246

Self-confidence, 97

Semprevivo, D., 83

Sengin, K. K., 46

Senior Nurse, 329

Serotonin reuptake inhibitors (SSRIs), 85

Settings for clinical practice, 38, 39

Sexual abuse among pregnant teen population, 336

Seyer-Hansen, H., 331

Shambaugh, B. F., 362

Shugars, D. A., 271

Sichel, D. A., 75, 76, 87

Siengsanor, C., 184

Sigma Theta Tau International, 91

Simmons College, 333

Simon, K., 84

Sinnott, M., 66, 281

Sipple, J. A., 220, 241, 333, 341, 362

Sirdumrong, N., 184

Skowronek, M. P., 338

Slovenia, 337

Smith, A. A., 278

Smith, M. C., 92, 177

Smith, M. L., 122, 137

Smith, N., 339

Sociocultural variables, 16, 307

Sohier, R., 54

Somder, H. H., 188

Southern College, 230

Spiritual Care Scale (SCS), 67

Spiritual variables, 16–17, 44, 46, 307

Spisak, D., 75

Spradley, B. W., 51

Sprague, A. E., 44, 66

Sproles, J. B., 51, 54, 69, 282

Squaires, M., 327

St. Olaf College, 333

St. Xavier College, 330

Stability through the use of systems, 7, 25–26, 38–40

Stanhope, M. K., 54

State Trait Anxiety Inventory, 151, 163

State University of North Dakota, 333

Steering committee and Emergis, Institute for Mental Health Care, 307

Stein, A., 81

Stevens, B., 55

Stevenson, M., 333

Stigma surrounding psychiatric disorders, 82

Stittich, E., 333

Stocks, J., 342

Story, E., 224, 239, 245, 331

Stowe, Z., 77

Strauss, A., 96, 116, 177

Strengths and wellness, focusing on, 97–98

Stressors, environmental
    administration of health care services, 290
    Assessment and Intervention Tool, Neuman Systems Model, 352–354
    community/aggregate clients, 51–52
    defining, 21
    education, nursing, 249–250
    guidelines, clinical practice, 39
    intrapersonal/interpersonal/extrapersonal, 22
    literature, review of the, 51–52
    Norway, 336
    nursing homes, 344
    postpartum mood disorders
        extrapersonal stressors, 82–83
        interpersonal stressors, 81–82
        intrapersonal stressors, 80–81
    research instruments, 152–155
    Thailand, nursing research in, 185–186
    variables affecting, client, 14

Strickland-Seng, V., 194, 220, 224, 241

Structure and systems perspective, 6, 9, 17